T0195310

UNEQUAL CITIES

HEALTH EQUITY IN AMERICA

Daniel E. Dawes, Series Editor

Unequal Cities

STRUCTURAL RACISM AND THE DEATH GAP IN AMERICA'S LARGEST CITIES

Edited by Maureen R. Benjamins and
Fernando G. De Maio

Foreword by Julie Morita

JOHNS HOPKINS UNIVERSITY PRESS | *Baltimore*

Johns Hopkins University Press
2715 North Charles Street
Baltimore, Maryland 21218-4363
www.press.jhu.edu

Library of Congress Cataloging-in-Publication Data

Names: Benjamins, Maureen R., editor. | De Maio, Fernando, 1976– editor.
Title: Unequal cities : structural racism and the death gap in America's Largest
    Cities / edited by Maureen R. Benjamins, Fernando G. De Maio ; foreword by
    Julie Morita.
Description: Baltimore : Johns Hopkins University Press, [2021] | Series: Health
    equity in America | Includes bibliographical references and index.
Identifiers: LCCN 2020033843 | ISBN 9781421440996 (hardcover ; alk. paper) |
    ISBN 9781421441009 (ebook)
Subjects: MESH: Health Equity | Urban Health | Health Status Disparities |
    Healthcare Disparities | Race Factors | United States
Classification: LCC RA418 | NLM W 76 AA1 | DDC 362.1/042—dc23
LC record available at https://lccn.loc.gov/2020033843

A catalog record for this book is available from the British Library.

*Special discounts are available for bulk purchases of this book. For more information,
please contact Special Sales at specialsales@jh.edu.*

To a visionary advocate for social justice,
Steve Whitman, PhD, in memoriam

You know, it's one thing to talk about data. But, I think, maybe it's possible to get lost in the data; remember that this is . . . literally a matter of life and death. I mean literally. Not as an expression.

—Steve Whitman, PhD
Address to the MacLean Center for Clinical Medical Ethics
at the University of Chicago, 2010

CONTENTS

While complying with Illinois's COVID-19 "Stay at Home" order during the spring of 2020, my heart sank as I listened to a report about the high percentage of COVID-19 deaths among Black Chicagoans. Specifically, while 29% of Chicago's population was Black, 70% of the recorded deaths were among Black residents. I was saddened by the news, but I was not surprised. This was not the first time that a public health emergency disproportionately affected Black residents of Chicago: during the 1989 measles epidemic, Black children made up more than 70% of Chicago's cases,[1] and during the 1995 heat wave, Black seniors over the age of 85 were twice as likely to die than their white counterparts.[2] In addition to Black Chicagoans having high poverty, unemployment, and uninsured rates, all of which limit their ability to comply with the public health measures recommended to prevent COVID-19 infections (e.g., avoid public transportation, work remotely), they have high rates of obesity, diabetes, and lung and heart disease, which are risk factors for severe illness or death from COVID-19. The COVID-19 pandemic and other public health crises expose the deep structural inequities that lead to the conditions that induce chronic, underlying poor health and contribute to dramatic disparities in morbidity and mortality.

As I listened to the COVID-19 story, the salience of the present volume was clear. This book details Black:white inequities in mortality, how these inequities vary across the 30 largest cities of the United States, and then dives deeper to examine inequities in the leading causes of death. Perhaps most importantly, the book is not just a description of the problem—it goes beyond, to describe a community-based approach in Chicago intended to reduce the life expectancy gap in the city.

During the two decades I served as Immunization Program Medical Director, Chief Medical Officer, and Commissioner of the Chicago Department of Public Health (CDPH), addressing racial and ethnic health disparities was among the department's top priorities. We were able to focus on these disparities because we had access to and the ability to analyze data that revealed the disparities. Shortly after starting at CDPH in 1999, I joined a team of public health workers and community members in a door-to-door survey designed to determine childhood immunization coverage levels in one of Chicago's South Side neighborhoods. The survey revealed a dramatic difference in immunization coverage levels of this predominately Black neighborhood when compared to citywide levels.[3] The survey results prompted us to analyze Chicago Public School data, which identified additional South and West Side neighborhoods with low vaccine coverage levels.[4] Although federal and state programs had eliminated financial barriers to vaccines, other barriers persisted. We used the neighborhood coverage levels to address these barriers strategically; we opened immunization-only clinics, ran public awareness campaigns, helped health care providers establish reminder systems, and operated case management programs in the areas with the lowest coverage levels. Granular data informed how and where we directed our resources.

The household survey made clear the immunization coverage disparities, and it also opened my eyes to other striking inequities among Chicago neighborhoods. It revealed the poverty, poor housing quality, lack of public transportation, and competing priorities experienced by many South Side parents compared to the experiences of my North Side neighbors. In subsequent years, we used city- and neighborhood-level data to inform HIV prevention efforts and to respond to meningococcal disease and hepatitis A outbreaks. And yet, few of our interventions addressed the structural or social factors that contributed to increased disease rates or disparities. Although our disease-specific interventions led to modest success in decreasing health disparities, city- and neighborhood-level data revealed persistent disparities in chronic health conditions.

This prompted the department to begin focusing on addressing health equity by eliminating systemic barriers to health such as poverty and lack of access to good jobs, quality education and housing, safe environments, and health care. In 2015, CDPH and our partners committed to addressing the social determinants of health in our community health improvement plan, Healthy Chicago 2.0.[5] This plan incorporated quantitative and qualitative data, highlighted the critical role that social and economic factors (e.g., housing, education, transportation) play in health, reflected evidence-based approaches for addressing health challenges, and utilized a process for cross-sector partners and community members to contribute to plan development and implementation.

Citywide and neighborhood-level data served CDPH well. We used maps comparing life expectancy among neighborhoods to raise awareness among key decision makers, including elected officials, about the inequity that exists in Chicago neighborhoods. We also used maps of neighborhoods with the lowest levels of socioeconomic opportunity for children and overlaid them on maps of neighborhoods with the poorest health outcomes for nontraditional partners in education, parks and recreation, housing, and transportation to demonstrate the relationship between their work and the health and well-being of Chicagoans. CDPH and our partners continuously tapped into city-level data to monitor progress toward achieving the Healthy Chicago 2.0 goals and to inform the next 5-year plan, Healthy Chicago 2025.[6] Unfortunately, not all cities have access to local data like Chicago does. For the largest cities in the United States, the Centers for Disease Control and Prevention (CDC) and other federal agencies provide important data on health behaviors, chronic conditions, and other health outcomes at the city level through initiatives like the National Immunization Survey and the Behavioral Risk Factor Surveillance System (for youth and adults). In addition, the largest US cities (e.g., New York, Los Angeles, and Chicago) have the resources to operate population-based surveys that provide city- and neighborhood-level estimates of health concerns and social, environmental, and neighborhood factors associated with health. Having access to local-level morbidity and mortality data allows public health agencies to identify and focus their resources on populations and communities at greatest risk for poor health outcomes. Unfortunately, as the COVID-19 pandemic underscored, there is wide variability in data quality and availability at the state, county, and city levels. This lack of consistently available, high-quality data contributed to inconsistent coordination and execution of public health responses.

Long-term commitments from government officials and cross-sector partners, as well as high levels of stable funding, are necessary to address the systemic and structural barriers to health that perpetuate the health inequities that plague our cities at baseline and are exacerbated during public health crises. High-quality, city-level data are needed to motivate, inform, and monitor these efforts. *Unequal Cities: Structural Racism and the Death Gap in America's Largest Cities* makes clear the need for, and value of, city-level data. Clearly, COVID-19 is a public health crisis. The disproportionate impact of COVID-19 on Black Americans should serve as a wake-up call that increased rates of chronic conditions like heart disease, cancer, and diabetes and the deep structural inequities that contribute to these increased rates among Black Americans are avoidable, unnecessary, unfair, and constitute a public health crisis in their own right. We need to establish systems to collect, analyze, and utilize city-level data now.

JULIE MORITA, MD
Former Commissioner,
Chicago Department of Public Health

References

1. Centers for Disease Control and Prevention. Epidemiologic Notes and Reports Update: Measles Outbreak—Chicago, 1989. *Morbidity and Mortality Weekly Report.* 1990;39(19):317–319.

2. Whitman S, Good G, Donoghue ER, Benbow N, Shou W, Mou S. Mortality in Chicago Attributed to the July 1995 Heat Wave. *American Journal of Public Health.* 1997;87(9):1515–1518.

3. Rosenthal J, Raymond D, Morita J, et al. African-American Children Are at Risk of a Measles Outbreak in an Inner-City Community of Chicago, 2000. *American Journal of Preventive Medicine.* 2002;23(3):195–199.

4. Ramirez E, Bulim ID, Kraus JM, Morita J. Use of Public School Immunization Data to Determine Community-Level Immunization Coverage. *Public Health Reports (Washington, DC: 1974).* 2006;121(2):189–196.

5. Dircksen J, Prachand N, Bocskay K, Sayer J, Schuh T. *Healthy Chicago 2.0: Partnering to Improve Health Equity (2016–2020).* Chicago: Chicago Department of Public Health; March 2016.

6. City of Chicago. Healthy Chicago 2025. 2020. https://www.chicago.gov/city/en/depts/cdph/provdrs/healthy_communities/svcs/healthy-chicago-2025.html.

ACKNOWLEDGMENTS

This book is based on research first conducted by Dr. Steve Whitman, the founding director of the Sinai Urban Health Institute (SUHI). SUHI is a unique public health research center based in a safety-net hospital system in Chicago. SUHI's mission is to achieve health equity through data-driven research like that presented in this book, as well as through interventions and evaluation. We are grateful to our colleague Bijou Hunt, who led many of the previous studies on mortality disparities across US cities and generously shared her insight and analytical expertise. We would also like to acknowledge the other SUHI researchers and collaborators who have contributed to this line of work over the years, particularly Jennifer Orsi, Summer Rosenstock, Jana Hirschtick, Michelle Hughes, and Marc Hurlbert.

We are extremely grateful to all of our SUHI colleagues for generously reviewing many chapters, prompting us to clarify our thoughts and consider the needs of different audiences. In particular, we appreciate the assistance of Christopher Ahmed and Uei Lei for helping us think through and create data visualizations. We also benefited from the support of fantastic colleagues at DePaul University: LaShawn Murray (Center for Community Health Equity) processed American Community Survey data to derive the Index of Concentration at the Extremes used in chapter 6, Nandhini Gulasingam (Faculty Scholarship and Support Center) applied her expertise in Geographic Information Systems to check our analysis plan, Preeya Waite (Center for Community Health Equity) provided careful proofreading, and Linda Levendusky (Faculty Scholarship and Support Center) offered amazing copy editing support. We would also like to acknowledge reviewers of early drafts, including Grace Budrys (DePaul University), Kimberly Elliott, Sharon Homan

(SUHI), and Sheri Cohen (Chicago Department of Public Health). Finally, we would like to thank our editor at Johns Hopkins University Press, Robin Coleman.

MAUREEN R. BENJAMINS

I am forever grateful for having had Steve (Whitman) as my mentor. His work and passion for social justice inspired me and so many others. He taught us that "if our data just sit on a shelf, we have failed" and that we always need to call out racism as a cause of health inequities. In my time at SUHI, I am thankful to have had a second mentor as well, Dr. Sharon Homan. She provided the perfect amount of support (pressure?) to get this book written. Thanks to our book "team," particularly Fernando De Maio, Abigail Silva, and Nazia Saiyed, who worked so diligently and collaboratively and made this process fun. (What should our next book be about?) On a personal level, I would like to thank my husband, Xander, for his unwavering support of my work, and my parents for modeling a commitment to the welfare of others. Finally, to my children, Nora, Reider, and Thomas, thank you for making me smile every day.

FERNANDO G. DE MAIO

I have held the work of SUHI in very high regard for a long time. Across its many articles and publications, there is a clear commitment to the principles of "radical statistics"—the idea that statistical analysis should be about not just describing the world but also changing it. When Maureen Benjamins generously invited me to work with her on this book, I, of course, could only jump at the opportunity. I am grateful to Maureen and everyone at SUHI for welcoming me as a visiting fellow in 2019.

I have a wonderful group of colleagues in Chicago and elsewhere who inspire me with their own work and support mine in all manner of ways. I cannot list them all here but would like to acknowledge a few in particular: Raj Shah, David Ansell, and many others at the Center for Community Health Equity; Deena Weinstein, Black Hawk Hancock, Roberta Garner, Tracey Lewis-Elligan, and others in the Department of Sociology; and Dan Schober and others at the Master of Public Health Program at DePaul University. My sincere thanks as well to colleagues at the Social Medicine Consortium and the American Medical Association. I am grateful for supportive friends, both old (Tom Anceski) and new (Emily Bergstrom). Last but certainly not least, I would like to thank my family, in both Toronto and Buenos Aires, and above all thank my daughters, Lucy and Joy, for everything.

UNEQUAL CITIES

A Path to Health Equity for Cities

MAUREEN R. BENJAMINS AND FERNANDO G. DE MAIO

T HE COVID-19 pandemic has brought public health to the forefront of national discourse and debates. As the death count rises,
COVID-19 has quickly become the third-leading cause of death in the
United States.[1] To our dismay, data reveal pronounced racial/ethnic inequities: Black people have died at a rate more than three times greater
than their white counterparts.[1] COVID-19 is a worldwide emergency,
with unprecedented health, social, and economic consequences. Yet from
a health equity perspective, COVID-19 follows a familiar pattern—a
cause of death that disproportionately harms communities of color. It
adds to an already unfair playing field in the United States, exacerbating
and reinforcing our country's deeply entrenched inequities.

We have also witnessed profound protests against police brutality and
institutional racism, triggered by the murder of George Floyd in May
2020—whose last words, "I can't breathe," tragically echoed those of
Eric Garner, who died from police violence in 2014. The Black Lives
Matter movement has forced many people in the United States to re-
consider their taken-for-granted notions of progress toward racial equality. As we write this book, there is a significant new reckoning of the
deadly toll of structural racism across the United States—a toll that is
vividly exposed in our health data.

These coinciding crises—COVID-19 and racism—heighten the need for us to better understand patterns of population health in the United States, particularly in our urban centers. It will come as no surprise that our country's health data reflect our social divisions. The elimination of racial and ethnic inequities—differences that are avoidable, unnecessary, and unfair—has been one of the overarching health-related goals of our country for several decades (as set forth and tracked through the federal government's Healthy People initiative). In 2020, racial health inequities became an even greater target of our national attention owing to the coinciding public health crisis of COVID-19 and racially motivated police violence. Yet differences in health outcomes between Blacks and whites persist. Nationally, a Black baby born today has a life expectancy of 75 years, compared to a white baby who could expect to live 79 years.[2] This gap exists not only at the national level but also within smaller geographic areas. For many outcomes, the gap widens as we zoom into those smaller areas. In Chicago, for example, the average life expectancy for Blacks is 8 years less than that of whites. And if we examine selected communities in the South Side of this city, we see that Black men have a 50% chance of dying between the ages of 16 and 65, mostly from early onset chronic disease.[3]

The reasons for these differences are myriad, but they are increasingly understood to originate *outside of the health care system*, in the social determinants of health. Often described as how "where we work, live, and play matters," the majority of deaths in the United States (most commonly estimated at 70%)[4] are attributed to these factors and not to genetics. This is critical because most, if not all, social determinants are theoretically modifiable. In other words, although we currently do not have the ability to change an individual's genetic code to prevent diseases or the progression of illness, we do have the ability to change some factors, including aspects of our built environment, policies that encourage harmful behaviors and restrict people's capacity to make healthy choices, and barriers to quality health care.

When you look at city data, like those presented in this book, you can see that the gaps between health outcomes for Blacks and whites are not inevitable or natural. They are the products of "economic, social, or environmental disadvantage," as defined by the Healthy People 2020 initiative.[5] For many years, these gaps have been labeled *health disparities*. Yet in recent years there has been an important shift in terminology among researchers toward the use of *health inequities*, emphasizing the idea that the data reflect not just numeric differences but also differences that are "unfair and unjust" (p. 5).[6] We must eliminate inequities to achieve *health equity*, where "everyone has a fair and just opportunity to be as healthy as possible" (p. 2).[7]

Although we highlight many racial inequities in mortality in this book, the data also show that health equity is achievable. Specifically, for each of the top causes of death, such as cancer, heart disease, and stroke, there are a few large cities in the United States in which Blacks and whites die at the same rate. This is a profound finding and signals to the rest of the nation what can be achieved. The equitable rates seen in these model cities stand in stark contrast to national rates, as well as the rates for many of our largest urban areas, where Black individuals die more frequently and at younger ages compared to whites.

The obvious next step is to look to these model cities and to the growing body of evidence-based best practices to create a road map for those still struggling. Recent initiatives involving screening, outreach, and navigation, for example, have shown reduced cancer mortality rates and the near elimination of cancer disparities over large areas.[8-10] Other research has demonstrated that a few US counties have eliminated racial inequities in all-cause mortality for African American men, as well as for specific causes of death such as ischemic heart disease, accidents, liver disease, and chronic lower respiratory disease.[11] There are important lessons to be drawn. Most importantly, these model cities demonstrate with clear epidemiological data that health equity is not an idealistic dream.

Our choice to focus on cities here was intentional. Four in five Americans (and an even higher proportion of Blacks) currently live in urban areas.[12,13] This number is expected to increase dramatically over the next three decades.[14] In addition, city-level information is critical to assist city officials, public health professionals, funders, and other organizations in making real, evidence-based decisions.[15] More specifically, it is the local departments of public health, as well as other city agencies and offices, that develop and enforce many health and social policies, provide health and social services, and allocate substantial funding for these initiatives. Cities also face constraints from policies and structures at the state and federal levels, but cities have power in themselves; much can be accomplished at this level if policies are directed toward health equity for all.

Currently, comprehensive data on mortality and related health inequities are available only at the national, state, and county levels, not at the city level. This data limitation is problematic because research has uncovered significant racial inequities in various health outcomes that become visible only at the local (e.g., subcounty) level.[16,17] In other words, bigger geographical units, such as counties, can hide important variations in health outcomes and social factors. If we limit research to only bigger geographical units (like counties and states), we risk overlooking the worst of the problems. This is why a recent call to action from the US Department of Health and Human Services included a demand for "timely, reliable, granular-level (i.e., sub-county), and actionable data" (p. 4) as one of their five recommendations for public health in the twenty-first century.[15] The World Health Organization's Commission on the Social Determinants of Health reached a similar conclusion, calling for innovation in the measurement of health inequities and advocating for the routine monitoring of health equity locally and nationally.[18] Yet, despite this clear and recognized need, our book is the first to provide comprehensive data on race-specific mortality rates and related measures of inequities at the city level across the United States.

The book addresses the increasing demand from cities and public health professionals for data that can be used to identify local issues, compare outcomes, and track progress.[19] However, information on mortality rates and measures of inequities for our largest cities is not sufficient to effect change on its own. We work from the position that a mere analysis of data and description of health inequities is not enough. Our challenge is to work concertedly and collaboratively toward the elimination of inequities within and between US cities—only by doing so can we clearly proclaim that Black Lives Matter. To advance that goal, public health professionals must communicate with diverse stakeholders, engage partners, and seek out evidence-based solutions. Given that past efforts have yet to be effective in eliminating the racial gap in health outcomes in our country, we call for a renewed approach that focuses on the upstream social determinants of health within the cities most at risk, integrates community engagement in all aspects, and is grounded in a social justice framework.

It is our hope that elected officials, researchers, clinicians, funders, and other health advocates will share our sense of alarm over the data presented in this book. The statistics, in most cities, are dire. May these data inform a call to action to address the structural barriers to achieving health equity in US cities.

References

1. APM Research Lab. The Color of Coronavirus: COVID-19 Deaths by Race and Ethnicity in the US. https://www.apmresearchlab.org/covid/deaths-by-race.

2. Kochanek K, Murphy S, Xu J, Aria E. Deaths: Final Data for 2017. *National Vital Statistics Reports.* 2019;68(9).

3. Geronimus AT, Bound J, Colen CG. Excess Black Mortality in the United States and in Selected Black and White High-Poverty Areas, 1980–2000. *American Journal of Public Health.* 2011;101(4):720–729.

4. McGinnis JM, Williams-Russo P, Knickman JR. The Case for More Active Policy Attention to Health Promotion. *Health Affairs.* 2002;21(2):78–93.

5. HealthyPeople.gov. Disparities. https://www.healthypeople.gov/2020/about /foundation-health-measures/Disparities.

6. Whitehead M. The Concepts and Principles of Equity and Health. *International Journal of Health Services.* 1992;22(3):429–445.

7. Braveman P, Arkin E, Orleans T, Proctor D, Plough A. *What Is Health Equity? And What Difference Does a Definition Make?* Princeton, NJ: Robert Wood Johnson Foundation; 2017.

8. Grubbs SS, Polite BN, Carney J Jr, et al. Eliminating Racial Disparities in Colorectal Cancer in the Real World: It Took a Village. *Journal of Clinical Oncology.* 2013;31(16):1928–1930.

9. Rust G, Zhang S, Yu Z, et al. Counties Eliminating Racial Disparities in Colorectal Cancer Mortality. *Cancer.* 2016;122(11):1735–1748.

10. Rust G, Zhang S, Malhotra K, et al. Paths to Health Equity: Local Area Variation in Progress toward Eliminating Breast Cancer Mortality Disparities, 1990–2009. *Cancer.* 2015;121(16):2765–2774.

11. Levine RS, Rust G, Aliyu M, et al. United States Counties with Low Black Male Mortality Rates. *American Journal of Medicine.* 2013;126(1):76–80.

12. Beadle MR, Graham GN. *National Stakeholder Strategy for Achieving Health Equity.* US Department of Health and Human Services; 2011.

13. US Census Bureau. American Fact Finder. 2020. https://data.census.gov/cedsci/.

14. US Conference of Mayors. *Metro Economies: Past and Future Employment Levels: Transportantion and the Cost of Congestion, Population Forecast.* Washington, DC; 2018.

15. DeSalvo KB, Wang YC, Harris A, Auerbach J, Koo D, O'Carroll P. Public Health 3.0: A Call to Action for Public Health to Meet the Challenges of the 21st Century. *Preventing Chronic Disease.* 2017;14:E78.

16. Boothe VL, Fierro LA, Laurent A, Shih M. Sub-county Life Expectancy: A Tool to Improve Community Health and Advance Health Equity. *Preventing Chronic Disease.* 2018;15:E11.

17. Whitman S, Shah AM, Benjamins MR, eds. *Urban Health: Combating Disparities with Local Data.* New York: Oxford University Press; 2011.

18. World Health Organization. *Closing the Gap in a Generation: Health Equity through Action on the Social Determinants of Health.* Geneva: World Health Organization; 2008.

19. Rothenberg R, Stauber C, Weaver S, Dai D, Prasad A, Kano M. Urban Health Indicators and Indices—Current Status. *BMC Public Health.* 2015;15:494.

PART I ENTRENCHED RACIAL HEALTH INEQUITIES IN THE UNITED STATES

Of all the forms of inequality, injustice in health is the most shocking and the most inhuman because it often results in physical death.
—Dr. Martin Luther King Jr.
Second National Convention of the
Medical Committee for Human
Rights, 1966

The United States has a history of racial inequities in health that decades of attention have not been able to eradicate. In part I, we provide the historical and theoretical context needed to understand how and why mortality experiences within the United States vary by race and place.

In chapter 1, "Context for Entrenched Racial Health Inequities," we review the historical background of health inequities in the United States and the attempts to promote greater racial equity through legislation, changes within the US health care system, and other health promotion initiatives. We provide a national overview of mortality disparities, including the relatively recent improvements in some indicators, as well as differences by geographic location. Finally, we summarize current sources of mortality data, which primarily exist at the national, state, and county levels. We discuss the pressing need for city-level data, where four in five US residents currently live. In particular, we highlight how larger geographic areas, even counties, can obscure important differences between groups, and we describe why we need data aligned with primary political jurisdictions (e.g., cities) to drive changes in health-related policies, programming, and funding.

In chapter 2, "Theorizing the Causes of Health Inequities," we explore different theoretical approaches for understanding the origins of health inequities, contrasting the traditional approach—"health is a personal responsibility"—with newer alternatives offered in the rapidly growing field of social epidemiology. We compare three influential models: one from a public health initiative in the San Francisco Bay area, one from the World Health Organization, and one from the sociological research literature. In doing so, we move from the *proximal* to the *distal*, from the *personal* to the *societal*. The causes of health inequities are complex and multifaceted, but they can roughly be categorized into two complementary schools of thought: the psychosocial and sociopolitical. After many decades of research, a consensus is emerging that points toward social and structural determinants as the root causes of health inequities. These theories offer a valuable lens through which to understand racial inequities in mortality across US cities.

ONE

Context for Entrenched Racial Health Inequities

MAUREEN R. BENJAMINS, FERNANDO G. DE MAIO,
AND RUQAIIJAH YEARBY

O N AVERAGE, individuals in the United States can expect to live to 79 years of age.[1] Our life expectancy has increased by almost 10 years in the past 5 decades.[2] However, it is well known that these advances have not been enjoyed equally by members of all social groups or by individuals living in all parts of the country, due to persistent inequalities in access to resources.[3] Thus, health inequities, or the differences in health outcomes between groups that stem from social, economic, or environmental disadvantage, continue to exist or even increase in the United States.[4-9] In particular, differential access to quality education, employment, housing, and health care has been linked to the striking gaps between the health of Blacks and whites.

Although the existence of health inequities has long been documented, the elimination of them only became one of our fundamental public health goals 30 years ago.[10] In recent years, many state and local public health departments across the country have also set equity-related goals, recognizing that it is not enough to measure overall population health without considering the inequities that can lurk undetected within aggregated data. Unfortunately, neither the well-documented history of disparate outcomes for different racial groups nor the relatively recent focus on this issue has resulted in health equity for all.[11] Much work remains to be done.

In this chapter, we review how the history of unequal access to resources is linked to racial inequities in health in the United States, focusing on differences in two of the most important indicators of population health: mortality and life expectancy. We first discuss the sociopolitical context of racial inequities and then briefly summarize past and current efforts to address them.

At the foundation of these efforts have been population health data, which are used to (1) describe the size of the difference between the best-off and worst-off groups, (2) set goals to reduce inequities, and (3) evaluate progress over time. We explore the existing sources of mortality data at the national, state, county, city, and neighborhood levels. Each level of analysis offers a different perspective on the nature of health inequities. However, we argue that city-level data reveal some of the most telling social patterns of avoidable mortality and are able to spur social and legislative efforts in particularly powerful ways. Despite this, until now, comprehensive data on mortality and inequities in mortality have not been available at the city level.

The US public health experience clearly shows that having rigorous data tailored to the needs of policy makers, funders, and public health practitioners is a critical piece of our country's efforts to eliminate health inequities.[12] Additionally, the experience also shows that concerted, data-driven action that addresses racial inequalities in the social determinants of health can solve seemingly intractable problems. Cities throughout the United States are testing and implementing effective structural solutions to improve health equity, from a task force in Chicago dedicated to overcoming the racial gap in breast cancer mortality to a state-wide initiative in Delaware to reduce cancer incidence, mortality, and disparities.[13,14] Although health inequities are deeply entrenched in US society, they vary from place to place. With the right combination of research, community mobilization, and political will to overcome historical and present-day racial inequalities in access to resources, they could be eliminated.

Health Inequities Defined

Acknowledging the numerous ways individuals and organizations talk about (and define) health inequities, we would like to clarify the terminology used in this book. We use the term *health inequities* to describe group-level differences in health outcomes that are "unnecessary and avoidable but, in addition, are also considered unfair and unjust" (p. 5).[15] A related term is *health disparities*, which is more generally used to label differences in health outcomes that are linked to social, economic, or demographic factors. The term *health disparities* differs from *health inequities* in a nuanced but important way. Specifically, the term *health inequities* adds a focus on the ethical dimension of the group differences and emphasizes that they are due to social disadvantage or exclusion.[16] Only by removing the social and structural obstacles to health and well-being, such as poverty and discrimination, can a society achieve *health equity*. *Health equity* means that "everyone has the opportunity to attain their highest level of health."[16] As the goal of this book is not just to document health inequities but also to move US cities toward equity, we stress that this work necessarily needs to focus on the structural issues that generate risk for marginalized populations (to be discussed in chapter 2). Efforts must also concentrate on the populations burdened with the highest risk of poor health owing to racism, socioeconomic marginalization, or other social processes—what Paul Farmer and others call "axes of oppression."[17,18] Finally, it is not uncommon for people to confuse discussions about health equity (related to unfair differences in health outcomes) with discussions of inequalities in health care access, utilization, and quality.[15] Here, we focus on the *health* outcomes, of which health care factors are just one of many potential determinants.

Throughout the book, we focus on comparisons specifically between Blacks and whites. Although we recognize the vast racial and ethnic diversity within this country, we did not include the other largest subpopulations for several reasons. In the United States, mortality inequities primarily afflict the Black population, while the other largest racial/ethnic subgroups, Hispanic and Asian populations, tend to have significantly lower mortality rates than both Blacks and whites.[19] At the same time, we recognize the important heterogeneity that exists within all of these very coarse groupings, including differences by nativity and length of time in the United States for immigrants. There are also significant mortality inequities for other groups, such as Native Americans. All of these inequities warrant attention and demand action. In addition, understanding inequities between any two groups requires a thorough appreciation of the specific historical and sociopolitical context of the relationship. Finally, logistically, the relatively smaller number of deaths for each cause of death within these other groups would greatly restrict how many cities we could include. Thus, this book will concentrate on health equity patterns between Black and white populations in the United States.

Sociopolitical Context of Health Equity

We have reliable data on health inequities between Blacks and whites going back to the nineteenth century.[20-22] After slavery ended, segregation and related discriminatory practices sustained stark differences in health into the 1900s and beyond. Blacks continued to fare worse than whites across a range of health indicators, including functional ability, chronic conditions, subjective well-being, and birth outcomes.[9,23-25] Given the huge variety of ways to assess health, it is useful to focus on all-cause mortality and life expectancy as summary measures that encapsulate all of the other components and clearly demonstrate the extent of health inequities.

Before addressing these inequities, we must first have a solid understanding of the factors that lead to the different health outcomes for Blacks and whites in our country. The issue is one not of biology but of the structural and social determinants of health, such as poverty and racial segregation.[26,27] A long history of research points to the "social seeds" of disease, perhaps most clearly stated in Friedrich Engels's *Condition of the Working Class in England* in 1845[28] and Rudolph Virchow's oft-cited analysis of typhus in Upper Silesia in 1848.[29] In the United States, the most important study in this vein was W. E. B. Du Bois's *The Philadelphia Negro* in 1899.[30] Du Bois used a wide range of data sources to implicate poverty and racism as the potential causes of racial disparities and concluded that differences in health outcomes between Black and white individuals resulted from a "social disease" as opposed to one based on race.[30]

Du Bois's research debunked the widely held assumption that any differences seen in health outcomes reflected inherent biological differences between "races."[31] Unfortunately, the utility of conceptualizing race as biologically based has enabled its persistence despite the preponderance of contrary evidence.[32,33] For example, many studies have shown that genetic variation *within* a racial group is greater than that seen *between* racial groups.[34,35] Not only is "race as biology" an inaccurate understanding, but it also presents a major stumbling block to equity, as those holding this view remain more tolerant of racial inequities and less inclined to seek or support efforts to address them.[36] Here we maintain the conceptualization of race as a social construct, which will be further supported by the findings presented in this book.

Since race is socially, not biologically, assigned, it follows that racial inequities in health reflect a broad constellation of factors, including lack of access to resources. In this chapter we examine how inequalities in access to housing and health care services are associated with mortality disparities between Blacks and whites. Additional social, economic, and environmental factors that contribute to health inequities, such as racism, are discussed in greater detail in chapter 2. Efforts to achieve health equity need to acknowledge all of these factors; more specifically, they need to incorporate multisector policy changes that address racial inequalities in access to resources, systemic changes within our health care system, and community-based initiatives that address social determinants of health. In the following section we summarize the laws and policies that fostered racial inequalities and led to different health outcomes for Blacks and whites.

The Jim Crow Era (1875–1968)

Understanding today's health inequities requires a historical perspective. During the Jim Crow era, the federal government enacted laws that either explicitly or implicitly supported the racially separate and unequal distribution of resources, including but not limited to education, employment, housing, and health care.[3] For example, in 1933, after the Federal Housing Administration (FHA) was created, it subsidized housing builders, but only as long as none of the homes were sold to Blacks, a practice that was called redlining.[37] The FHA also published an underwriting manual that stated that housing loans to Blacks would not be insured by the federal government.[37] Private lenders followed suit, providing conventional mortgages to whites while drastically limiting the number of conventional mortgages to Blacks. Due to the FHA and its policies, only 2.3% of FHA-insured mortgages and 5.0% of conventional mortgages outstanding in 1950 were for nonwhites.[38] As a result, Blacks were often excluded from the burgeoning suburbs and relegated to inner-city housing projects.

This pattern of inequality was also seen in health care. With the passage of the Hospital Survey and Construction Act of 1946, better known as the Hill-Burton Act, the government allotted funding for the construction of hospitals and nursing homes, granting states the authority to regulate this construction.[39] The act also provided that adequate health care facilities be made available to all state residents without discrimination of color, but "an exception shall be made in cases where separate hospital facilities are provided for separate population groups, if the plan makes equitable provision on the basis of need for facilities and services of like quality for each such group."[39] Thus, the act allowed states to supervise, regulate, and maintain the placement of racially segregated hospital and nursing home facilities throughout their territory, which limited Blacks' access to health care.[40]

Blacks fought to obtain the rights of full citizenship in the United States, such as equal access to health care, throughout the Jim Crow era.[41] As Gamble noted, "For much of the twentieth century, the color line in medicine was so rigidly drawn that hospitals and medical institutions could, and routinely did, exclude Blacks" (p. 99).[42] It took a concerted effort of combined political action and research to begin setting a new course. For example, in 1930 the US Public Health Service instituted National Negro Health Week to draw attention to minority health issues; 2 years later, the Office of Negro Health Work was established.[42] At that point, broader federal initiatives also began to gain ground, driven by "medical civil rights activists," who were a part of the civil rights movement that focused on equality of rights in every area of life.

In 1954, the US Supreme Court ruled in *Brown v. Board of Education* that separate and unequal education violated the Constitution because separate is inherently unequal. Seven years after the *Brown* decision, a group of Black physicians, dentists, and patients filed a similar lawsuit targeting racially segregated hospitals. Specifically, the lawsuit was filed against two hospitals in North Carolina that received federal funding for their construction but denied access to Black patients and physicians.[40] The federal government joined the case in support of the Black litigants, and as a result, the hospitals' racial discriminatory practice was found unconstitutional in 1963.[43] One year later, Congress enacted the Civil Rights Act of 1964, prohibiting racial discrimination in voting, education, health care, and employment. In 1968, Congress passed the Fair Housing Act, which banned racial discrimination in the sale and rental of housing.[3]

Given policies such as these, it is not surprising that there were latent health inequities in all-cause mortality and life expectancy between Blacks and whites at this time. In fact, whites have enjoyed a longer life expectancy than Blacks since record keeping began. In 1850, whites could expect to live to age 40, on average, while Blacks could only expect to live to age 23.[22] While this gap varied throughout the 1900s, the inequities in mortality rates did not substantially improve during the Jim Crow era,[44–46] or even worsened depending on the measure of disparity (e.g., relative vs. absolute)[47] or years of study.[23]

After Jim Crow (1969–Present)

Although laws passed during the civil rights era prohibited racial discrimination in access to resources, racial inequalities persist as illustrated by inequalities in housing and health care. Mortgage lending discrimination against Blacks was not outlawed until 1974, while discrimination against lending and reinvestment in Black neighborhoods was only prohibited in 1977.[48] Despite the changes in the law, Blacks have never achieved equal home ownership compared to whites, and thus many neighborhoods remain racially segregated. In 1976, only 44% of Blacks owned homes, compared to 69% of whites.[49] In 2014, the rate of Black homeownership was 43% compared to 72% for whites. This inequality in homeownership is present even when Blacks have a high income or a college education. For example, homeownership for college-educated Blacks is 58% compared to 76% for college-educated whites.[49]

From 2004 to 2009, several banks, including Countrywide and Wells Fargo, charged Black borrowers more than similarly qualified white borrowers for their loans.[3] Banks steered Blacks into subprime loans even though they qualified for conventional loans.[3] Subprime loans generally carried less favorable terms, such as prepayment penalties and adjustable interest rates that significantly increased after the first few years. A 2018 report by the Center for Investigative Reporting showed that discriminatory practices limiting Blacks' access to home ownership persisted "in 61 metro areas—from Detroit and Philadelphia to Little Rock and Tacoma, Washington—even when controlling for applicants' income, loan amount and neighborhood."[50]

As a result of these discriminatory practices, many American neighborhoods remain racially segregated, which negatively impacts Blacks' access to health care and other resources. For example, in racially segregated neighborhoods, Blacks are disproportionately likely to undergo surgery in low-quality hospitals, whereas in more integrated areas, Blacks and whites undergo surgery at low-quality hospitals at the same rate.[51] This is significant because among Medicare patients most of the racial disparities in risk-adjusted death rates for major surgery are a result of the location of care.[51] Where one lives also influences access to healthy food, with food choices being more limited for people living in racially segregated neighborhoods.[52] The poor nutritional quality of food available in these "food deserts" has been shown to lead to obesity, a risk factor for cancer and cardiovascular disease.[53,54]

Although Title VI of the Civil Rights Act of 1964 prohibits the exclusion from, participation in, and denial of benefits based on race by those receiving federal financial assistance,[55] such as Medicare and Medicaid, it has only been applied to the racial segregation of hospital patients. The desegregation of hospitals has been linked to significant improvements in health for Black populations, particularly in infant mortality rates.[56,57] Unfortunately, the federal government failed to apply Title VI to hospital closures or other health care providers, such as nursing homes and physicians.[3,43] For example, a report of 190 urban community hospitals found that the percentage of Black residents in the neighborhood was the most significant factor in hospital closures between 1980 and 1987. As the percentage of Black residents increased in the neighborhood, hospital closures increased.[43] Another study showed that 45% of hospitals open in 1970 had closed by 2010, and 60% of these hospitals were in predominately Black neighborhoods.[3] Detroit is a poignant example of these race-based hospital closures; in 1960, it had 42 hospitals open in predominately Black neighborhoods; by 2010, only 4 were still open.[3]

Much research also documents discriminatory practices by providers, which lead to racial inequities in mortality and life expectancy. For example, researchers found that physicians provided less comprehensive treatment to Black Medicare patients than to white ones, resulting in Blacks having higher mortality rates (even after controlling for income).[58] Likewise, another study found that Blacks were less likely than whites to receive curative surgery for early-stage lung cancer, which is linked to increased Black mortality rates.[59] And, according to a study conducted by Harvard researchers, Black Medicare patients received poorer basic care than white Medicare patients who were treated for the same illnesses, including treatments linked to lower death rates.[60,61]

The Patient Protection and Affordable Care Act of 2010

A review of efforts to improve our nation's health equity would be incomplete without discussing the Patient Protection and Affordable Care Act (ACA) of 2010.[62] This act overhauled the US health care system to expand access to care, limit health care costs, and improve quality of care.[63] It included changes to insurance coverage that expanded Medicaid eligibility, increased subsidies, and transformed individual insurance markets. Although the Supreme Court struck down mandatory Medicaid expansion, many states chose to expand Medicaid anyway.[64] The ACA also attempted to reduce racial and ethnic health inequities through provisions that addressed the following: (1) data collection and reporting by race, ethnicity, and language; (2) workforce diversity; (3) cultural competence of health care providers; (4) disparities research; and (5) specific initiatives directed at disparities in prevention.[65]

The ACA mandated that the secretary of the US Department of Health and Human Services (DHHS) develop a national strategy to improve the quality of health care to reduce health inequities. It also created the Patient-Centered Outcomes Research Institute, which is required to identify a national research agenda, including health and health care inequities. The ACA provided for the creation of quality measures to improve the assessment of health inequities and additional payment bonuses for Medicare providers rectifying health inequities through changes such as increased staffing in long-term care facilities. It also provided technical assistance grants to health care providers to address health inequities and expanded access to primary health care by investing $11 billion in the Health Resources and Services Administration's community health centers.

In addition to measures to address racial health inequities, Section 1557 of the ACA prohibits racial discrimination, fixing the gaps of Title VI of the Civil Rights Act and adding new protections. This section applies to almost all health care providers, including hospitals, physician offices, community health centers, nursing homes, home health agencies, and health insurers.[66] It also prohibits sex discrimination in health care for the first time.

By providing nondiscrimination requirements and expanding insurance coverage, the ACA has the potential to increase access to health care for minorities.[67] In fact, initial evaluations reveal that the ACA has increased the percentage of Americans with health insurance, particularly for young adults, the relatively poor, populations with the most serious health challenges, and people of color.[63,68] More research is still needed to document the impact of the ACA on health outcomes and health care costs beyond descriptive studies.

Patterns of Health Inequities

Although both Black and white populations have experienced improved overall mortality rates and life expectancy over the past 50 years, a large gap between the two groups can still be seen (see figure 1.1). Racial inequities in mortality rates actually increased during the last decades of the twentieth century, with the first signs of improving equity appearing at the beginning of the twenty-first century. At that point, inequities in mortality narrowed as a result of mortality rates declining more sharply among Blacks than whites.[19,69]

The racial gap is still sizable, however. In 2017, the age-adjusted mortality rate for Blacks was 881 per 100,000, compared to 755 for whites.[2] Thus, the rate for Blacks was 1.2 times that for whites. Throughout the book we will use this number—the Black:white mortality rate ratio—as one critical metric for measuring racial inequities. It provides the relative disparity between the two groups. Following the mortality pattern, the average life expectancy in 2017 for a Black baby was 75 years, while a white baby could expect to live until age 79.[2] The gap in life expectancy

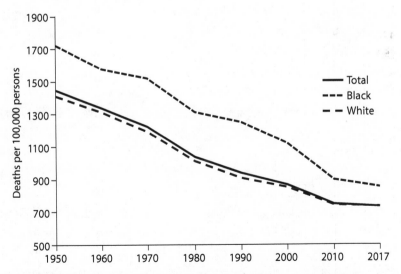

Figure 1.1. Mortality Rates in the United States by Race, 1950–2017.
Notes: Mortality rates are age-adjusted. Black and white groups include Hispanics. *Source:* National Center for Health Statistics, National Vital Statistics System.

between whites and Blacks generally narrowed through the end of the century and during the early 2000s (similar to mortality rates). For instance, between 1990 and 2009 the Black:white difference in life expectancy at birth shrank nearly 3 years for males (from 8 to 5 years) and nearly 2 years for females (from 6 to 4 years).[70]

Looking at trends within different causes of death provides additional insight into our country's progress (or lack of) in achieving health equity in mortality. As we will see in later chapters, mortality inequities vary across causes of death, with Blacks having a mortality disadvantage for some, but not all, causes compared to whites. In the case of heart disease, the racial disparity in mortality increased over the second half of the twentieth century owing to slower improvements in rates for Blacks compared to whites. Improvements since then have been modest.[9,71,72] Data shown in chapter 4 indicate that heart disease mortality rates are still 30% higher for Blacks than for whites. Cancer mortality, which, together with heart disease, accounts for 44% of deaths in the United States, also reveals changing levels of racial inequity. For example, in the early 1950s Blacks had lower cancer mortality rates than whites, but since the 1960s cancer mortality has been significantly higher for Blacks than whites.[73] Our data show that Black cancer mortality rates are still 20% higher than those for whites. Inequities also continue to exist within deaths due to stroke, diabetes, and influenza and pneumonia. In contrast, a few causes of death (e.g., accidents, chronic lower respiratory disease, and Alzheimer's disease) show no racial inequities or a higher mortality rate for whites than for Blacks at the national level.[2]

Importance of Place

During this time, health has increasingly been linked with place. Sayings such as "Your zip code matters more than your genetic code" reflect the growing awareness of the importance of place in determining individual health outcomes (figure 1.2).[26,27,74] Not only do geographic differences in mortality exist, but there are also differences in the levels of racial inequities at the regional, state, and county levels.[2] For example, life expectancy

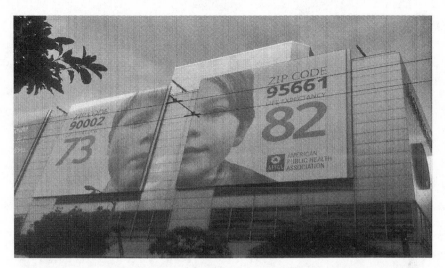

Figure 1.2. Your Zip Code Should Not Predict How Long You Will Live, but It Does. *Note:* San Francisco, October 27, 2012; American Public Health Association annual conference.

varies more between Black and white Americans on the West Coast, in the Midwest, and in the Southeast than it does in New England.[70]

Looking at life expectancy at the state level reveals gaps hidden within national data.[70,75] For example, overall life expectancy varied among states from a high of 80 years in Hawaii to a low of 74 years in Mississippi.[75] When comparing inequities between Blacks and whites, the largest gap in life expectancy was seen in Washington, DC (with a 9-year gap for women and a 14-year gap for men), while 10 states had either no disparity or a Black advantage.[76] Some states have shown substantial improvements over the past 30 years, such as New York, where the gap has decreased from 8 to 2 years for men and from 4 to 1 year for women.[70]

Zooming in further, evidence uncovers even more variation when you measure life expectancy at the county level. Overall, there is a 35-year difference in life expectancy between people living in the healthiest and the unhealthiest counties in the United States, as seen in figure 1.3. Racial inequities at the county level also exist for specific causes of death, such as overall cancer[77] and colorectal cancer.[78] At an even smaller level of analysis, a study of differences in life expectancy across census tracts in US cities

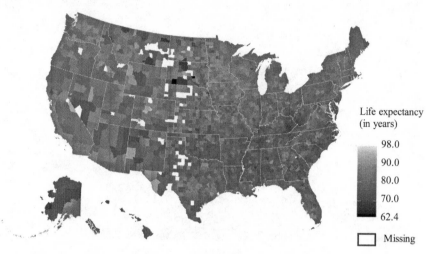

Life expectancy (in years)

98.0
90.0
80.0
70.0
62.4

☐ Missing

Figure 1.3. Life Expectancy at Birth by County. *Note:* US county-level data from County Health Rankings, computed using National Center for Health Statistics Mortality Data (2015–2017), https://www.countyhealthrankings.org/. *Source:* Christopher L. Ahmed, 2019.

reveals the largest gaps in Chicago, followed by New York, New Orleans, and Baltimore.[79] Note that both the county and census tract analyses used small area estimation methodology, instead of calculating actual mortality rates from death certificate data, like we do here with city-level data.

Over the long term, national mortality trends reveal some progress. However, that progress, when it exists, is not necessarily linear, universal, or automatic. The country's experience in the past few decades reveals how much more still needs to be done. The long-standing racial inequities in mortality and life expectancy have been created, reinforced, and, more recently, attenuated by many national policies, legislation, and initiatives.

Documenting and Assessing Progress in Eliminating Racial Health Inequities

Data are still needed to motivate, sustain, and evaluate current efforts to advance health equity. In the United States, government agencies are the primary source of health data at the national and state levels. Data for smaller geographic areas are becoming increasingly available from a variety of sources as well. Here we describe the efforts made over time to collect, analyze, and disseminate data on racial health inequities in the United States. We then summarize the various sources of data and information specifically related to life expectancy, mortality, and inequities within.

National Initiatives to Measure Racial Health Inequities

Annual reports to the president and Congress on the health of the nation have been required since the Public Health Service Act of 1944. These routine health reports were elevated in 1977 when the Office of Disease Prevention and Health Promotion was created within DHHS (formerly known as the US Department of Health, Education, and Welfare). The new office was tasked with creating goals and metrics for evaluating the New Deal and Great Society programs, including Medicare and Medicaid. To this end, a report that is considered to be the first of the *Healthy People* reports was released in 1979,[80] and the *Health, United States* reports began to annually track health outcomes.

Both of these reports were critical for monitoring the overall health of US residents, as well as for setting targets and providing influential definitions of key variables. However, given the huge amount of data available to document the health of a population, disparities within outcomes could be easily overlooked, ignored, or even concealed. For that reason, Secretary of Health Margaret Heckler created a task force in 1984 to report specifically on the health of minorities in the United States. Known as the *Malone-Heckler Report*, this document highlighted the discrepancy between overall improvements in population health and the persistence of significant racial and ethnic inequities. Although hailed as a critical first step in recognizing the extent of inequities in our country, the report was also criticized for focusing on individual-level solutions, rather than historical and social determinants of inequities.[81]

In 1986, DHHS created the Office of Minority Health (OMH) to design and seek policy and programmatic solutions to health disparities (see table 1.1). In 1993, the Office of Research on Minority Health was created within the National Institutes of Health (NIH) and tasked with

Table 1.1. Examples of National Initiatives to Measure and Eliminate Health Disparities in the Past Three Decades

Description	Purpose	Lead(s)	Year
Creation of the Task Force on Black and Minority Health	Coordinate efforts to specifically examine minority health	DHHS	1984
Creation of the Office of Minority Health	Focus on policy and programmatic solutions to disparities	DHHS	1986
Reduction of health disparities added to the Healthy People goals	Prioritize health equity work by adding the reduction of disparities as one of the main objectives for Healthy People 2000	DHHS	1990
Creation of the Office of Research on Minority Health	Create a research agenda on minority health within NIH	DHHS	1993
Creation of Center for Linguistic and Cultural Competence in Health Care	Collaborate with public and private organizations to help the health care system to deliver better care	OMH	1995
Launch of Racial and Ethnic Approaches to Community Health (REACH)	Fund local initiatives to reduce health disparities	CDC	1999
Elimination of health disparities added to the *Healthy People* goals	Elevate national attention to disparities through the more ambitious goal of achieving health equity in Healthy People 2010	DHHS	2000
Creation of the National Center of Minority Health and Health Disparities	Bring increased national attention to health disparities through programs, a research agenda, funding, and collaboration within and across federal agencies	NIH	2000
New National Standards for Culturally and Linguistically Appropriate Services (CLAS) in Health and Health Care	Enhance existing standards to improve quality of care and to address health care disparities	OMH	2000
Unequal Treatment: Confronting Racial and Ethnic Disparities in Health Care	Delineate racial and ethnic disparities in health care and their determinants	IOM	2002
National Healthcare Disparities Report first mandated by Congress	Measure trends in aspects of care (such as quality and safety) and disparities within	AHRQ	2003
Launch of the National Health Plan Collaborative to Reduce Disparities and Improve Quality	Provide recommendations for policy initiatives to address health disparities	AHRQ, RWJF, health plans	2004
National Leadership Summit on Eliminating Racial and Ethnic Disparities	Coordinate national efforts related to reducing health disparities	OMH	2006
Creation of the National Partnership for Action to End Health Disparities	Mobilize a nationwide, comprehensive, community-driven, and sustained approach toward achieving health equity	OMH	2007

Table 1.1. (Continued)

Description	Purpose	Lead(s)	Year
Elevation of NCMHHD to an Institute (now known as the National Institute on Minority Health and Health Disparities)	Increase focus on, and funding for, research, education, training, and outreach programs related to minority health and health disparities	NIH	2010
Passage of the Patient Protection and Affordable Care Act	Overhaul the US health care system in an effort to expand access to care, limit health care costs, and improve quality of care	US Congress	2010
National Stakeholder Strategy for Achieving Health Equity	Assess and provide recommendations related to awareness, leadership, health systems, cultural and linguistic competency, and data, research, and evaluation	OMH	2011
HHS Action Plan to Reduce Racial and Ethnic Health Disparities	Outline plan for reducing disparities in health care	DHHS	2011
Compendium of Federal Datasets Addressing Health Disparities	List of data sets and data-related resources developed, maintained, or funded by federal agencies	Multiple	2016
Healthy People 2020 Health Disparities Data Widget	Provide a new data search function to find health disparities data related to the HP2020 objectives	ODPHP, NCHS, OMH	2017
Launch of HD*Pulse* website	Provide data on health disparities from public health surveillance systems, as well as a library of evidence-based interventions	NIMHD	2017
A Blueprint to Help Communities Promote Equity	Draw policy makers' attention to the broad determinants of disparities, such as discrimination, segregation, and disparities in political power	RWJF and ChangeLab Solutions	2019

Notes: NIH = National Institutes of Health; OMH = Office of Minority Health; AHRQ = Agency for Healthcare Research and Quality; DHHS = Department of Health and Human Services; IOM = Institute of Medicine; ODPHP = Office of Disease Prevention and Health Promotion; RWJF = Robert Wood Johnson Foundation; NIMHD = National Institute of Minority Health and Health Disparities.

developing a minority health research agenda. Building on this national focus on disparities, NIH created the National Center on Minority Health and Health Disparities in 2000 (later promoted to an institute) to guide scientific advancements in this area through the funding of research, training, and outreach initiatives. Around the same time, OMH developed enhanced National Standards for Culturally and Linguistically Appropriate Services in Health and Health Care (CLAS) to improve quality of care and address health care disparities.

To coordinate efforts such as these, OMH convened several thousand experts and leaders in 2006 for the National Leadership Summit for Eliminating Racial and Ethnic Disparities. This meeting led to the formation of the National Partnership for Action to End Health Disparities, a group dedicated to increasing the effectiveness of health equity programs across the country.[82] This collaborative group produced the *National Stakeholder Strategy for Achieving Health Equity*, a comprehensive report and list of recommendations related to awareness; leadership; health system and life experience; cultural and linguistic competency; and data, research, and evaluation.[83]

DHHS continues to document health inequities through the Healthy People initiative, which was designed to provide a framework for national public health activities by setting goals and monitoring progress each decade. As a sign of the federal government's higher prioritization of health equity, DHHS included the reduction of health disparities as an overarching goal of Healthy People 2000 (along with increasing healthy life span and improving access to preventive services). Specific objectives to improve outcomes for specific subpopulations and directly reduce disparities in outcomes were created. Although many of the objectives in this area were not met (or outcomes even regressed), the next iteration of Healthy People had an even more ambitious goal—the total elimination of health disparities.[84] To facilitate the tracking of this, a data widget was added to the Healthy People website (www.healthy people.gov) in 2017 to help people find data and information related to health disparities.

As a complement to the Healthy People initiative, in 2003 Congress mandated the Agency for Healthcare Research and Quality (AHRQ; part of DHHS) to prepare an annual *National Healthcare Quality and Disparities Report*. The report provides a summary of measures related to health care quality and access to care, with a special focus on disparities based on race/ethnicity, income, and other social factors.[85] Simultaneously, the Institute of Medicine, part of the National Academy of Sciences, released a widely read report entitled *Unequal Treatment: Confronting Racial and Ethnic Disparities in Health Care*, which, like

W. E. B. Du Bois's *The Philadelphia Negro*, highlighted the social causes of health inequities.[86] This report not only emphasized the link between racial inequalities in access to resources and health disparities but also delineated racial and ethnic disparities in health care that were not due to access to care or other "known factors." Written by an expert panel, the report presented specific recommendations to promote equity within health care, including addressing residential racial segregation. Although *Unequal Treatment* greatly increased awareness of racial inequalities and health inequities, the recommendations it offered were criticized for not identifying the organizations responsible for carrying out the recommended changes and for not being aligned with existing federal policies and structures.[81]

In addition to the policy changes included in the ACA (discussed previously), it also influenced the availability of data related to measuring racial health inequities. The secretary of DHHS is now required to collect data to track health disparities under Medicaid and Medicare; to evaluate data collection approaches "that allow for the ongoing, accurate, and timely collection and evaluation of data on disparities in health care services and performance on the basis of race, ethnicity, sex, primary language, and disability status"; and to analyze the data to detect and monitor trends in health disparities.[62] The ACA also made OMH a part of the Office of the Secretary, increasing the authority and stature of the office, and created individual offices of minority health throughout DHHS, including within the Centers for Disease Control and Prevention, AHRQ, and the Centers for Medicare & Medicaid Services. Finally, it created the National Institute on Minority Health and Health Disparities (NIMHD), which launched the HD*Pulse* website. Billing itself as "an ecosystem of health disparities and minority health resources," HD*Pulse* offers both a data portal that curates and visualizes data from public health surveillance systems and an intervention portal to provide evidence-based support for those working toward health equity. DHHS has released an action plan focused on health care and health care disparities as a result of the creation of these new offices and has increased data collection requirements to measure racial health disparities.[87]

Numerous national groups are also working on racial disparities specifically within health care, such as the National Health Plan Collaborative to Reduce Disparities and Improve Quality, a cooperative of large health plans, researchers, government institutions, and funders.[88] Furthermore, considering the vast range of potential actions to address inequities, various partnerships and organizations have put together recommendations for policy initiatives (at any level of government) to guide future efforts. One recent example, funded by the Robert Wood Johnson Foundation (RWJF), helped draw policy makers' attention to the broad determinants of inequities, such as structural discrimination, racial segregation, and disparities in political power.[89]

While not a comprehensive list of historical and current initiatives, this brief summary provides insight into the increasingly robust national framework available for monitoring and advocating for health equity. Yet as we document in this book, focusing only on the national picture often hides critical equity problems.

State and Local Initiatives to Measure Racial Health Inequities

There are also, of course, many state and local efforts to document and reduce inequities. In 2018, a report from OMH entitled *State and Territorial Efforts to Reduce Health Disparities* provided state profiles with standardized data on health disparities, as well as detailed descriptions of each state's existing initiatives to reduce health disparities.[90] The findings showed that 23 of the 56 states and territories included had a plan for addressing health equity or minority health. Other helpful reviews focus on state-level policies, finding a wide range of related activities, with efforts accelerating in the 2000s. The most commonly enacted policies create government structures (such as new offices, task forces, or committees), support research and data collection efforts, and fund specific minority health initiatives.[91,92] In fact, a 2017 survey found that almost all (94%) state health departments collect and track data on disparities.[93]

Numerous examples of county- and city-level initiatives to monitor and address inequities can be found, although they are less universal. As one example, the Louisville Metro Department of Public Health &

Wellness has a Center for Health Equity, which functions across the department to monitor progress in meeting the needs of all residents. Similarly, the Los Angeles County Health Department has a Center for Health Equity to increase the use of health equity best practices and coordinate health-equity-related work around their county, Baltimore has an Equity Assessment program, and Austin has an Office of Equity. Health equity is also a central pillar of the strategic planning efforts of the Chicago Department of Public Health, in our home city.[94] The National Association of County and City Health Officials (NACCHO), which supports local health departments, has a Health Equity and Social Justice program specifically designed to support local health departments like these in their efforts to address inequities. An increasing number of cities also have initiatives to track disparities and monitor their impact. New York City's series of reports entitled *Health Disparities in New York City*, the Chicago Health Atlas, and Louisville's *Center for Health Equity* reports are all examples of the various ways that cities have documented racial inequities in a range of health outcomes. Other data initiatives are discussed in the following section as we turn our attention to sources of mortality data.

Availability of Mortality Data

The data needed to calculate mortality rates and life expectancies come from death certificates. In the United States, these forms are completed by the attending physician at the time of death. They include information on the decedent (name, sex, date of birth, race/ethnicity, marital status, address, birthplace, occupation, and education level) and details about the death (immediate and underlying causes, date, and location), among other variables. Deaths are first registered at the local level (city or county), then reported to the state, and finally compiled by the National Vital Statistics System (NVSS), which is part of the CDC. Once these data are aggregated by the NVSS, they are made available to the public through the systems described below, or by request to individual researchers under particular conditions. Note that the NVSS restricts access to data that might compromise confidentiality. For microdata files, such as those including geographic units of states or cities, the NVSS requires an approved research proposal and data use agreement.

Mortality data are then combined with population data to calculate mortality rates, which can be used as is (crude) or age-adjusted. Mortality rates for each specific age group can then be used to calculate the average life expectancy at birth for a population. They can also be calculated for specific causes of death (e.g., stroke). Numerous sources provide the raw data, as well as race-specific data for various geographies, as summarized in table 1.2 and described below. While not an exhaustive catalog, it calls attention to the wide range of sources and sponsoring organizations (both government and otherwise) and highlights current limitations.

Mortality data are consistently available at the national, state, and county levels, offering different insight into the nature of health inequities. The national level, for example, is typically used to set benchmarks, but the state, county, and local levels introduce variability, detailing large-scale differences that can be hidden in the national picture.

National Mortality and Life Expectancy Data

Anyone interested in mortality data for the United States can download the public-use data through the NVSS website or the CDC's Wide-ranging Online Data for Epidemiologic Research (WONDER) system (table 1.2). In addition to the raw data, both sources provide detailed mortality tables, often by age, race, sex, and cause of death. For example, life expectancy data for the United States have been estimated decennially since 1900 and annually since 1945 by the NVSS.[95] The HD-*Pulse* website also provides national death rates for all-cause mortality and the leading causes of death (calculated using NVSS public-use data and SEER*Stat programs) and helps users focus on health disparities by providing links to other data sources and evidence-based interventions.

National-level data and information on mortality and life expectancy are also routinely available through government-sponsored websites, reports, and publications (e.g., *Healthy People*; *Health, United States*; *Morbidity and Mortality Weekly Reports*; Surveillance, Epidemiology,

Table 1.2. Notable Sources of Data on Mortality (and Racial Disparities within) at Different Geographic Levels in the United States

Source	Description	Level of Data					Mortality Data Available			Sponsoring Organization(s)
		National	State	County	City	Local	Raw Data	Rates by Race/Ethnicity	Measures of Racial Disparities	
US National Mortality Files	Raw mortality data files available upon request (with a data use agreement).	✓	✓	✓	✓	✓	✓			National Vital Statistics System (NCHS)
HD*Pulse*	Data portal designed to increase access to minority health and health disparities data. Includes all-cause and cause-specific mortality data, by race/ethnicity, sex, and age.	✓	✓	✓				✓	✓	National Institute for Minority Health and Health Disparities (NIH)
Wide-ranging Online Data for Epidemiologic Research (WONDER)	Online system designed to make public health information from the CDC publicly available. Mortality data available by age, gender, race, and ethnicity.	✓	✓	✓			✓	✓*		CDC
Healthy People	Data to track national health goals. Website provides measures and data, including many mortality outcomes. Health Disparities widget highlights equity in selected outcomes.	✓	✓				✓	✓	✓*	Office of Disease Prevention and Health Promotion (DHHS)

(continued)

Table 1.2. (Continued)

| Source | Description | Level of Data | | | | | | Mortality Data Available | | | Sponsoring Organization(s) |
		National	State	County	City	Local	Raw Data	Rates by Race/Ethnicity	Measures of Racial Disparities	
Health, United States	Annual reports on national health outcomes, including life expectancy, all-cause mortality, leading causes of death, infant and child mortality, drug overdose deaths, suicide, and liver disease mortality. Online Data Finder for access to tables and figures.	✓	✓*					✓*	✓*	CDC
Surveillance, Epidemiology, and End Results (SEER)	Provides mortality data (for all causes) and cancer-specific statistical reports. Data use agreements needed for state and county data. SEER-Explorer allows users to query information, and a Health Disparities Calculator helps analyze disparities.	✓	✓	✓			✓	✓	✓*	National Cancer Institute

Measure	Description					Data source
Global Burden of Disease project	International data source, including US and state-level data on overall and cause-specific mortality, life and healthy life expectancy, and premature mortality.		✓	✓	✓	Institute for Health Metrics and Evaluation
America's Health Rankings	Ranks states for the following mortality outcomes: premature deaths, infant mortality, and deaths due to cancer, cardiovascular disease, suicide, injury, and drugs.	✓*	✓	✓	✓	United Health Foundation
County Health Rankings	Ranks all US counties across a wide variety of measures. Includes years of potential life lost, premature mortality, child mortality, and infant mortality, as well as mortality from alcohol-impaired driving, motor vehicle crashes, injury, homicides, firearms, and drug overdoses.	✓*	✓*	✓	✓	RWJF, University of Wisconsin Population Health Institute

(continued)

Table 1.2. (Continued)

Source	Description	Level of Data					Mortality Data Available			Sponsoring Organization(s)
		National	State	County	City	Local	Raw Data	Rates by Race/Ethnicity	Measures of Racial Disparities	
City Health Dashboard	Displays mortality data for breast cancer, colorectal cancer, cardiovascular disease, and opioid overdose, as well as premature deaths and life expectancy.				✓	✓*		✓*		New York University Langone Health; RWJF
Big Cities Health Coalition Data Platform	Posts data from the 30 largest US cities on overall mortality, life expectancy, and infant mortality, as well as deaths from opioid overdose, cancer, breast cancer, lung cancer, diabetes, heart disease, HIV, influenza/ pneumonia, firearm, motor vehicle, homicide, and suicide.				✓			✓*		Big Cities Health Coalition
United States Small-Area Life Expectancy Estimate Project (USALEEP)	Life expectancy estimates for all census tracts in the United States.					✓	✓			RWJF, NAPHSIS, and NCHS

Notes: An asterisk indicates that it is only provided for selected outcomes. CDC = Centers for Disease Control and Prevention; NIH = National Institutes of Health; RWJF = Robert Wood Johnson Foundation; NACCHO = National Association of County and City Health Officials; NAPHSIS = National Association for Public Health Statistics and Information Systems; NCHS = National Center for Health Statistics; DHHS = Department of Health and Human Services.

and End Results [SEER]). In addition, foundation-supported efforts (e.g., *Cancer Statistics*) and peer-reviewed publications often provide national-level mortality information.

State Mortality Data

Given the well-known variance in health outcomes by region of the country, as well as the preponderance of state-level legislation that impacts health, having specific mortality data for all 50 states is critical. Many of the resources discussed above also provide state-level mortality data obtained from the NVSS, including CDC WONDER and HD*Pulse*. For example, anyone can view or download data on overall mortality for any (or all) states through CDC WONDER. This includes the number of overall deaths and the crude and age-adjusted mortality rates for different groups defined by age, sex, and race and ethnicity. More specific data, such as data on underlying or multiple causes of death by state, are available upon request. In addition, state departments of public health further disseminate this information through their own reports and websites.

Numerous efforts have been made to compile, summarize, and disseminate state-level mortality data (from the NVSS) across the United States. America's Health Rankings (AHR) is one of the longest-running compilations of health data at the state level. AHR reports regularly highlight pronounced state-level variations in all categories.[96] The strengths of this initiative are that it presents mortality rates separately by race/ethnicity and shows trends over the past 5 years. Many other notable efforts to document state-level health outcomes exist, including the Global Burden of Disease studies, which incorporate state-level mortality rates for most summary (not cause-specific) measures.[97] Similarly, the Health of the States initiative provides state-level information (and rankings) for 39 health outcomes, including all-cause mortality, life expectancy, years of life lost, and mortality due to 14 specific causes of death.[98] The *State and Territorial Efforts to Reduce Health Disparities* report mentioned earlier also includes overall and infant mortality rates by race/ethnicity for 56 states and territories.[90] Still other efforts, such as the state snapshots based on the *National Healthcare Quality and Disparities* report from AHRQ or the County Health Rankings (CHR), also include state-level mortality rates for a variety of conditions.[99,100]

Importantly, none of these sources systematically include any measures of racial/ethnic disparities, such as mortality rate ratios or excess deaths. Without a clear metric for quantifying the extent of inequities, we risk overlooking one of the most crucial stories these data can tell— the glaring health inequities.

County Mortality Data

Counties have historically been the smallest geographic unit for which vital statistics data (and other selected outcomes) are routinely collected and reported. Like the national- and state-level mortality data, the primary source for county-level data is the CDC WONDER website. HD-*Pulse* also provides both the raw data and tables for each county.

Several additional groups use and disseminate these mortality data in different forms. Using data from CDC WONDER, the CHR initiative provides a snapshot of overall health and determinants of health for every county in the United States.[100] CHR has ranked all counties within each state annually according to a broad range of health-related factors since 2010. The core mortality measure, premature death, is provided separately by race/ethnicity when numbers permit, but no measures of disparities are included to help counties address issues of equity. This model can compare counties across (and within) states. These rankings (and CHR) get widespread attention from the media and public. In addition, the SEER program provides mortality data (for all causes, not just cancer) at the county level.

Of course, individual research efforts have also expanded our knowledge related to mortality at the county level. For example, researchers using data from the NVSS and small area estimation methodology have comprehensively examined mortality from the leading causes of death at the county level between 1980 and 2014,[101] as well as cancer-specific mortality disparities.[77] Others have studied premature morbidity[102,103] and life expectancy by county.[104]

City Mortality Data

Traditionally, much less data and information are available for mortality at the city level (compared to national, state, and county). However, the significance of documenting health outcomes at the city level was recently acknowledged (and elevated) by two new initiatives. First, the CDC, in cooperation with the RWJF and the CDC Foundation, launched the 500 Cities Project in 2015 to provide health data for the 500 largest US cities. This initiative provides data on 27 chronic disease outcomes at the city and census tract levels (using small area estimation). While it does not include any data on mortality, it does highlight the growing need for city-level data.

A second city-level initiative, the City Health Dashboard, grew out of the 500 Cities Project.[105] This project's user-friendly website provides city-level data from multiple national sources on 37 indicators for the largest 500 US cities. The Dashboard provides life expectancy estimates and premature mortality rates, as well as a handful of cause-specific rates. Currently, the Dashboard provides data points for each outcome, based on multiyear rolling averages. It is a valuable one-stop data resource for city leaders and public health professionals. However, it does have several notable limitations for those interested in health equity at the city level. To begin, county-level data are sometimes used instead of city-level data to calculate mortality rates, particularly for specific race/ethnic groups (Asian, Black, Hispanic, and white, when numbers permit). Given the amount of variation possible within even a single county or city, these estimates may obscure racial inequities. In addition, no measures of inequities, such as rate ratios or rate differences, are available as of this writing. Furthermore, since the Dashboard was created to assist individual cities, it is difficult to compare all cities at once (unlike the rankings available for states and counties). Finally, the site provides only estimates (using small area estimation methodology), not actual calculations of life expectancy for each city.

A precursor to both of these, and an early indicator of cities' need for data specific to their jurisdictions, is the data platform of the Big Cities Health Coalition (BCHC). A project of NACCHO, the BCHC offers a forum for the leaders of America's 30 largest metropolitan health departments to exchange strategies and jointly address issues to promote and protect the health of the 55 million people it serves. The organization curates the Big Cities Health Inventory, which provides 18,000 data points for its member cities. The platform provides data on overall mortality and life expectancy, as well as numerous cause-specific rates. Although this is another great source of information for cities, the limitations must be noted. Certain outcomes are missing data for more than half of the cities. For some cities, results reflect county, not city, data. The website provides race- and ethnicity-specific rates, but only for a limited number of cities (or counties). Like other data sources, there are no disparity measures. Also, the BCHC has specifically chosen not to compare or rank the cities. Finally, the data are provided by each city and submitted to the BCHC, making it difficult to ensure standardization of the calculations.

Neighborhood Mortality Data

Although city-level data are generally the smallest unit aligned with government jurisdictions (and thus most relevant for guiding and motivating policy changes), data for even smaller geographic units are increasingly being collected or calculated. This information, on neighborhoods or census tracts, is valuable for identifying inequities within cities, targeting city-level resources, and galvanizing groups within large urban areas. One impressive example of this type of work is the U.S. Small-area Life Expectancy Estimates Project (USALEEP), which began providing life expectancy estimates at the census tract level for almost all US tracts in 2018.[106] This huge undertaking provides important data never before available at such a local level. Despite this, we still lack critical information to drive racial equity efforts. For example, USALEEP data are not available at a meaningful neighborhood level and do not include measures of disparity. Although the USALEEP project does not specifically focus on inequities, the Mapping Life Expectancy effort pioneered by Virginia Commonwealth University and funded by the RWJF does.[107] This initiative calculated neighborhood-level life expectancies and mapped them according to familiar landmarks, subway routes, and highways to highlight the substantial inequities existing within cities (see figure 1.4).

Although few national efforts have examined mortality in areas smaller than cities, several local efforts have. Within Chicago, for example, researchers have investigated mortality from selected causes of death (as well as life expectancy) across the city's 77 officially designated community areas.[108–110] These studies highlighted striking racial/ethnic and geographic disparities. Other cities and counties, such as Los Angeles County, CA, King County, WA, and New York City, NY, have focused

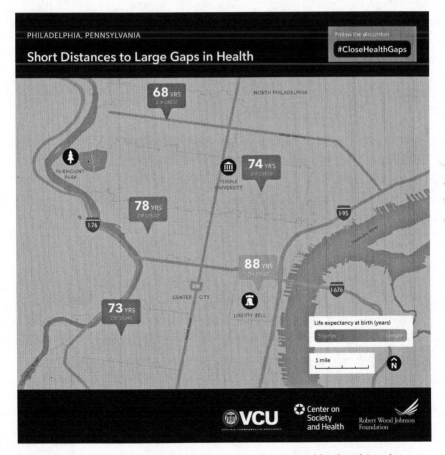

Figure 1.4. Example of City-Level Figure Visualizing Neighborhood-Level Disparities in Life Expectancy. *Source:* VCU Center on Society and Health.

on census tract, neighborhood, or borough-level disparities in life expectancy and mortality. Clearly there is value in analyzing data at this level as well. Zooming into lower levels of geography, moving from the national to the state to the city or even to communities—we gain greater insight into social divisions and health inequities.

Summary of Existing Mortality Data

Recognition of the importance of local data has produced increasingly focused data collection efforts. Much attention is being directed to state- and county-level data, resulting in numerous initiatives providing high-quality comparisons and rankings. *However, we still do not have comprehensive city-level data on mortality.* Importantly, no source provides race-specific mortality rates for all of the leading causes of death, and little or no information on mortality inequities at the city-level is available. These shortcomings limit the ability of urban leaders and other stakeholders to understand (and subsequently address) their cities' overall levels of health and health equity.[111] More broadly, this information also allows us to compare cities—identifying cities that have relatively good mortality outcomes and equity among racial groups, as well as those that may need support to improve outcomes and advance health equity.

Why Cities? The Importance of Local Data

We have mentioned the importance of city-level data throughout this chapter, but now we would like to make our rationale more explicit. The choice to focus on cities goes beyond logistics, although those numbers are quite marked. For example, four in five Americans currently live in urban areas. The percentage of urban (versus rural) residents has steadily grown since the start of the twentieth century, and that figure is expected to increase dramatically over the next three decades.[112-114] Furthermore, people of color are even more likely than whites to live in urban areas; for the period from 2006 to 2008, 88% of the US Black population was living in an urban area, compared to 73% of whites.[83]

We focus on cities for two even more crucial reasons: larger geographic areas (even counties) can obscure significant differences between groups, and data aligned with political jurisdictions are critical for driving change.

Larger Geographic Units Hide Variation

We have seen that, in the United States, high-quality data document mortality and inequities at the national, state, and county levels. However, research has demonstrated the "profound" inequities revealed when health outcomes are examined at subcounty levels.[115,116] In other words, the smaller the geographical unit, the more variations in outcomes and social factors emerge. Without city-level data, we risk overlooking the most critical public health challenges. This is why a recent call to action based on listening sessions hosted by DHHS included a demand for "timely, reliable, granular-level (i.e., subcounty), and actionable data" as one of their five recommendations for improving public health in the twenty-first century.[117] Similarly, a working group of the National Committee on Vital and Health Statistics recently created a framework for increasing the availability of subcounty data to guide local, multisectoral health improvement initiatives.[118] Data for areas smaller than counties are clearly needed.

Informing Policy and Programming

Even city-level data hide variation across neighborhoods;[116] however, policy change is most likely to occur at the city, not the neighborhood, level. Thus, it is essential to match the level of data with the primary political jurisdictions in order to make the data most relevant and actionable. City officials, public health professionals, health care providers, community leaders, and other stakeholders need city-level information to support evidence-based changes in policies, services, and funding.[117] For instance, local departments of public health, in partnership with city agencies and government offices, are at the front line for creating health-related policies. They also control large budgets. On average, local health departments serving areas with 500,000 to 999,999 residents spend an estimated $47 million annually, and departments serving areas with more than 1 million residents spend $174 million annually.[119]

Data comparing cities may also be valuable to individuals working to improve health (or health equity) at the state, regional, or national levels. In particular, data comparing cities can guide regional or national stakeholders looking to target larger efforts to the neediest areas. As recognized by the World Health Organization, "information that shows the gaps between cities or within the same city is a crucial requirement to trigger appropriate local actions to promote health equity" (p. 727).[120]

City Spotlight: Chicago

Throughout this book we highlight our home city of Chicago to provide an example of how individual cities can understand the unique history and context of health and health equity within their jurisdiction. In parts II and III, which present large amounts of city-specific data, the spotlights offer a template for the interpretation of the mortality and equity numbers. These examples of Chicago data provide a foundation for the final section of the book (part IV), which offers a social justice framework for health equity work, as well as specific "case studies" from Chicago to help public health advocates, civic leaders, and other stakeholders envision the steps needed to improve on their own city's current health outcomes and levels of equity.

Nearly 3 million people live in Chicago, making it the third-largest US city. Chicago is known for the Cubs, chilly winters, deep-dish pizza, and, unfortunately, extreme levels of racial segregation. Numerous researchers have detailed the blatant socioeconomic, geographic, and racial inequities in Chicago over time.[121] This gap—between rich and poor, North and South, Black and white—is still vividly apparent as one travels from the famous "Magnificent Mile" of high-end stores along the northern part of Michigan Avenue down to the equally infamous "South Side," which has been devastated by failed public housing efforts like the Robert Taylor Homes (now gone). Robert Sampson has eloquently described this journey through the diverse and disparate Chicago communities in much greater detail.[121] Data also support these racial and geographic divides in the city; for example, 30% of Black adults lived in poverty in 2017, while only 10% of whites did.[122] Across Chicago's 77 community areas, levels of poverty ranged from 2% to 66%.[122]

Stemming from these socioeconomic inequities, Chicago also has well-documented health inequities between communities and racial groups.[123] More specifically, research has documented Chicago's racial inequities in mortality over the past several decades. This work shows that racial inequities in all-cause mortality in Chicago tend to be larger than the national averages, and that the gap worsened between 1990 and 2005.[9] In this book we highlight findings that reveal that these inequities have not been eliminated (chapters 3–5), despite the city health department's recent focus on health equity and the work of other local organizations (such as the work of West Side United, highlighted in chapter 9).

Conclusion

For well over 100 years, the United States has experienced glaring racial inequities in mortality, due in large part to racial inequalities in access to resources. Over time, efforts to both document and address these inequities have grown, reflecting an increased focus on health equity from our government, academic institutions, philanthropists, and community members and organizations. *Yet these efforts have not succeeded in bringing health equity to all Americans.* This compels us to identify new avenues for intervention, and city-centered initiatives represent one of our most promising opportunities. To date, city-level efforts have been uneven, likely hampered by a lack of relevant data to motivate stakeholders, convince funders, and guide actions. In this book we provide the much-needed data on city-level mortality outcomes and inequities, shining a light on striking variations across race and place. The presentation of these findings is intended to help keep urban equity issues at the forefront in order to build awareness, stimulate partnerships, and pressure leaders to take concrete steps to equality.

Before presenting these city-level mortality data, we need to first understand the broad range of individual, social, and structural factors that impact mortality (and other health outcomes) at the population level. The following chapter provides a useful lens to help readers think about the differences among health outcomes across cities and across racial groups. We offer several theoretical frameworks for identifying the city characteristics, far upstream from individual health outcomes, which have led to the mortality inequities still seen across our country.

References

1. Xu J, Murphy SL, Kochanek KD, Arias E. *Mortality in the United States, 2018.* Hyattsville, MD: National Center for Health Statistics; January 2020.

2. Kochanek K, Murphy S, Xu J, Arias E. Deaths: Final Data for 2017. *National Vital Statistics Reports.* 2019;68(9).

3. Yearby R. Racial Disparities in Health Status and Access to Healthcare: The Continuation of Inequality in the United States due to Structural Racism. *American Journal of Economics and Sociology.* 2018;77(3–4):1113–1152.

4. Singh GK, Siahpush M. Widening Socioeconomic Inequalities in US Life Expectancy, 1980–2000. *International Journal of Epidemiology.* 2006;35(4):969–979.

5. Pool LR, Ning H, Lloyd-Jones DM, Allen NB. Trends in Racial/Ethnic Disparities in Cardiovascular Health among US Adults from 1999–2012. *Journal of the American Heart Association.* 2017;6(9).

6. Singh GK, Jemal A. Socioeconomic and Racial/Ethnic Disparities in Cancer Mortality, Incidence, and Survival in the United States, 1950–2014: Over Six Decades of Changing Patterns and Widening Inequalities. *Journal of Environmental and Public Health.* 2017;2017:2819372.

7. Yedjou CG, Tchounwou PB, Fonseca DD, et al. Assessing the Racial and Ethnic Disparities in Breast Cancer Mortality in the United States. *International Journal of Environmental Research and Public Health.* 2017;14(5).

8. National Center for Health Statistics. *Health, United States, 2017: With Special Feature on Mortality.* Hyattsville, MD: National Center for Health Statistics; 2018.

9. Orsi JM, Margellos-Anast H, Whitman S. Black–White Health Disparities in the United States and Chicago: A 15-Year Progress Analysis. *American Journal of Public Health.* 2010;100(2):349–356.

10. US Department of Health and Human Services. About Healthy People. Foundation Health Measures: Disparities. 2018. http://www.healthypeople.gov /2020/about/disparitiesAbout.aspx.

11. Wallerstein NB, Yen IH, Syme SL. Integration of Social Epidemiology and Community-Engaged Interventions to Improve Health Equity. *American Journal of Public Health.* 2011;101(5):822–830.

12. National Center for Health Statistics. *Healthy People 2010 Final Review.* Hyattsville, MD: National Center for Health Statistics; 2012.

13. Grubbs SS, Polite BN, Carney J Jr, et al. Eliminating Racial Disparities in Colorectal Cancer in the Real World: It Took a Village. *Journal of Clinical Oncology.* 2013;31(16):1928–1930.

14. Ansell D, Grabler P, Whitman S, et al. A Community Effort to Reduce the Black/White Breast Cancer Mortality Disparity in Chicago. *Cancer Causes Control.* 2009;20(9):1681–1688.

15. Whitehead M. The Concepts and Principles of Equity and Health. *International Journal of Health Services.* 1992;22(3):429–445.

16. American Public Health Association. Health Equity. https://www.apha.org/topics-and-issues/health-equity.

17. Braveman P, Arkin E, Orleans T, Proctor D, Plough A. *What Is Health Equity? And What Difference Does a Definition Make?* Princeton, NJ: Robert Wood Johnson Foundation; 2017.

18. Farmer P. *Pathologies of Power.* Berkeley: University of California Press; 2003.

19. Xu J, Murphy SL, Kochanek KD, Bastian B, Arias E. Deaths: Final Data for 2016. *National Vital Statistics Reports.* 2018;67(5):1–76.

20. Byrd WM, Clayton LA. *An American Health Dilemma.* New York: Routledge; 2000.

21. Washington HA. *Medical Apartheid: The Dark History of Medical Experimentation on Black Americans from Colonial Times to the Present.* New York: Anchor Books; 2008.

22. Haines MR. Ethnic Differences in Demographic Behavior in the United States: Has There Been Convergence? *Historical Methods.* 2003;36(4):157–195.

23. Hummer RA. Black-White Differences in Health and Mortality: A Review and Conceptual Model. *Sociological Quarterly.* 1996;37(1):105–125.

24. Centers for Disease Control and Prevention. *CDC Health Disparities and Inequalities Report—United States, 2013.* Atlanta, GA: US Department of Health and Human Services, Centers for Disease Control and Prevention; 2013.

25. Barr DA. *Health Disparities in the United States: Social Class, Race, Ethnicity, and Health.* Baltimore: Johns Hopkins University Press; 2008.

26. Ansell D. *The Death Gap: How Inequality Kills.* Chicago: University of Chicago Press; 2017.

27. Krieger N. *Epidemiology and the People's Health: Theory and Context.* Oxford: Oxford University Press; 2011.

28. Engels F. *The Condition of the Working Class in England.* Leipzig, Germany: Otto Wigand; 1887.

29. Taylor R, Rieger A. Medicine as Social Science: Rudolf Virchow on the Typhus Epidemic in Upper Silesia. *International Journal of Health Services.* 1985;15(4):547–559.

30. Du Bois WEB. *The Philadelphia Negro.* Philadelphia: University of Pennsylvania Press; 1899.

31. Krieger N. Shades of Difference: Theoretical Underpinnings of the Medical Controversy on Black/White Differences in the United States, 1830–1870. *International Journal of Health Services.* 1987;17(2):259–278.

32. Cooper R, David R. The Biological Concept of Race and Its Application to Public Health and Epidemiology. *Journal of Health Politics Policy and Law.* 1986;11(1):97–116.

33. Goodman AH. Why Genes Don't Count (for Racial Differences in Health). *American Journal of Public Health.* 2000;90(11):1699–1702.

34. Templeton AR. Biological Races in Humans. *Studies in History and Philosophy of Biological and Biomedical Sciences.* 2013;44(3):262–271.

35. Templeton AR. Human Races: A Genetic and Evolutionary Perspective. *American Anthropologist.* 1998;100(3):632–650.

36. Williams MJ, Eberhardt JL. Biological Conceptions of Race and the Motivation to Cross Racial Boundaries. *Journal of Personality and Social Psychology.* 2008;94(6):1033–1047.

37. Rothstein R. *The Color of Law.* New York: Liveright; 2017.

38. Gordon A. The Creation of Homeownership: How New Deal Changes in Banking Regulation Simultaneously Made Homeownership Accessible to Whites and out of Reach for Blacks. *Yale Law Journal.* 2005;115:186–224.

39. Hospital Survey and Construction Act. In 42 U.S.C. § 291e(F) 2020.

40. *Simkins v. Moses H. Cone Memorial Hospital.* F2d 323, 959 (Court of Appeals for the 4th Circuit 1963).

41. Bell DA. Brown v. Board of Education and the Interest-Convergence Dilemma. *Harvard Law Review.* 1980;93(3):518–533.

42. Gamble VN, Stone D. U.S. Policy on Health Inequities: The Interplay of Politics and Research. *Journal of Health Politics, Policy and Law* 2006;31(1):93–126.

43. Smith D. *Health Care Divided: Race and Healing a Nation.* Ann Arbor: University of Michigan Press; 1999.

44. Keppel KG, Pearcy JN, Heron MP. Is There Progress toward Eliminating Racial/Ethnic Disparities in the Leading Causes of Death? *Public Health Reports.* 2010;125(5):689–697.

45. Satcher D, Fryer GE, McCann J, Troutman A. What If We Were Equal? A Comparison of the Black-White Mortality Gap in 1960 and 2000. *Health Affairs.* 2005;24(2):459–464.

46. Sloan FA, Ayyagari P, Salm M, Grossman D. The Longevity Gap between Black and White Men in the United States at the Beginning and End of the 20th Century. *American Journal of Public Health.* 2010;100(2):357–363.

47. Levine RS, Foster JE, Fullilove RE, et al. Black-White Inequalities in Mortality and Life Expectancy, 1933–1999: Implications for Healthy People 2010. *Public Health Reports.* 2001;116(5):474–483.

48. Massey DS. The Legacy of the 1968 Fair Housing Act. *Sociological Forum (Randolph, NJ).* 2015;30(Suppl 1):571–588.

49. Parker K, Horowitz J, Mahl B. On Views of Race and Inequality, Blacks and Whites Are Worlds Apart. *Pew Research Center Report.* 2016:1–107.

50. Jan T. The Senate Rolls Back Rules Meant to Root Out Discrimination by Mortgage Lenders. *Washington Post.* March 14, 2018. https://www .washingtonpost.com/news/wonk/wp/2018/03/14/the-senate-rolls-back-rules -meant-to-root-out-discrimination-by-mortgage-lenders/.

51. Dimick J, Ruhter J, Sarrazin MV, Birkmeyer JD. Black Patients More Likely Than Whites to Undergo Surgery at Low-Quality Hospitals in Segregated Regions. *Health Aff (Millwood).* 2013;32(6):1046–1053.

52. Lang ME, Bird CE. Understanding and Addressing the Common Roots of Racial Health Disparities: The Case of Cardiovascular Disease and HIV/AIDS in African Americans. *Health Matrix.* 2015;25:109–138.

53. Walker RE, Keane CR, Burke JG. Disparities and Access to Healthy Food in the United States: A Review of Food Deserts Literature. *Health and Place.* 2010;16(5):876–884.

54. Larson NI, Story MT, Nelson MC. Neighborhood Environments: Disparities in Access to Healthy Foods in the U.S. *American Journal of Preventive Medicine.* 2009;36(1):74–81.

55. Civil Rights Act of 1964. In 42 U.S.C.A. § 2000d 2020.

56. Krieger N, Chen JT, Coull B, Waterman PD, Beckfield J. The Unique Impact of Abolition of Jim Crow Laws on Reducing Inequities in Infant Death Rates and Implications for Choice of Comparison Groups in Analyzing Societal Determinants of Health. *American Journal of Public Health.* 2013;103(12):2234–2244.

57. Almond D, Chay KY, Greenstone M. Civil Rights, the War on Poverty, and Black-White Convergence in Infant Mortality in the Rural South and Mississippi. MIT Department of Economics Working Paper; 2006.

58. Gornick ME, Eggers PW, Reilly TW, et al. Effects of Race and Income on Mortality and Use of Services among Medicare Beneficiaries. *New England Journal of Medicine.* 1996;335(11):791–799.

59. Bach PB, Cramer LD, Warren JL, Begg CB. Racial Differences in the Treatment of Early-Stage Lung Cancer. *New England Journal of Medicine.* 1999;341(16):1198–1205.

60. Ayanian JZ, Weissman JS, Chasan-Taber S, Epstein AM. Quality of Care by Race and Gender for Congestive Heart Failure and Pneumonia. *Medical Care.* 1999;37(12):1260–1269.

61. Daniel P, Rodrigo C, McKeever TM, Woodhead M, Welham S, Lim WS. Time to First Antibiotic and Mortality in Adults Hospitalised with

Community-Acquired Pneumonia: A Matched-Propensity Analysis. *Thorax.* 2016;71(6):568–570.

62. Patient Protection and Affordable Care Act. In 42 USC § 18001 2010.

63. Blumenthal D, Abrams M, Nuzum R. The Affordable Care Act at 5 Years. *New England Journal of Medicine.* 2015;372(25):2451–2458.

64. *National Federation of Independent Business v. Sebelius.* U.S. 567, 519 (Supreme Court of the United States 2012).

65. Andrulis DP, Siddiqui NJ, Purtle JP, Duchon L. *Patient Protection and Affordable Care Act of 2010: Advancing Health Equity for Racially and Ethnically Diverse Populations.* Washington, DC: Joint Center for Political and Economic Studies; 2010.

66. Watson SD. Lessons from Ferguson and Beyond: Bias, Health, and Justice. *Minnesota Journal of Law, Science and Technology.* 2017;18:111–142.

67. Yearby R. Breaking the Cycle of "Unequal Treatment" with Health Care Reform: Acknowledging and Addressing the Continuation of Racial Bias. *Connecticut Law Review.* 2012;44:1281–1324.

68. French MT, Homer J, Gumus G, Hickling L. Key Provisions of the Patient Protection and Affordable Care Act (Aca): A Systematic Review and Presentation of Early Research Findings. *Health Services Research.* 2016;51(5):1735–1771.

69. Cunningham TJ, Croft JB, Liu Y, Lu H, Eke PI, Giles WH. Vital Signs: Racial Disparities in Age-Specific Mortality among Blacks or African Americans—United States, 1999–2015. *MMWR Morbidity and Mortality Weekly Report.* 2017 May 5;66(17):444–456.

70. Harper S, MacLehose RF, Kaufman JS. Trends in the Black-White Life Expectancy Gap among U.S. States, 1990–2009. *Health Affairs.* 2014;33(8):1375–1382.

71. Van Dyke M, Greer S, Odom E, et al. Heart Disease Death Rates among Blacks and Whites Aged ≥35 Years—United States, 1968–2015. *MMWR Surveillance Summaries.* 2018;67(5):1–11.

72. Singh GK, Siahpush M, Azuine RE, Williams SD. Widening Socioeconomic and Racial Disparities in Cardiovascular Disease Mortality in the United States, 1969–2013. *International Journal of MCH and AIDS.* 2015;3(2):106–118.

73. Singh GK, Jemal A. Socioeconomic and Racial/Ethnic Disparities in Cancer Mortality, Incidence, and Survival in the United States, 1950–2014: Over Six Decades of Changing Patterns and Widening Inequalities. *Journal of Environmental and Public Health.* 2017;2017:19.

74. Kawachi I, Berkman LF. *Neighborhoods and Health.* Oxford: Oxford University Press; 2003.

75. Wei R, Anderson RN, Curtin LR, Arias E. U.S. Decennial Life Tables for 1999–2001: State Life Tables. *National Vital Statistics Reports.* 2012;60(9):1–66.

76. Bharmal N, Tseng C-H, Kaplan R, Wong MD. State-Level Variations in Racial Disparities in Life Expectancy. *Health Services Research.* 2012;47(1pt2).

77. Mokdad AH, Dwyer-Lindgren L, Fitzmaurice C, et al. Trends and Patterns of Disparities in Cancer Mortality among US Counties, 1980–2014. *Journal of the American Medical Association.* 2017;317(4):388–406.

78. Rust G, Zhang S, Malhotra K, et al. Paths to Health Equity: Local Area Variation in Progress toward Eliminating Breast Cancer Mortality Disparities, 1990–2009. *Cancer.* 2015;121(16):2765–2774.

79. Spoer B. Powerful Open Data Tool Illustrates Life Expectancy Gaps Are Larger in More Racially Segregated Cities. Build Healthy Places Network; 2019.

80. *Healthy People: The Surgeon General's Report on Health Promotion and Disease Prevention.* Rockville, MD: US Public Health Service; 1979.

81. Gamble VN, Stone D. U.S. Policy on Health Inequities: The Interplay of Politics and Research. *Journal of Health Politics Policy and Law.* 2006;31(1):93–126.

82. US Department of Health and Human Services. National Partnership for Action: About the NPA. https://minorityhealth.hhs.gov/npa/files/Plans/Toolkit/NPA_Toolkit.pdf.

83. Beadle MR, Graham GN. *National Stakeholder Strategy for Achieving Health Equity.* Hyattsville, MD: US Department of Health and Human Services; 2011.

84. US Department of Health and Human Services. *Healthy People 2000 Final Review.* Hyattsville, MD: US Department of Health and Human Services; 2001.

85. Agency for Healthcare Research and Quality. *National Healthcare Quality and Disparities Reports.* Rockville, MD: Agency for Healthcare Research and Quality; 2019.

86. Smedley BD, Stith AY, Nelson AR, Institute of Medicine Committee on Understanding and Eliminating Racial and Ethnic Disparities in Health Care. *Unequal Treatment: Confronting Racial and Ethnic Disparities in Health Care.* Washington, DC: National Academies Press; 2003.

87. US Department of Health and Human Services. *HHS Action Plan to Reduce Racial and Ethnic Health Disparities.* Hyattsville, MD: US Department of Health and Human Services; 2011.

88. Lurie N, Fremont A, Somers SA, et al. The National Health Plan Collaborative to Reduce Disparities and Improve Quality. *Joint Commission Journal on Quality and Patient Safety.* 2008;34(5):256–265.

89. ChangeLab Solutions. *Blueprint for Changemakers: Achieving Health Equity through Law and Policy.* 2019. https://www.changelabsolutions.org/product/blueprint-changemakers.

90. US Office of Minority Health. *State and Territorial Efforts to Reduce Health Disparities: Findings of a 2016 Survey by the U.S. Department of Health and Human Services Office of Minority Health.* Rockville, MD: US Department of Health and Human Services, Office of Minority Health; 2018: https://minorityhealth.hhs.gov/assets/PDF/OMH-Health-Disparities-Report-State-and-Territorial-Efforts-October-2018.pdf.

91. Ladenheim K, Groman R. State Legislative Activities Related to Elimination of Health Disparities. *Journal of Health Politics Policy and Law*. 2006;31(1):153–183.

92. Young JL, Pollack K, Rutkow L. Review of State Legislative Approaches to Eliminating Racial and Ethnic Health Disparities, 2002–2011. *American Journal of Public Health*. 2015;105:S388–S393.

93. Association of State and Territorial Health Officials. *Forces of Change Survey Report*. 2017. https://www.astho.org/Research/Forces-of-Change/Report /2017-Full/.

94. Dircksen J, Prachand NG, Adams D, et al. *Healthy Chicago 2.0: Partnering to Improve Health Equity (2016–2020)*. Chicago: Chicago Department of Public Health; March 2016.

95. Arias E, Xu JQ, Kochanek KD. United States Life Tables, 2016. *National Vital Statistics Reports*. 2019;68(4). Hyattsville, MD: National Center for Health Statistics; 2019.

96. United Health Foundation. *America's Health Rankings Annual Report 2018*. 2018. https://www.americashealthrankings.org/.

97. Mokdad AH, Ballestros K, Echko M, et al. The State of U.S. Health, 1990–2016: Burden of Diseases, Injuries, and Risk Factors among U.S. States. *Journal of the American Medical Association*. 2018;319(14):1444–1472.

98. Woolf SH, Aron L, Chapman DA, et al. *The Health of the States: How U.S. States Compare in Health Status and the Factors That Shape Health— Summary Report*. Richmond, VA: Center on Society and Health, Virginia Commonwealth University; 2016.

99. Agency for Health Care Research and Quality. State Snapshots 2019. https://www.ahrq.gov/data/state-snapshots.html.

100. University of Wisconsion Population Health Institute. County Health Rankings. 2020. www.countyhealthrankings.org.

101. Dwyer-Lindgren L, Bertozzi-Villa A, Stubbs RW, et al. US County-Level Trends in Mortality Rates for Major Causes of Death, 1980–2014. *Journal of the American Medical Association*. 2016;316(22).

102. Cullen MR, Cummins C, Fuchs VR. Geographic and Racial Variation in Premature Mortality in the U.S.: Analyzing the Disparities. *PLOS One*. 2012;7(4):e32930.

103. Kiang MV, Krieger N, Buckee CO, Onnela JP, Chen JT. Decomposition of the US Black/White Inequality in Premature Mortality, 2010–2015: An Observational Study. *BMJ Open*. 2019;9(11):e029373.

104. Dwyer-Lindgren L, Bertozzi-Villa A, Stubbs RW, et al. Inequalities in Life Expectancy among US Counties, 1980 to 2014: Temporal Trends and Key Drivers. *JAMA Internal Medicine*. 2017;177(7):1003–1011.

105. Gourevitch MN, Athens JK, Levine SE, Kleiman N, Thorpe LE. City-Level Measures of Health, Health Determinants, and Equity to Foster

Population Health Improvement: The City Health Dashboard. *American Journal of Public Health.* 2019;109(4):585–592.

106. Arias E, Escobedo L, Kennedy J, Fu C, Cisewski J. U.S. Small-Area Life Expectancy Estimates Project: Methodology and Results Summary. *Vital Health Statistics.* 2018;2(181).

107. Virginia Commonwealth University Center on Society and Health. Mapping Life Expectancy. 2019. https://societyhealth.vcu.edu/work/the-projects /mapping-life-expectancy.html.

108. Hunt BR, Deot D, Whitman S. Stroke Mortality Rates Vary in Local Communities in a Metropolitan Area: Racial and Spatial Disparities and Correlates. *Stroke.* 2014;45(7):2059–2065.

109. Hunt BR, Tran G, Whitman S. Life Expectancy Varies in Local Communities in Chicago: Racial and Spatial Disparities and Correlates. *Journal of Racial and Ethnic Health Disparities.* 2015;2(4):425–433.

110. Hunt BR, Whitman S, Henry CA. Age-Adjusted Diabetes Mortality Rates Vary in Local Communities in a Metropolitan Area: Racial and Spatial Disparities and Correlates. *Diabetes Care.* 2014;37(5):1279–1286.

111. Booske BC, Rohan AM, Kindig DA, Remington PL. Grading and Reporting Health and Health Disparities. *Preventing Chronic Disease.* 2010;7(1):A16.

112. US Conference of Mayors. *Metro Economies: Past and Future Employment Levels: Transportantion and the Cost of Congestion, Population Forecast.* Washington, DC; 2018.

113. US Census Bureau. American Fact Finder. 2019. https://data.census.gov /cedsci/.

114. Fields A, Holder KA, Burd C. *Life Off the Highway: A Snapshot of Rural America.* 2016. https://www.census.gov/newsroom/blogs/random -samplings/2016/12/life_off_the_highway.html.

115. Boothe VL, Fierro LA, Laurent A, Shih M. Sub-county Life Expectancy: A Tool to Improve Community Health and Advance Health Equity. *Preventing Chronic Disease.* 2018;15:E11.

116. Whitman S, Shah AM, Benjamins MR, eds. *Urban Health: Combating Disparities with Local Data.* New York: Oxford University Press; 2011.

117. DeSalvo KB, Wang YC, Harris A, Auerbach J, Koo D, O'Carroll P. Public Health 3.0: A Call to Action for Public Health to Meet the Challenges of the 21st Century. *Preventing Chronic Disease.* 2017;14:E78.

118. National Committee on Vital and Health Statistics, US Department of Health and Human Services. *NCVHS Measurement Framework for Community Health and Well-Being, V4.* 2017. https://ncvhs.hhs.gov/wp-content/uploads /2018/03/NCVHS-Measurement-Framework-V4-Jan-12-2017-for-posting -FINAL.pdf.

119. National Association of County and City Health Officials. *National Profile of Local Health Departments.* 2020. https://www.naccho.org/uploads

/downloadable-resources/Programs/Public-Health-Infrastructure/NACCHO
_2019_Profile_final.pdf.

120. Kumaresan J, Prasad A, Alwan A, Ishikawa N. Promoting Health
Equity in Cities through Evidence-Based Action. *Journal of Urban Health*.
2010;87(5):727–732.

121. Sampson RJ. *Great American City: Chicago and the Enduring Neighborhood Effect*. Chicago: University of Chicago Press; 2012.

122. City of Chicago. Chicago Health Atlas, Indicators. 2020. https://www
.chicagohealthatlas.org/indicators.

123. De Maio F, Shah RC, Mazzeo J, Ansell DA, eds. *Community Health
Equity: A Chicago Reader*. Chicago: University of Chicago Press; 2019.

TWO

Theorizing the Causes of Health Inequities

FERNANDO G. DE MAIO AND MAUREEN R. BENJAMINS

EXPLAINING BLACK:WHITE gaps in mortality across large US cities is a complex task. For many, it is uncomfortable—a task that re-quires grappling with deep-rooted social divisions and assumptions about "race" in US society. Acknowledging the large inequities between Black and white people seen in some of the most critical population health indicators, including premature and infant mortality, forces us to come to grips with a kind of inequality that contemporary color-blind discourse attempts to mask from public view.[1] Health inequities reveal patterns that many people would prefer to ignore, particularly when one goes beyond the national statistics and examines, as we do in this book, inequities in specific places. It is difficult to comprehend that our neigh-bors in our own cities may have dramatically higher chances of dying prematurely simply because of the color of their skin. To understand why this is the case, we must expose the health effects associated with economic inequality, residential segregation, and racism.[2-5]

Yet, as one might expect, Black:white gaps in population health in-dicators can be understood in different ways, just as race and the causes of poverty or economic inequality can be. For us, however, it is clear: race is a socially constructed phenomenon, not a biological reality.[5-7] When we think about "racial" differences in health, we understand them as the products of rac*ism*, not race. In other words, we are confronting the effects of the social process of racism, which operates on several levels, from interpersonal to structural. Similarly, we recognize that levels of poverty and economic inequality—along with correlated issues like residential racial segregation—are themselves created by public policy and private actions (and are thus amendable to change). There is nothing inevitable about the patterns of inequality that shape our cities.

In this chapter, we explore the causes of health inequities from different theoretical approaches. We contrast the traditional approach, whereby "health is a personal responsibility," with newer alternatives emerging from the rapidly growing research literature on health inequities. These alternatives draw particularly from the field of social epidemiology.[8,9] We compare three influential "big picture" models—one from a public health initiative in the San Francisco Bay Area, one from the World Health Organization (WHO), and one from the sociological research literature—to move from the *proximal* to the *distal*, from the *personal* to the *societal*. The causes of health inequities may be complex and multifaceted, but they are composed of two complementary schools of thought: the psychosocial and the sociopolitical theoretical explanations.[9] After many decades of research, a consensus is emerging that points toward social and structural determinants as the root causes of health inequities. In this chapter, we argue that these theories add a valuable lens through which to interpret statistical data measuring inequalities in mortality across our cities.

Why We Need Theory to Understand Health Inequities

Theories help make sense of the world. They call attention to particular patterns and causal pathways to provide different explanations for why the world is the way it is. For example, Marxist theories use concepts like social class, class consciousness, and capitalist exploitation to make us look at the means of production in a society. Feminist theories emphasize patriarchy and focus our gaze on gender inequality.[10,11] Behavioral theories often highlight individuals and their attitudes, beliefs, and behaviors.[12] Much like politics, theory shapes the questions we ask and the data we seek. Ultimately, theory can guide our actions to change the world for the better.

The Traditional Approach: Health Is a Personal Responsibility

The traditional approach to understanding health and health inequities emphasizes personal responsibility. Indeed, society often portrays poor health pejoratively, as an individual's *fault*.[11–13] In this way, diabetes, obesity, and cancer are the logical (and possibly even deserved) by-products of poor lifestyle choices. Solutions thus revolve around improving people's personal habits through targeted health promotion, health literacy improvements, or advancements in general health education. This approach focuses on the "beliefs, behaviors, and biology" of individuals.[14] To be sure, effective programs that intervene in this way, helping people to make healthier choices and ultimately live longer lives, abound. But when taken to an extreme, in isolation from a social analysis, this perspective overemphasizes personal responsibility, while neglecting the constraints that limit personal choices.[15]

The prominent social epidemiologist Nancy Krieger calls this the "medical and lifestyle" explanation of health inequities.[9] Its focus is on biological explanations of disease that are amenable to intervention through health care and public health outreach. In the language of public health, these are the "proximal" causes of disease; they exist and can be measured, and potentially modified, at the individual level.[16] Taking some of the leading causes of death—heart disease, cancer, stroke, chronic lower respiratory diseases—we can identify proximal risk factors, including high blood pressure, elevated blood glucose, and obesity. Moving farther "away" from the disease outcome, we can name common modifiable risk factors, such as unhealthy diet, physical inactivity, or tobacco use, and target these as issues addressable through education and health promotion.[12] Arguably, this is the dominant theoretical framework for understanding poor health in society today.[5,9] While important in recognizing that individuals can and do impact their own health, this neglects to consider place (where we live, work, and play) and social structure and glosses over external factors (including racism, xenophobia, economic exploitation, and gender inequality) that inhibit people from making healthy choices in their lives.

Social Epidemiologic Alternatives: The Structural and Social Determinants of Health

When we look for patterns among social groups (which could be defined in terms of socioeconomic status, race/ethnicity, or other social characteristics) and variation between places, a different picture emerges. This demands an entirely different theoretical perspective, one that examines the "distal" causes of disease.[16] Turning our attention to what public health recognizes as upstream factors expands our understanding of the causes of health inequities in ways that the traditional "health is a personal responsibility" model alone cannot. Many models of this kind can be found in the public health literature.[5,9,11,17] Here, we contrast three influential versions—one from a public health initiative in the San Francisco Bay Area, one from the WHO, and one from the sociological research literature (see figure 2.1).

The three panels in figure 2.1 correspond to different (but complementary) theories of health inequities. Figure 2.1a illustrates the perspective of the Bay Area Regional Health Inequities Initiative (BARHII), a coalition of the San Francisco Bay Area's 11 public health departments.[18] It exemplifies the "upstream-downstream" spectrum particularly well, showing the movement from grand social inequities (class, race/ethnicity, immigration status, gender, and sexual orientation) and "institutional power" (describing the roles of corporations and businesses, government agencies, schools, and other institutions) on the left to living conditions and then to individual risk behaviors, disease and injury, and mortality on

Figure 2.1. *(opposite)* Three Alternative Models for Thinking about the Social Determinants of Health. *Sources:* (a) Bay Area Regional Health Inequities Initiative. *Applying Social Determinants of Health Indicators to Advance Health Equity: A Guide for Local Health Department Epidemiologists and Public Health Professionals.* Oakland, CA; 2015. (b) Solar O, Irwin A. *A Conceptual Framework for Action on the Social Determinants of Health.* Geneva: World Health Organization; 2007. (c) Coburn D. Beyond the Income Inequality Hypothesis: Class, Neo-liberalism, and Health Inequalities. *Social Science and Medicine.* 2004;58(1):41–56.

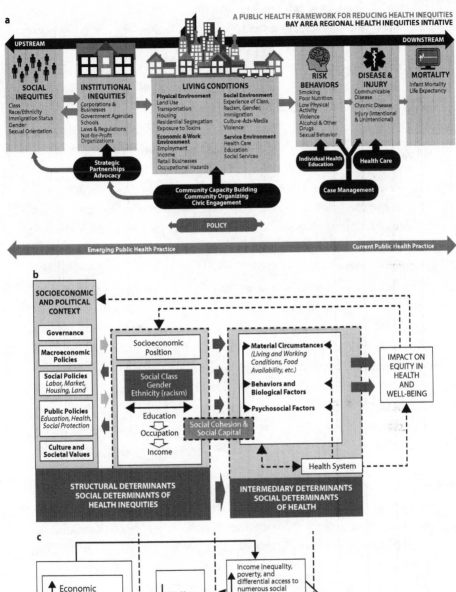

a

A PUBLIC HEALTH FRAMEWORK FOR REDUCING HEALTH INEQUITIES
BAY AREA REGIONAL HEALTH INEQUITIES INTIATIVE

UPSTREAM → DOWNSTREAM

SOCIAL INEQUITIES
Class
Race/Ethnicity
Immigration Status
Gender
Sexual Orientation

INSTITUTIONAL INEQUITIES
Corporations & Businesses
Government Agencies
Schools
Laws & Regulations
Not-for-Profit Organizations

LIVING CONDITIONS

Physical Environment
Land Use
Transportation
Housing
Residential Segregation
Exposure to Toxins

Economic & Work Environment
Employment
Income
Retail Businesses
Occupational Hazards

Social Environment
Experience of Class, Racism, Gender, Immigration
Culture-Ads-Media
Violence

Service Environment
Health Care
Education
Social Services

RISK BEHAVIORS
Smoking
Poor Nutrition
Low Physical Activity
Violence
Alcohol & Other Drugs
Sexual Behavior

DISEASE & INJURY
Communicable Disease
Chronic Disease
Injury (Intentional & Unintentional)

MORTALITY
Infant Mortality
Life Expectancy

Strategic Partnerships Advocacy

Community Capacity Building
Community Organizing
Civic Engagement

Individual Health Education

Health Care

Case Management

POLICY

← Emerging Public Health Practice   Current Public Health Practice →

b

SOCIOECONOMIC AND POLITICAL CONTEXT

Governance

Macroeconomic Policies

Social Policies
Labor, Market, Housing, Land

Public Policies
Education, Health, Social Protection

Culture and Societal Values

Socioeconomic Position

Social Class
Gender
Ethnicity (racism)

Education
⇩
Occupation
⇩
Income

Social Cohesion & Social Capital

Material Circumstances
(Living and Working Conditions, Food Availability, etc.)

Behaviors and Biological Factors

Psychosocial Factors

Health System

IMPACT ON EQUITY IN HEALTH AND WELL-BEING

**STRUCTURAL DETERMINANTS
SOCIAL DETERMINANTS OF HEALTH INEQUITIES**

**INTERMEDIARY DETERMINANTS
SOCIAL DETERMINANTS OF HEALTH**

c

↑ Economic Globalization

↑ Neo-liberalism

↑ Power of Capital

Welfare Regimes

↑ Markets

Income inequality, poverty, and differential access to numerous social resources including work type, education, health care, housing, transportation, nutrition, etc.

↓ Social Cohesion[1] (Trust)

↓ Health & Well-Being

↓ Economic Wealth

the right. The utility of this model is that it places traditional public health interests in a much wider context, linking individual behaviors with social conditions. It situates health care in an important but downstream role that acknowledges the importance of individual health education and case management. The model signals the underlying role and importance of policy (although remaining abstract and undefined). Developed by a regional public health initiative, this rich model uses a level of analysis that we find particularly useful in thinking about city-level change, be it through community organizing, civic engagement, or advocacy (themes we will return to in chapters 7–9). Yet, as with any model, it has gaps. One of the most crucial points of debate is over what it identifies as the fundamental cause of mortality, *how far* upstream it takes us. To understand this limitation, we will present and contrast the BARHII model with two alternatives.

In figure 2.1b, we see the much more global perspective offered by the WHO. Developed as part of the widely cited *Commission on the Social Determinants of Health*, this conceptual framework presents an important way of thinking about health inequities that emphasizes socioeconomic and political contexts as the fundamental causes of health and well-being in populations.[19] The WHO model lists many of the same factors as the BARHII model but reorders the causal chain, leading to different emphases and interpretations. Critically, however, the WHO model identifies very different factors on the upstream side of the model (the left side of the figure). Notice the issues on the far left: governance, macroeconomic policies, social policies (labor market, housing, and land), and public policies (education, health, and social protection). In the WHO model, *these* are the fundamental causes of health. While the BARHII model identifies "housing" as part of the physical environment, a key element under living conditions, the WHO model lists it under "social policies" and also, implicitly, under "material circumstances." The WHO model shows that housing is not just something to be measured as a social determinant of health, but is the result of social policies that themselves must be understood as determinants of health. The difference is subtle but important. Both models have utility, showing casual chains at the local (BARHII) and global (WHO) levels. So it is not surprising that they illustrate causal chains differently.

In figure 2.1c we reproduce an important model put forth by David Coburn, a sociologist whose work focuses on the political and economic determinants of health.[20] Here the "upstream" and "downstream" language is eschewed in favor of a very different terminology that on the surface may appear to be divorced from the more applied perspective of the BARHII model. Coburn's model is perhaps best seen as a more abstract version of the WHO model, incorporating concepts like "neoliberalism" and "welfare regimes" into the WHO's more generic use of "governance" to give particular meaning to those concepts. To be sure, these are concepts far removed from traditional public health work and are not commonly referenced in popular health care debates. For Coburn (and other researchers who emphasize the political determinants of health, including Vicente Navarro and Carles Muntaner), a model of health inequities must focus on the political and economic factors that drive the social determinants of health.[21–23] Thus, this model emphasizes the degree to which market relations dominate social life, with concepts like "welfare regimes," a term coined by political scientists to describe how public policies buttress populations from the effects of market forces.[24] In this tradition, researchers distinguish the "social democratic" welfare regime of the Scandinavian countries (characterized by universalistic programs that promote equality and relatively large state involvement in the economy) from the "liberal" welfare regime characteristic of the United States (with means-tested, and stigmatized, assistance targeted at low-income populations and the promotion of so-called market solutions to social problems).[23–26] Arguably, this model places more traditional social determinants of health (i.e., education, housing, transportation, nutrition) in a somewhat more marginal position; it shifts our attention to a very different part of the causal process that links society to health. As we will see below, this particular model calls for us to reevaluate how we conceptualize city-specific social determinants of health such as income inequality.

There are many other models we could consider, employing different categories of factors and relationships. Our interest here is not to pit one against another, or to evaluate the utility of any one particular model in any given context. Rather, we introduce these models as distinct but complementary "big picture" ways of thinking about the causes of health inequities. Clearly, there is overlap between the models in figure 2.1; all illustrate some type of causal chain, from the distal to the proximal, culminating in health outcomes. All three models also attempt to integrate social characteristics (features of the places where we live, work, and play) with personal outcomes (health), yet they differ in how they frame the overall process, what factors they emphasize, and, perhaps most importantly, what issues they identify as the fundamental causes of health in society.

The basic idea behind these models is similar: to fully understand the causes of health inequities, we need to go beyond the individualistic analysis offered by the "health is a personal responsibility" framework and look at factors that influence groups and specific populations.[27] There are many names for this idea in the literature; "fundamental causes," the "causes of the causes," "root causes," and others. However, the idea itself is clear. When applied to cities, it puts the focus on income inequality, racial residential segregation (and the dramatic disinvestment that is associated with it in the United States), poverty, housing instability, and a host of other social issues as the fundamental causes of health inequities.[28-30]

These "big picture" models are just the starting point for a theory of health inequities. Digging deeper into the literature reveals at least two distinct theoretical traditions embedded in these models: the psychosocial and the sociopolitical frameworks.[9] Perhaps the best way to think about them is as different ways to consider the connections between the varying boxes in figure 2.1. What links income inequality to health? How does residential segregation influence life expectancy? The psychosocial and sociopolitical frameworks are theories that emphasize different relationships and offer unique insights on why health inequities may vary by city and by cause of death:

1. The *psychosocial tradition* emphasizes psychologically mediated social determinants of health, often with a focus on individual-

level stress pathways. The resulting research often emphasizes the relationship between different social stressors (e.g., economic inequality, discrimination, unemployment) and particular health outcomes, usually using data from a single institution, community, or city.

2. The *sociopolitical tradition*, in contrast, focuses primarily on power, politics, economics, and rights as the key determinants of health, often invoking a structural analysis (instead of the individual-level focus of the psychosocial tradition). Research guided by this theoretical perspective often concentrates on associations between characteristics of places and population health outcomes, typically using ecological data or combinations of individual- and ecological-level data from many communities or cities at once.

The Psychosocial Tradition: Linking Social Status to Health

The first approach, the psychosocial tradition, is a long-standing pillar of health inequities work, exemplified by the landmark Whitehall studies of the 1970s that tracked the health of British civil servants.[5,12,27] Those studies offered the clearest documentation to date of the *social gradient* in health, finding an improvement in health outcomes as one moved up the socioeconomic ladder, from the least to the most advantaged.[5] The Whitehall studies revealed important differences by employment grade (what some call occupational prestige). Employees near, but not at, the top of the occupational ladder had worse health than those at the very top. The pattern was consistent as one moved down the ladder for a wide range of health outcomes, including mortality in studies that followed Whitehall participants over time. The Whitehall studies found threefold differences in death rates between unskilled workers and high-level executives, with the gradient in mortality running across the whole hierarchy.

From these data, researchers developed a series of psychosocial explanations for the connection between social status and different stress responses in the body.[12] These models include the influential "allostatic load" model, which describes the long-term effects of the physiological responses to chronic, low-level stress, and the "fight or flight" syndrome, which focuses on the body's responses to acute stressors.[5,12] These models have become part of popular discourse, deeply influencing how we think about the links between social conditions and health outcomes.

But as important as the Whitehall studies were to the development of health inequities research, they had significant blind spots. To begin, they did not incorporate any information on *place*, nor did they focus on racial/ethnic inequities. Their aim was to document the social gradient in health as measured by occupational prestige and social status. Understanding health inequities across large US cities requires overcoming these blind spots. A theory of health inequities in the United States must address city-to-city variability and racial gaps in health arising from our country's history of racism.

In the 1990s, social epidemiologist Richard Wilkinson and others widened the psychosocial model to explore the health effects of income inequality, opening a new branch of research that connected population-level characteristics to disease processes in the body.[11,31] Wilkinson hypothesized a potential psychosocial effect associated with living in unequal *places* that applied across the population, effectively bringing the Whitehall studies into the real world of communities and neighborhoods. Our interest in this approach is not only the characteristics of a social hierarchy typifying a workplace but also the social and economic characteristics of the places where individuals live, work, and play.[32] Wilkinson argued that the main driver of population health in the advanced industrialized countries of the world is not overall income (e.g., how rich, on average, a place is) but the level of income inequality (i.e., how income is distributed across the population) in that place. While initially developed to account for differences in health across countries, Wilkinson's model quickly gained attention as a possible framework for understanding health inequities in the United States using state-, city-, and even census-tract-level data.[33–36]

Statistical tests of the Wilkinson hypothesis generated considerable controversy.[37–39] Strongest support has been found in studies using mortality data. In a particularly influential analysis, Nancy Ross and colleagues explored the association between the level of income inequality and all-cause mortality rates within that city.[40] They found that even a very small change in income inequality, say, increasing the proportion of income of the poorest half of households by 1%, was associated with significant reductions in overall mortality. Across US cities, income inequality explained more than one-third of the variability in working-age mortality rates.[40] Black:white differences in mortality rates were not examined.

Not all studies support the income inequality hypothesis, signaling the complexity underlying causal patterns in population health. Studies using other indicators of health (e.g., self-rated health status) provide less conclusive support, sometimes finding no association between a city's level of inequality and the subjective health of its residents.[35,37,38,41] Methodological debates over the most appropriate statistical analysis approach, the interpretation of cross-sectional versus longitudinal patterns, and even the most appropriate geographical level for studying the hypothesis have yet to be settled.[37,41] One of the most important debates has concerned how to account for *both* income inequality and racial segregation (which are often entwined and are thus difficult to pry apart in the same statistical model), an issue that we explore in chapter 6 using a relatively new concept called the index of concentration at the extremes (ICE).[42,43] And while debates continue over the best way to measure and theorize about income inequality as a determinant of health across US cities, there is growing consensus that place matters, and that at least some of the relationship is due to the psychosocial effects of living in an unequal place.

On a more critical level, it must be acknowledged that much of the Wilkinson-inspired literature failed to take race and racism into account. But around the same time that he was developing his psychosocial model for the health effects of income inequality, other researchers were developing psychosocial explanations for the health effects of racism and discrimination. A critical study in this area was that of neonatologists Richard David and James Collins, who explored low birth weight inequalities by race and nativity.[44] They found no difference in the distributions of low birth weight among infants of US-born white and African-born Black mothers, while infants of US-born Black mothers had a higher prevalence of low birth weight. Their work debunked hypotheses centered on genetic explanations for poorer birth outcomes for Black infants; it argued for a psychosocial model linking women's exposure to racial discrimination as a lifelong stressor that affected pregnancy outcomes, an idea since confirmed in many other studies.[45–48] Black:white inequities in infant mortality remain a priority in health equity research.[49]

Perhaps the most influential theoretical breakthrough in this area was Arlene Geronimus's formulation of the *weathering* hypothesis, which argued that the Black:white health gap seen in many studies is the result of cumulative exposure to socioeconomic disadvantage and racism.[50–52] According to this perspective,

> Blacks experience early health deterioration as a consequence of the cumulative impact of repeated experience with social or economic adversity and political marginalization. On a physiological level, persistent, high-effort coping with acute and chronic stressors can have a profound effect on health. The stress inherent in living in a race-conscious society that *stigmatizes and disadvantages* Blacks may cause disproportionate physiological deterioration, such that a Black individual may show the morbidity and mortality typical of a White individual who is significantly older. Not only do Blacks experience poor health at earlier ages than do Whites, but this deterioration in health *accumulates*, producing ever-greater racial inequality in health with age through middle adulthood.[50] (p. 826; emphasis added)

Within the psychosocial paradigm, much of the work has focused on understanding individuals' *perceptions* of inequality and racism/discrimination and how these perceptions alter physiological processes. These distinct strands of scholarship all rely on psychosocial explanations for how society "gets under our skin," often invoking physiological models describing stress responses in the body.[50]

The psychosocial tradition is widely cited in contemporary health equity research. Yet much of the psychosocial literature has not been grounded in *place*, in *context*. City data may be used, as they were in the influential study on income inequality by Ross and colleagues discussed above, but the focus of this line of research has arguably not been cities or inequities between cities. What if *place* takes a more central role in our theorizing?

The Sociopolitical Tradition: Theorizing Place

A related but different perspective is offered by what Krieger describes as the sociopolitical framework. This approach has deep roots in social theory, beginning with the classic works of Friedrich Engels and his contemporary, Rudolf Virchow, who documented the structural causes of health for working-class people in Europe in the 1840s.[11] Engels and Virchow ascribed the root causes of health to social and economic systems, not the behaviors or attitudes of individuals.

This theoretical orientation provides new insight into the idea that a city's level of income inequality could influence the health of its residents. As we saw earlier in this chapter, the income inequality hypothesis is best described as a psychosocial explanation of health inequities; it theorizes that exposure to inequality has adverse health effects. The more inequality in our city, the worse off we all will be.[31,32,53] Importantly, some studies suggest that this effect extends throughout the socioeconomic ladder, affecting the health of poor and rich, as all are exposed to psychosocial stressors associated with living in unequal places.[11,54]

An alternative interpretation of the relationship between income inequality and population health comes from researchers working within the sociopolitical framework, as illustrated in figure 2.1C. This tradition accepts the validity of the link between income inequality and population health but asserts that the psychosocial explanation unnecessarily and inappropriately focuses on individuals at the expense of the true root causes.[55,56] From this perspective, income inequality is acknowledged as important, even critical, for understanding public health. But it is not the *cause* of poor health; it is the consequence of earlier political and economic processes that should be our true focus.[26,55-57] For Coburn, "income inequality is itself the consequence of fundamental changes in class structure which have produced not only income inequality but also numerous other forms of health-relevant social inequalities. . . . Income inequality is a *consequence*, not the *determinant*" (p. 43; emphasis added).[20] This raises important questions about the focus of public health policy and practice. If Coburn is right, do we shift even further upstream than suggested by the more frequently applied BARHII model of social determinants of health?

The theoretical framework of Coburn and others in this tradition is very abstract and quite a departure from traditional public health perspectives. It is more removed from the everyday personal lives of individuals. Instead, it reflects the public issues within which our lives play out. While not discounting the psychosocial effects of inequality and discrimination, the theoretical viewpoint offered by the sociopolitical framework directs our attention to power, politics, history, and economics, the issues the WHO reinforces in its theoretical model (see figure 2.1). The idea is powerful and is echoed in the contemporary "Health in All Policies" approach to public policies.[58,59]

The psychosocial and sociopolitical theoretical approaches are not, of course, mutually exclusive. Applied to the income inequality hypothesis, they give us different lenses for examining empirical findings and lead us to different kinds of interpretations. The literature on the health effects of racism and discrimination is similar. We saw earlier in this chapter that the foundational work in that area invoked the psychosocial pathways featured in the Whitehall studies and Wilkinson's income inequality model. Developments like Geronimus's weathering framework were based on similar ideas and foregrounded the lived experience of racism and discrimination. The latest work in this area has taken a more structural focus. The term *structural racism*—conceptually very different from interpersonal racism—began to take hold in research studies in the 1990s and 2000s, largely through the scholarship of Camara Jones.[3,6,60] Studies that followed go beyond the psychosocial effects of perceived discrimination to delve into the sociopolitical context that drives racialized inequalities in health.[3,61,62]

Recently, Javier Rodriguez described this as "the politicization of public health . . . [changing] the conceptualization of politics as a powerful predecessor, in the causal chain, of the social determinants of health."[63] One recently published comparison of low birth weight inequities across cities reveals important differences. In Toronto, Canada, no association was found between factors that most public health researchers would label "social determinants," including unemployment, lack of high school graduation, and community racial/ethnic composition, and low birth weight prevalence. Yet the same study found significant associations between those social determinants and low birth weight prevalence among communities in Boston, Baltimore, Chicago, and Philadelphia in the United States.[64] The reasons for the difference are complex, but they revolve around the concept of structural racism, or "the totality of ways in which societies foster racial discrimination through mutually reinforcing systems of housing, education, employment, earnings, benefits, credit, media, health care, and criminal justice" (p. 1453).[3] New studies in this area are also exploring the legacy effects of structural racism, recognizing that the health of any individual is influenced by exposure to stressors across their life course (and also influenced by effects that may echo for generations). For example, studies like Sara Jacoby et al.'s analysis of the effect of redlining and structural racism on present-day urban violence in Philadelphia feature a theoretical argument very different from the "health is a personal responsibility" model that started off our chapter.[65] From this perspective, we focus on social and political arrangements that harm populations— what many people now refer to as structural violence.[66]

One promising approach to studying structural racism as a determinant of health in US cities has revolved around the ICE metric.[67] This simple measure quantifies the proportion of a population that is concentrated in the most disadvantaged and most advantaged groups. Specifically, the ICE quantifies the extent to which a community's residents are concentrated in the extremes of distributions, typically measured in terms of income inequality and racial segregation (often used to quantify their combined influence on population health). Chambers et al. described the ICE as an indicator of structural racism, which "involves systematic laws and processes used to differentiate access to services, goods, and opportunities in society by racial groups" (p. 160).[68] For Chambers et al., "ICE measures the extent to which structural racism persists by examining how concentrated deprived versus privileged groups are in neighborhoods" (p. 167).[68] Their exploration of both pre-term birth and infant mortality found that across all ICE measures (income, race, and income + race) Black women residing in disadvantaged neighborhoods experienced worse outcomes compared to women living in more advantaged neighborhoods. Their results echo similar findings from New York City for preterm birth and infant mortality,[69] Boston for preterm birth,[70] and Chicago for premature mortality.[71] Studies like these shed light on the sociopolitical framework, pointing to the deep structural roots underpinning health inequities.

Much of the literature using the ICE concerns community differences within a single city, yet the full value of the index may be realized in comparative work across cities. Use of the ICE to understand patterns of mortality across the 30 largest US cities will be explored in chapter 6.

A Synthesis

The psychosocial and sociopolitical frameworks emphasize different causal factors for explaining health inequities. The former identifies social determinants of health, like social status, to gain insight into how those social determinants affect bodily processes. The latter takes an even more upstream focus, recognizing health inequities to highlight structural and political factors. A synthesis of the two has recently taken the form of "ecosocial" theory, as developed by Nancy Krieger.[9] This approach builds on and extends psychosocial and sociopolitical theories to analyze what Krieger calls the "embodied population distributions of disease and health." From the psychosocial tradition, it focuses on identifying physiological pathways that link stress to bodily processes, while simultaneously examining the larger political and structural factors in which our lives play out. Krieger's ecosocial theory is clear in its questioning, urging us to investigate, "who and what drive current and changing patterns of social inequalities in health?"

Conclusion

These theoretical frameworks are critical for understanding health inequities in the United States today. The psychosocial tradition reminds us of the psychologically mediated mechanisms by which inequality and racism "get under our skin." The sociopolitical paradigm calls out the root causes underlying our perceptions of inequality and experiences of racism/discrimination. It reminds us that health inequities can vary from place to place, depending on context. It is a major reason why we must examine health inequities across US cities.

These theoretical traditions can be best regarded as lenses that allow us to concentrate on different patterns and different interpretations of the processes depicted in our "big picture" models (figure 2.1). Their utility lies in their ability to describe and explain patterns of health inequities and in their capacity to advance our discussion from the overly reductionist "health is a personal responsibility" model. Across the analyses presented in this book, we are clear that there are no biological reasons why Black individuals in our country can expect to live fewer years than whites. The health inequities evident in the United States are not the product of biology, nor are they natural and static. They vary from place to place and can change over time. The substantial inequities in life expectancy and mortality rates shown in the following chapters are in many ways the sum product of the pathways illustrated in these theories—from stress responses to income inequality to structural racism and, more broadly, structural violence. Documenting how these inequities *vary* across major US cities is a critical step toward understanding and addressing the root causes of these inequities.

References

1. Bonilla-Silva E. *Racism without Racists: Color-Blind Racism and the Persistence of Racial Inequality in the United States*. 3rd ed. Lanham, MD: Rowman & Littlefield; 2006.

2. Massey DS, Denton NA. *American Apartheid: Segregation and the Making of the Underclass*. Cambridge, MA: Harvard University Press; 1998.

3. Bailey ZD, Krieger N, Agenor M, Graves J, Linos N, Bassett MT. Structural Racism and Health Inequities in the USA: Evidence and Interventions. *Lancet*. 2017;389(10077):1453–1463.

4. Krieger N. Living and Dying at the Crossroads: Racism, Embodiment, and Why Theory Is Essential for a Public Health of Consequence. *American Journal of Public Health.* 2016;106(5):832–833.

5. Barr DA. *Health Disparities in the United States: Social Class, Race, Ethnicity, and Health.* Baltimore: Johns Hopkins University Press; 2008.

6. Jones CP. Levels of Racism: A Theoretic Framework and a Gardener's Tale. *American Journal of Public Health.* 2000;90(8):1212–1215.

7. Jones CP. Invited Commentary: "Race," Racism, and the Practice of Epidemiology. *American Journal of Epidemiology.* 2001;154(4):299–304; discussion 305–306.

8. O'Campo P, Dunn JR, eds. *Rethinking Social Epidemiology: Towards a Science of Change.* Dordrecht: Springer; 2012.

9. Krieger N. *Epidemiology and the People's Health: Theory and Context.* Oxford: Oxford University Press; 2011.

10. Cockerham WC, ed. *Medical Sociology on the Move: New Directions in Theory.* Heidelberg: Springer; 2013.

11. De Maio F. *Health and Social Theory.* Basingstoke: Palgrave Macmillan; 2010.

12. Bartley M. *Health Inequality: An Introduction to Theories, Concepts and Methods.* London: Polity Books; 2016.

13. Mills CW. *The Sociological Imagination.* New York: Oxford University Press; 1959.

14. Ansell D. *The Death Gap: How Inequality Kills.* Chicago: University of Chicago Press; 2017.

15. Lang ME, Bird CE. Understanding and Addressing the Common Roots of Racial Health Disparities: The Case of Cardiovascular Disease and HIV/AIDS in African Americans. *Health Matrix.* 2015;25:109–138.

16. Link BG, Phelan J. Social Conditions as Fundamental Causes of Disease. *Journal of Health and Social Behavior.* 1995;Spec No:80-94.

17. Krieger N. Ladders, Pyramids and Champagne: The Iconography of Health Inequities. *Journal of Epidemiology and Community Health.* 2008;62(12):1098–1104.

18. Bay Area Regional Health Inequities Initiative. *Applying Social Determinants of Health Indicators to Advance Health Equity: A Guide for Local Health Department Epidemiologists and Public Health Professionals.* Oakland, CA; 2015.

19. Solar O, Irwin A. *A Conceptual Framework for Action on the Social Determinants of Health.* Geneva: World Health Organization; 2007.

20. Coburn D. Beyond the Income Inequality Hypothesis: Class, Neo-liberalism, and Health Inequalities. *Social Science and Medicine.* 2004;58(1):41–56.

21. Navarro V, Shi L. The Political Context of Social Inequalities and Health. *Social Science and Medicine.* 2001;52(3):481–491.

22. Navarro V. Neoliberalism as a Class Ideology; or, The Political Causes of the Growth of Inequalities. *International Journal of Health Services.* 2007;37(1):47–62.

23. Muntaner C, Borrell C, Ng E, et al. Politics, Welfare Regimes, and Population Health: Controversies and Evidence. *Sociology of Health and Illness.* 2011;33(6):946–964.

24. Brennenstuhl S, Quesnel-Vallee A, McDonough P. Welfare Regimes, Population Health and Health Inequalities: A Research Synthesis. *Journal of Epidemiology and Community Health.* 2012;66(5):397–409.

25. Esping-Andersen G. *The Three Worlds of Welfare Capitalism.* Princeton, NJ: Princeton University Press; 1990.

26. Coburn D. Income Inequality, Welfare, Class and Health: A Comment on Pickett and Wilkinson, 2015. *Social Science and Medicine.* 2015;146:228–232.

27. Marmot M. *The Health Gap.* New York: Bloomsbury; 2015.

28. Williams DR, Collins C. Racial Residential Segregation: A Fundamental Cause of Racial Disparities in Health. *Public Health Reports.* 2001;116(5):404–416.

29. Landrine H, Corral I. Separate and Unequal: Residential Segregation and Black Health Disparities. *Ethnicity and Disease.* 2009;19(2):179–184.

30. Adler NE, Glymour MM, Fielding J. Addressing Social Determinants of Health and Health Inequalities. *Journal of the American Medical Association.* 2016;316(16):1641–1642.

31. Wilkinson RG. *Unhealthy Societies.* London: Routledge; 1996.

32. Wilkinson RG, Pickett K. *The Inner Level.* London: Penguin; 2018.

33. Pickett KE, Wilkinson RG. Income Inequality and Health: A Causal Review. *Social Science and Medicine.* 2015;128:316–326.

34. Wilkinson RG, Pickett KE. Income Inequality and Socioeconomic Gradients in Mortality. *American Journal of Public Health.* 2008;98(4):699–704.

35. Wilkinson RG, Pickett KE. Income Inequality and Population Health: A Review and Explanation of the Evidence. *Social Science and Medicine.* 2006;62(7):1768–1784.

36. Lobmayer P, Wilkinson RG. Inequality, Residential Segregation by Income, and Mortality in US Cities. *Journal of Epidemiology and Community Health.* 2002;56(3):183–187.

37. Lynch J, Smith GD, Harper S, et al. Is Income Inequality a Determinant of Population Health? Part 1. A Systematic Review. *Milbank Quarterly.* 2004;82(1):5–99.

38. Lynch J, Harper S, Smith GD. Commentary: Plugging Leaks and Repelling Boarders—Where to Next for the SS Income Inequality? *International Journal of Epidemiology.* 2003;32(6):1029–1036; discussion 1037–1040.

39. De Maio F. Advancing the Income Inequality Hypothesis. *Critical Public Health.* 2012;22(1):39–46.

40. Ross NA, Wolfson MC, Dunn JR, Berthelot JM, Kaplan GA, Lynch JW. Relation between Income Inequality and Mortality in Canada and in the United States: Cross Sectional Assessment Using Census Data and Vital Statistics. *British Medical Journal.* 2000;320(7239):898–902.

41. Lynch J, Smith GD, Harper S, Hillemeier M. Is Income Inequality a Determinant of Population Health? Part 2. U.S. National and Regional Trends in Income Inequality and Age- and Cause-Specific Mortality. *Milbank Quarterly.* 2004;82(2):355–400.

42. Deaton A, Lubotsky D. Income Inequality and Mortality in U.S. Cities: Weighing the Evidence. A Response to Ash. *Social Science and Medicine.* 2009;68(11):1914–1917.

43. Deaton A, Lubotsky D. Mortality, Inequality and Race in American Cities and States. *Social Science and Medicine.* 2003;56(6):1139–1153.

44. David RJ, Collins JW Jr. Differing Birth Weight among Infants of U.S.-Born Blacks, African-Born Blacks, and U.S.-Born Whites. *New England Journal of Medicine.* 1997;337(17):1209–1214.

45. Love C, David RJ, Rankin KM, Collins JW Jr. Exploring Weathering: Effects of Lifelong Economic Environment and Maternal Age on Low Birth Weight, Small for Gestational Age, and Preterm Birth in African-American and White Women. *American Journal of Epidemiology.* 2010;172(2):127–134.

46. Wallace M, Crear-Perry J, Richardson L, Tarver M, Theall K. Separate and Unequal: Structural Racism and Infant Mortality in the US. *Health and Place.* 2017;45:140–144.

47. Willis E, McManus P, Magallanes N, Johnson S, Majnik A. Conquering Racial Disparities in Perinatal Outcomes. *Clinics in Perinatology.* 2014;41(4):847–875.

48. Wise PH. Confronting Racial Disparities in Infant Mortality: Reconciling Science and Politics. *American Journal of Preventive Medicine.* 1993;9(6 Suppl):7–16.

49. Mehra R, Boyd LM, Ickovics JR. Racial Residential Segregation and Adverse Birth Outcomes: A Systematic Review and Meta-analysis. *Social Science and Medicine.* 2017;191:237–250.

50. Geronimus AT, Hicken M, Keene D, Bound J. "Weathering" and Age Patterns of Allostatic Load Scores among Blacks and Whites in the United States. *American Journal of Public Health.* 2006;96(5):826–833.

51. Geronimus AT. Understanding and Eliminating Racial Inequalities in Women's Health in the United States: The Role of the Weathering Conceptual Framework. *Journal of the American Medical Women's Association.* 2001;56(4):133–136, 149–150.

52. Geronimus AT. The Weathering Hypothesis and the Health of African-American Women and Infants: Evidence and Speculations. *Ethnicity and Disease.* 1992;2(3):207–221.

53. Kawachi I, Subramanian SV. Income Inequality. In: Berkman LF, Kawachi I, Glymour MM, eds. *Social Epidemiology*. Oxford: Oxford University Press; 2014:126–152.

54. Kawachi I, Kennedy BP, Wilkinson RG, eds. *The Society and Population Health Reader: Income Inequality and Health*. New York: Free Press; 1999.

55. Muntaner C, Rai N, Ng E, Chung H. Social Class, Politics, and the Spirit Level: Why Income Inequality Remains Unexplained and Unsolved. *International Journal of Health Services*. 2012;42(3):369–381.

56. Muntaner C, Lynch J, Oates GL. The Social Class Determinants of Income Inequality and Social Cohesion. *International Journal of Health Services*. 1999;29(4):699–732.

57. Muntaner C, Lynch J. Income Inequality, Social Cohesion, and Class Relations: A Critique of Wilkinson's Neo-Durkheimian Research Program. *International Journal of Health Services*. 1999;29(1):59–81.

58. Guglielmin M, Muntaner C, O'Campo P, Shankardass K. A Scoping Review of the Implementation of Health in All Policies at the Local Level. *Health Policy*. 2018;122(3):284–292.

59. Shah RC, Kamensky SR. Health in All Policies for Government: Promise, Progress, and Pitfalls to Achieving Health Equity. *DePaul Law Review*. 2020;69.

60. Jones C. The Impact of Racism on Health. *Ethnicity and Disease*. 2002;12(1):S2-10-13.

61. Geronimus AT. To Mitigate, Resist, or Undo: Addressing Structural Influences on the Health of Urban Populations. *American Journal of Public Health*. 2000;90(6):867–872.

62. Schulz AJ, Mullings L, eds. *Gender, Race, Class, and Health: Intersectional Approaches*. New York: Wiley; 2005.

63. Rodriguez JM. The Politics Hypothesis and Racial Disparities in Infants' Health in the United States. *SSM Population Health*. 2019;8:100440.

64. De Maio F, Ansell D, Shah RC. Racial/Ethnic Minority Segregation and Low Birth Weight in Five North American Cities. *Ethnicity and Health*. 2020;25(7): 915–924.

65. Jacoby SF, Dong B, Beard JH, Wiebe DJ, Morrison CN. The Enduring Impact of Historical and Structural Racism on Urban Violence in Philadelphia. *Social Science and Medicine*. 2018;199:87–95.

66. De Maio F, Ansell D. "As Natural as the Air around Us": On the Origin and Development of the Concept of Structural Violence in Health Research. *International Journal of Health Services*. 2018;48(4):749–759.

67. Krieger N, Waterman PD, Spasojevic J, Li W, Maduro G, Van Wye G. Public Health Monitoring of Privilege and Deprivation with the Index of Concentration at the Extremes. *American Journal of Public Health*. 2016;106(2):256–263.

68. Chambers BD, Baer RJ, McLemore MR, Jelliffe-Pawlowski LL. Using Index of Concentration at the Extremes as Indicators of Structural Racism to

Evaluate the Association with Preterm Birth and Infant Mortality—California, 2011–2012. *Journal of Urban Health*. 2019;96(2):159–170.

69. Huynh M, Spasojevic J, Li W, et al. Spatial Social Polarization and Birth Outcomes: Preterm Birth and Infant Mortality—New York City, 2010–14. *Scandinavian Journal of Public Health*. 2018;46(1):157–166.

70. Krieger N, Waterman PD, Batra N, Murphy JS, Dooley DP, Shah SN. Measures of Local Segregation for Monitoring Health Inequities by Local Health Departments. *American Journal of Public Health*. 2017;107(6):903–906.

71. Lange-Maia BS, De Maio F, Avery EF, et al. Association of Community-Level Inequities and Premature Mortality: Chicago, 2011–2015. *Journal of Epidemiology and Community Health*. 2018;72(12):1099–1103.

PART II   RACIAL INEQUITIES IN US CITIES: AN ANALYSIS OF MORTALITY DATA

In considering the health statistics of the Negroes, we seek first to know their absolute condition . . . we want to know what their death rate is, how it has varied and is varying and what its tendencies seem to be; with these facts fixed we must then ask, What is the meaning of a death rate like that of the Negroes of Philadelphia? Is it, compared with other races, large, moderate or small; and in the case of nations or groups with similar death rates, What has been the tendency and outcome? Finally, we must compare the death rate of the Negroes with that of the communities in which they live and thus roughly measure the social difference between these neighboring groups; we must endeavor also to eliminate, so far as possible, from the problem disturbing elements which would make a difference in health among people of the same social advancement. Only in this way can we intelligently interpret statistics.

—W. E. B. Du Bois
The Philadelphia Negro, 1899

In part I, we observed that glaring racial inequities in mortality have persisted in the United States for well over 100 years. For Americans, mortality depends on the color of your skin and the city you live in. Race matters. Place matters. In part II, we dig into the epidemiology of mortality, life expectancy, and premature death to understand the magnitude of racial inequities in these outcomes and in specific causes of death, within and across US cities. Chapter 3 compares overall mortality experiences of US residents by race and geography and identifies the best- and worst-performing cities. In chapters 4 and 5, we investigate the racial inequities revealed within the leading causes of death and selected other causes, respectively. These analyses illustrate the substantial geographic and racial inequities that exist across causes of death. These city-level data provide city planners and public health leaders with the information necessary to advance policies and implement evidence-informed programs.

Chapter 3, "Inequities in All-Cause Mortality, Life Expectancy, and Premature Mortality," presents new data on city-level disparities in three critical mortality outcomes for the largest US cities. We introduce all-cause mortality rates, life expectancy, and premature mortality for each city, as well as show outcomes separately for Blacks and whites. We then highlight the wide range of geographic and racial disparities found within these summary measures of mortality. For example, a baby born in San Francisco or San Jose had a life expectancy that was more than 10 years longer than a baby born in other big cities. Racial differences in life expectancy were shown within almost all the major cities, but nowhere more than in Washington, DC, where a Black baby's life expectancy was more than 12 years less than a white baby's. Together, these data allow us to identify the few cities that have both better-than-average mortality outcomes and high levels of equity, as well as the larger group of cities that fall below national averages for both the mortality outcomes and the equity measures. These unique data points provide a nuanced look at equity among our most populous urban areas.

In chapter 4, "Inequities in the 10 Leading Causes of Death," we see data for the same big cities for the 10 leading causes of death—heart disease, cancer, chronic lower respiratory diseases, accidents, stroke, Alzheimer's disease, diabetes, influenza and pneumonia, kidney disease, and suicide. Black mortality rates are significantly higher than those for whites for many causes, including heart disease, cancer, stroke, diabetes, and kidney disease, while white rates are higher than Black rates for Alzheimer's disease, accidents, suicide, and chronic lower respiratory diseases. The size of the inequity varies among cities, however. Notably, for almost all causes, some cities have achieved equity between races. For example, in Boston and Columbus, Blacks and whites are equally as likely to die of heart disease even though Blacks have a 30% higher heart disease mortality rate nationally. These differences in cause-specific mortality rates and levels of disparities can help direct public health actions to the right places to improve equity within and across cities.

Three additional causes of death demand our immediate attention. Chapter 5, "Inequities in Selected Causes of Death," shifts the focus to mortality rates and measures of inequities for HIV, homicide, and opioid-related mortality. The data here reveal huge racial disparities and wide variation in disparities by city; the inequities in these conditions are even greater than those seen for the leading causes of death discussed in chapter 4. Across the United States, Blacks are more than eight times more likely to die from homicide than whites. However, across cities, the Black rate ranges from 2.5 (El Paso) to 26.4 (Chicago) times the white rate. Although these selected causes of death affect fewer people, the lack of equity across these outcomes presents a major social justice issue within our urban areas.

[THREE]

Inequities in All-Cause Mortality, Life Expectancy, and Premature Mortality

MAUREEN R. BENJAMINS, NAZIA SAIYED, ABIGAIL SILVA, AND FERNANDO G. DE MAIO

CIVILIZATIONS HAVE ATTEMPTED to track and understand when (and why) people die since ancient times.[1,2] In the United States, measures of mortality have been documented since at least 1850,[3] and they have been a primary focus of our nation's health goals since the advent of the Healthy People initiative in 1979.[4] Calculated by dividing the number of deaths in an area by the population size, mortality rates can be used to describe all deaths or deaths within specific age groups (e.g., infant mortality) or causes (e.g., cancer mortality). All-cause mortality is a useful starting point for summarizing the health of those living in the largest US cities. With this information, government agencies and other urban stakeholders can assess the burden of death, prioritize resources, and monitor trends over time.

Building on mortality rates, one can calculate life expectancy at birth. This may be the best single indicator of overall health since it summarizes mortality from all diseases and injuries, across all ages. Life expectancy at birth represents the number of years a person can expect to live based on current mortality rates for each specific age group. Because the unit of measurement—years of life—is something everyone can appreciate, life expectancy is easier to interpret than mortality rates. It also captures the public interest more than most other health outcomes. In the United States, public health agencies and researchers routinely calculate life expectancy for the nation, as well as for all states and counties.[5,6] Numerous recent stories about life expectancy have garnered widespread attention, including a downward trend in life expectancy in the United States,[7-9] double-digit disparities in life expectancy among neighborhoods or census tracts within a single city,[5,10,11] and startling comparisons of life expectancies between specific US groups and less developed countries that indicate that groups in the United States lag behind seemingly poorer places.[12]

Finally, we believe that it is also useful to include a measure of premature death to round out our picture of mortality in the United States. Specifically, we present Years of Life Lost (YLL), which reflects the number of years of life lost due to premature death (here, before age 75). Importantly, this measure takes into account the timing of the death, not just the death itself. Thus, it gives more weight to the deaths of younger people, as opposed to the measurement of mortality rates, which are dominated by deaths experienced in older age.[13] YLL was first added to US reports on mortality in 1982 to help highlight the burden of premature mortality for certain racial and socioeconomic groups.[14]

Unfortunately, government data sources (including reports and online data warehouses) generally do not provide these types of mortality data at the city level or information on city-level racial inequities in mortality. More broadly, although many government sources of data and individual studies include race-specific mortality rates (and other health outcomes), they commonly neglect the important next step of quantifying potential racial differences with rate ratios or estimates of excess deaths. This chapter addresses these critical gaps in our national mortality data, as summarized below.

Racial and Geographic Variations in Mortality, Life Expectancy, and Years of Life Lost

All-cause mortality rates and life expectancies have steadily, but inconsistently, improved in the United States over the course of the twentieth century and the beginning of the twenty-first.[15] Although YLL has only been tracked more recently, it improved significantly between 1990 and 2016.[16,17] Despite this progress, the United States experienced an unprecedented increase in mortality rates (and a corresponding decline in life expectancy) from 2014 to 2017.[7] These worsening health outcomes were particularly seen for Black and white males and white females, partially explained by increases in deaths due to accidents, drug overdoses, and suicide.[7,18]

Black Americans have been burdened with higher death rates and lower life expectancies than whites for as long as our country has kept records of race-specific mortality.[3] In 1950, the Black mortality rate was 1,722 per 100,000 and the white rate was 1,411.[19] These racial inequities generally narrowed through the end of the twentieth century and the early 2000s,[20,21] but they remain a significant concern today. When the CDC started tracking YLL in 1982, Black rates were nearly twice white rates.[13] YLL rates for Blacks compared to whites have improved significantly since then.[16] This presumably reflects the recent increases in deaths from specific causes, such as opioid use and suicide, that have disproportionately affected white (and younger) individuals.[22] Although the national racial inequity in YLL has narrowed, it still persists.

Substantial research also documents geographic variations at the state, county, and local levels. For example, in 2016, the age-adjusted overall death rate at the state level ranged from 492 per 100,000 in California to 768 in Mississippi.[17] Huge variations can also be seen in mortality and life expectancy at the county level.[6,23] For 2017, the state of New York reported varying all-cause mortality rates from a low of 474 per 100,000 in New York County (which includes Manhattan) to 929 in Hamilton County, the state's least populated county.[6] Data also reveal a 20-year difference in life expectancy between people living in the healthiest and the unhealthiest counties in the United States.[24] County differences are also evident in YLL. County Health Rankings data show YLL rates for 2015–2017 in Texas counties ranging from 4,000 to 14,600.[23] At an even more local level, estimates for life expectancy varied substantially by census tract across the country (based on small area estimates), ranging from a low of 56 years to a high of 98 years.[5] However, finding statistics like these at the city level has been much more challenging.

Examining Mortality at the City Level

Across the globe, researchers are increasingly in search of local data to identify inequities and inform place-based initiatives. Although high-quality data at the national, state, and county levels are available (as seen in the previous examples), comprehensive mortality data are still needed at the city level. First, it is clear that larger geographic areas, even counties, can obscure important differences between groups.[25] Secondly, elected officials and other urban stakeholders need data that are aligned with political jurisdictions to motivate and guide steps toward health equity. Moreover, four in five people in the United States currently live in urban areas,[26] a number that continues to grow.[27] Finally, we have seen that cities are often the leading edge in innovative policy development.

Despite all of this, we still lack a comprehensive source for race-specific mortality rates, life expectancies, and years of life lost for the largest US cities or for racial inequities within these measures of city-level mortality. Here we address this gap by providing up-to-date data on three mortality outcomes, as well as the inequities within, for the most populous US cities. Individuals and organizations with a national perspective will find critical information about the country's urban health and health equity outcomes. At the city level, leaders and advocates will have the targeted data they need to understand their issues, empower and motivate partners, and begin exploring ways to address any identified mortality or equity challenges.

Here we analyzed the nearly 13.5 million deaths that occurred in the United States between 2013 and 2017. A little over 1.4 million of these deaths were within the 30 largest cities. Details on the data and analyses are provided in the appendix, along with potential data limitations. Note that calculations for Las Vegas have been removed due to concerns related to unreliable death certificate data for that city. Briefly, we calculated 5-year average annual outcomes for the non-Hispanic white (white), non-Hispanic Black (Black), and total populations of the United States, as well as for each of the 29 most populous cities. We used mortality data from the National Vital Statistics System and population data from the American Community Survey (ACS). Rates were age-adjusted using the 2000 standard US population. All data are for 2013–2017. Table 3.1 contains a summary of the mortality outcomes and related measures of inequity.

All-Cause Mortality

As seen in figure 3.1, the all-cause mortality rate for the United States was 762 per 100,000 total population. In other words, an average of 762 people per 100,000 died each year in our country during this period. This rate was not consistent across our country's largest cities; some cities had rates nearly *two times higher* than others. San Francisco had the lowest rate (559 per 100,000), a rate 27% lower than the national average. Several cities on the west coast (i.e., San Jose, Los Angeles, San Diego, and Seattle) as well as New York, had rates under 650. Of the 29 largest cities included here, 12 had all-cause mortality rates lower than the national average. On the other end of the spectrum, three cities had rates more than 25% higher than the national average (Memphis, Detroit, and Baltimore). These important findings begin to reveal the significant inequalities that exist across US cities—but as we will see below, it is critically important to examine inequalities both between and within cities.

Given that the overall mortality rates include the total population, race-specific rates are needed to start identifying potential subpopulation disparities. The all-cause mortality rate for Blacks in the United States was 958 per 100,000 (indicated by the dark vertical line in figure 3.1). Across the largest cities, the Black rate ranged from 739 (Boston) to 1,242 (Louisville). High rates were also seen in cities like Houston, Portland, and Baltimore. Three of the large cities had Black mortality rates lower than the national white rate. This rate, the number of white individuals who died annually in the United States, was 776 per 100,000 (shown by the gray vertical line in figure 3.1). This rate showed even more variation than the Black rate across cities, ranging from 464 (Washington, DC) to 1,172 (Louisville). The white rate was also elevated in cities such as Indianapolis, Baltimore, and San Antonio.

Table 3.1. Mortality and Equity Outcomes

	Mortality Outcomes		
	All-Cause Mortality Rate	Life Expectancy at Birth	Years of Life Lost (YLL)
Description	Number of deaths each year per 100,000 population	Average number of years from birth a person can expect to live, according to the population's current age-specific death rates	Number of years of life lost due to premature death each year per 100,000 population
Calculation	$\dfrac{\text{Number of deaths in a population}}{\text{Population}} \times 100{,}000$	Calculated with Chiang II methodology, based on life table with 13 age-specific mortality rates	$\dfrac{\text{Number of years of life lost before age 75}}{\text{Population under age 75}} \times 100{,}000$
Example	All-cause mortality rate in Baltimore was 1,052 per 100,000 population (2013–2017)	During 2013–2017, the life expectancy for a baby born in Phoenix was 80 years	In Los Angeles, there were 5,039 years of life lost each year (2013–2017)
Equity Outcomes	*Rate Ratio*: Black mortality rate / white mortality rate *Rate Difference*: Black mortality rate – white mortality rate *Excess Deaths*: No. Blacks deaths based on Black mortality rate – no. expected Black deaths if white rate was applied to Black population	*Absolute Difference*: white life expectancy – Black life expectancy	*Absolute Difference*: Black YLL – white YLL

Notes: All outcomes shown in chapter 3 are 5-year averages using 2013–2017 data. Mortality data are from the National Vital Statistics System, and population data are from the American Community Survey. Mortality rates are age-adjusted using US 2000 standard population.

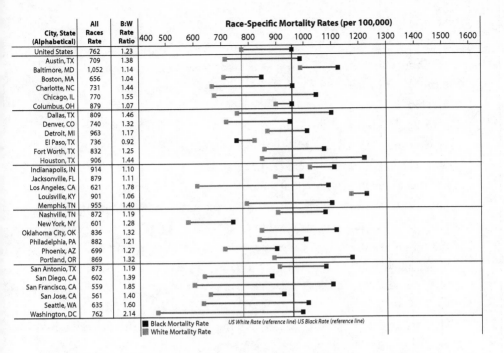

City, State (Alphabetical)	All Races Rate	B:W Rate Ratio
United States	762	1.23
Austin, TX	709	1.38
Baltimore, MD	1,052	1.14
Boston, MA	656	1.04
Charlotte, NC	731	1.44
Chicago, IL	770	1.55
Columbus, OH	879	1.07
Dallas, TX	809	1.46
Denver, CO	740	1.32
Detroit, MI	963	1.17
El Paso, TX	736	0.92
Fort Worth, TX	832	1.25
Houston, TX	906	1.44
Indianapolis, IN	914	1.10
Jacksonville, FL	879	1.11
Los Angeles, CA	621	1.78
Louisville, KY	901	1.06
Memphis, TN	955	1.40
Nashville, TN	872	1.19
New York, NY	601	1.28
Oklahoma City, OK	836	1.32
Philadelphia, PA	882	1.21
Phoenix, AZ	699	1.27
Portland, OR	869	1.32
San Antonio, TX	873	1.19
San Diego, CA	602	1.39
San Francisco, CA	559	1.85
San Jose, CA	561	1.40
Seattle, WA	635	1.60
Washington, DC	762	2.14

Figure 3.1. All-Cause Mortality Rates and Mortality Inequities in the United States and the 29 Largest Cities. *Notes:* Age-adjusted 5-year average (2013–2017) mortality rates per 100,000 population. B:W = Black:white. All rate ratios were statistically significant (p < 0.05).

The race-specific rates make it clear that racial differences in mortality rates exist at both the national and city levels. More significant to note is the extent to which these differences vary among cities. Here we quantify local health inequities using both relative and absolute measures. To better assess the overall burden of the mortality inequities on the Black population, we also calculate the number of excess Black deaths.

The relative difference between races, measured by rate ratios, shows that the Black all-cause mortality rate in the United States was 1.23 times that of the white mortality rate. Across the largest cities, 28 had rate ratios above 1, indicating that the Black rates were higher than the white rates in each city. The rate ratios ranged from 1.04 (Boston) to 2.14 (Washington, DC). Sixteen cities had rate ratios significantly higher than the United States as a whole. Only one city (El Paso) showed a Black advantage, where the Black all-cause mortality rate was lower than the white rate (RR = 0.92). Note that this city has an unusual racial/ethnic distribution, with 3% of the population being Black, 15% white, and 80% Hispanic (appendix, table A.1). All of the rate ratios were statistically significant.

Absolute differences between the Black and white rates were measured with rate differences. In figure 3.1, the gray lines connecting the two squares for each location (that is, the race-specific mortality rates) represent the absolute difference. For the United States, subtracting the white rate from the Black rate resulted in a rate difference of 181 per 100,000. Across the cities, all cities had significant rate differences, with 28 indicating a higher Black than white rate. Again, only in El Paso was the white rate higher than the Black rate. Variation among cities was substantial, with the rate difference ranging from −67 (El Paso) to 531 (Washington, DC) per 100,000. The three cities with the largest rate differences (Washington, DC, San Francisco, and Los Angeles) had differences that were at least five times higher than those of the three cities with the lowest (positive) rate differences (Boston, Columbus, and Louisville).

Next, we look at excess, or preventable, deaths, a measure that reflects both race-specific mortality rates and the size of the area's Black population. Based on our analysis (2013–2017), over 70,000 excess deaths occur in the United States each year as a result of the higher Black mortality rates compared to white rates. That is the equivalent of 192 potentially preventable Black deaths a day (or eight additional Black deaths *every single hour*). At the city level, El Paso had no excess Black deaths because the Black mortality rate was lower than the white mortality rate. Four cities (El Paso, Boston, San Jose, and Portland) had fewer than 100 excess Black deaths (figure 3.2). For San Jose and Portland, the low numbers reflect the cities' small Black populations. The other two cities have few excess Black deaths because of their relatively high levels of equity.

However, at the other end of the spectrum, the number of excess deaths was extremely high in Chicago and New York, cities that each had over 3,000 excess deaths each year. In both cities (which have large Black

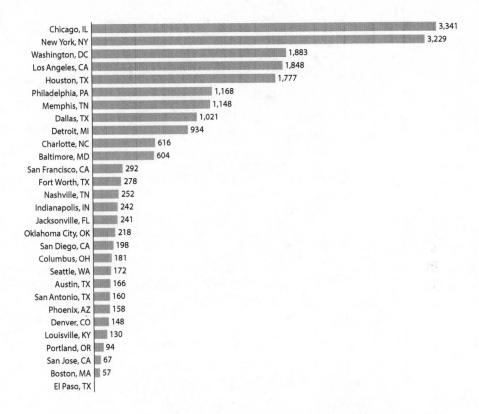

Chicago, IL	3,341
New York, NY	3,229
Washington, DC	1,883
Los Angeles, CA	1,848
Houston, TX	1,777
Philadelphia, PA	1,168
Memphis, TN	1,148
Dallas, TX	1,021
Detroit, MI	934
Charlotte, NC	616
Baltimore, MD	604
San Francisco, CA	292
Fort Worth, TX	278
Nashville, TN	252
Indianapolis, IN	242
Jacksonville, FL	241
Oklahoma City, OK	218
San Diego, CA	198
Columbus, OH	181
Seattle, WA	172
Austin, TX	166
San Antonio, TX	160
Phoenix, AZ	158
Denver, CO	148
Louisville, KY	130
Portland, OR	94
San Jose, CA	67
Boston, MA	57
El Paso, TX	

Figure 3.2. Annual Excess Black Deaths Due to Unequal Mortality Rates.
Notes: Excess deaths represent the average number of excess Black deaths annually due to the higher Black mortality rate compared to the white rate (2013–2017). El Paso had no excess Black deaths (due to a higher white mortality rate).

populations and medium to high levels of inequities), an average of nine Black people died each day because of inequities in mortality. Six other cities had more than 1,000 excess Black deaths per year.

Life Expectancy

The findings for life expectancy logically follow these same general trends. The life expectancy for a baby born in the United States between 2013 and 2017 was 78.6 years, as seen in figure 3.3. However, wide variability among cities was seen again, with 10 years separating

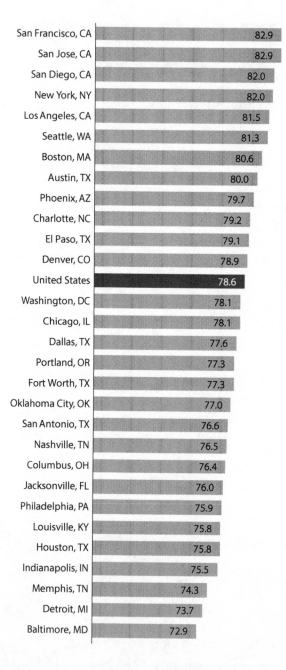

San Francisco, CA — 82.9
San Jose, CA — 82.9
San Diego, CA — 82.0
New York, NY — 82.0
Los Angeles, CA — 81.5
Seattle, WA — 81.3
Boston, MA — 80.6
Austin, TX — 80.0
Phoenix, AZ — 79.7
Charlotte, NC — 79.2
El Paso, TX — 79.1
Denver, CO — 78.9
United States — 78.6
Washington, DC — 78.1
Chicago, IL — 78.1
Dallas, TX — 77.6
Portland, OR — 77.3
Fort Worth, TX — 77.3
Oklahoma City, OK — 77.0
San Antonio, TX — 76.6
Nashville, TN — 76.5
Columbus, OH — 76.4
Jacksonville, FL — 76.0
Philadelphia, PA — 75.9
Louisville, KY — 75.8
Houston, TX — 75.8
Indianapolis, IN — 75.5
Memphis, TN — 74.3
Detroit, MI — 73.7
Baltimore, MD — 72.9

Figure 3.3. Life Expectancy in the United States and the 29 Largest Cities. *Note:* Life expectancy at birth in years; 5-year averages (2013–2017).

the city with the lowest versus the highest life expectancy. More specifically, life expectancy at the city level ranged from a low of 72.9 in Baltimore to a high of 82.9 years in both San Francisco and San Jose. Of the largest cities, 12 had life expectancies significantly above the national average, and 17 had life expectancies significantly below the average. At the extremes, four cities had a life expectancy more than 3 years higher than the US average, while four cities were 3 or more years lower than the US average. To put the lowest city-level life expectancies into context, the life expectancies in the three bottom cities over this period were lower than several countries in the global south, such as Mexico and Nicagua.[28] They are also equal to or lower than the US life expectancy nearly 40 years prior.[19]

The life expectancy for a Black baby born in the United States during this period was 74.4 years (table 3.2). Across the largest cities, Black life expectancy ranged from 70.2 years in Houston to 78.7 years in New York—a difference of 8.5 years between the two.

Not surprisingly, the life expectancy for a white baby born in the United States during the same period was higher, at 78.4 years. The range across cities (10.6 years) was slightly larger in magnitude than that seen for Black life expectancy, ranging from a high of 85.5 years (Washington, DC) to under 75 years in Baltimore.

At the national level, the absolute difference between Black and white life expectancies was 4.1 years. Only one city (El Paso) had a longer life expectancy for Blacks compared to whites. At the other extreme, there was a difference of more than 12 years between Black and white life expectancies in Washington, DC. Twenty-five of the large cities had a difference of 3 or more years between their Black and white rates.

Years of Life Lost

Finally, we examine premature mortality. From 2013 to 2017, an average of 6,694 years of life were lost annually per 100,000 population as a result of premature mortality (i.e., deaths before age 75; table 3.3).

Table 3.2. Racial Differences in Life Expectancy in the United States
and the 29 Largest Cities

City, State (Sorted by Difference)	Black Life Expectancy	White Life Expectancy	Black:White Difference
United States	74.4	78.4	4.1
Washington, DC	73.4	85.5	12.1
San Francisco, CA	71.8	82.3	10.5
Los Angeles, CA	72.3	81.8	9.5
Chicago, IL	72.3	80.5	8.3
Seattle, WA	73.5	81.6	8.1
Dallas, TX	72.1	79.0	6.8
Houston, TX	70.2	76.8	6.6
Memphis, TN	71.8	77.8	6.0
Charlotte, NC	75.0	80.8	5.8
Oklahoma City, OK	71.4	77.2	5.7
Austin, TX	74.4	80.1	5.6
Portland, OR	71.5	77.2	5.6
Denver, CO	74.2	79.7	5.5
San Diego, CA	76.1	81.4	5.2
San Jose, CA	76.3	81.0	4.6
Fort Worth, TX	72.8	77.1	4.3
Phoenix, AZ	75.3	79.6	4.3
New York, NY	78.7	82.6	4.0
Louisville, KY	72.2	76.2	4.0
Nashville, TN	73.3	77.2	3.9
Indianapolis, IN	72.2	76.0	3.8
Baltimore, MD	71.1	74.9	3.8
San Antonio, TX	72.4	76.2	3.8
Philadelphia, PA	73.4	77.1	3.8
Detroit, MI	72.7	75.8	3.1
Columbus, OH	74.0	76.5	2.5
Jacksonville, FL	73.6	76.0	2.5
Boston, MA	78.5	79.9	1.5
El Paso, TX	78.4	77.8	−0.6

Notes: Age-adjusted 5-year averages (2013-2017). Black:white difference shown in years.

As with the other measures of mortality, huge differences were seen across the 29 largest US cities. The YLL per 100,000 population ranged from 4,052 in San Jose to 12,518 in Detroit. Two other cities (Baltimore and Memphis) also had over 10,000 YLL annually during this period.

Premature mortality varied by race and geography. The YLL for Black individuals in the United States was 10,701. This ranged from 7,668 in New York to 14,877 in Houston. As could be expected, the YLL for US whites was much lower than that for Blacks, at 6,743 per 100,000.

Washington, DC, had the least YLL for whites (2,635), while Detroit and Louisville both had more than 10,000 YLL.

An analysis of equity outcomes reveals that racial disparities in premature mortality were even more striking than those observed in the other mortality measures (table 3.3). The data showed that Blacks had more years of life lost than whites in the United States and in all of the largest cities. Absolute differences ranged from a low of 1,802 in Detroit (where the white rate was nearly twice as high as the national average) to a high of 9,856 years of life lost in Washington, DC.

Table 3.3. Years of Life Lost (<75 Years) in the United States and the 29 Largest Cities

City, State (Sorted by Rate Difference)	Total Rate	Black Rate	White Rate	Rate Difference
United States	6,694	10,701	6,743	3,958
Washington, DC	7,787	12,491	2,635	9,856
San Francisco, CA	4,453	13,780	4,416	9,364
Chicago, IL	7,580	13,398	5,134	8,264
Los Angeles, CA	5,156	12,435	4,605	7,830
Seattle, WA	4,921	11,303	4,553	6,750
Houston, TX	8,882	14,877	8,151	6,726
Portland, OR	6,730	13,385	6,671	6,715
Dallas, TX	7,422	12,572	6,352	6,220
Oklahoma City, OK	8,165	13,995	7,943	6,052
Denver, CO	6,602	11,604	5,864	5,740
Baltimore, MD	12,215	14,724	9,376	5,348
Memphis, TN	11,091	13,315	7,987	5,328
Austin, TX	5,113	10,326	5,080	5,246
Phoenix, AZ	6,514	11,150	6,443	4,707
San Antonio, TX	8,005	12,620	8,150	4,469
Fort Worth, TX	7,307	11,623	7,259	4,363
Charlotte, NC	6,107	9,214	4,973	4,242
San Diego, CA	4,510	8,835	4,809	4,026
Indianapolis, IN	9,405	13,809	9,845	3,964
Columbus, OH	8,241	11,426	7,738	3,688
Philadelphia, PA	9,339	11,795	8,156	3,639
San Jose, CA	4,052	8,313	4,731	3,582
New York, NY	4,904	7,668	4,153	3,515
Louisville, KY	9,178	14,722	11,208	3,514
Nashville, TN	8,134	11,264	8,020	3,244
Jacksonville, FL	9,090	11,617	8,906	2,711
Boston, MA	5,688	7,806	5,489	2,317
El Paso, TX	6,171	9,407	7,160	2,247
Detroit, MI	12,517	13,494	11,692	1,802

Notes: Age-adjusted 5-year averages (2013–2017). Years of life lost = [(75 – age at death) / (population under 75)] × 100,000.

Best- and Worst-Performing Cities

Simultaneously assessing a city's mortality outcome and level of disparity reveals that those with the *best* equity in mortality outcomes often had the *worst* overall outcomes (figure 3.4). For example, Detroit was one of the top five cities for greatest equity in life expectancy between Blacks and whites, but it was in the bottom five cities for overall life expectancy. The opposite results were seen as well; San Francisco and Los Angeles were both in the bottom five cities for equity in life expectancy, but in the top five cities for longest life expectancy overall. This does not necessarily mean, however, that cities can only excel in one dimension or that there is an automatic trade-off between overall outcome and level of inequity.

For life expectancy, the best-performing cities (i.e., those with life expectancy above the national average and racial inequities below the national average) were El Paso, Boston, and New York (the latter not as convincingly as El Paso and Boston, with results closer to the national inequity). Conversely, eight cities struggled to achieve both an average life expectancy and minimal health inequities. Within this group, Washington, DC, stands out for having the largest inequities, along with below-average life expectancy. Similar trends occur with the other measures. For all-cause mortality, El Paso and Boston continued to perform well, while eight cities performed worse than the national average for the overall outcome and corresponding equity. El Paso, Boston, and New York were all in the "best performing" category for premature mortality as well (along with San Jose), while Washington, DC, again fell below the national levels for the overall outcome and for racial equity within it (along with 10 other cities).

Fully understanding mortality at the city level requires not only access to city-level outcome data or even race-specific outcome data; we must take the additional step of documenting and assessing the data to determine the existence and size of the racial inequities. This will enable us to distinguish between cities doing well in overall health outcomes and those faring well in health equity.

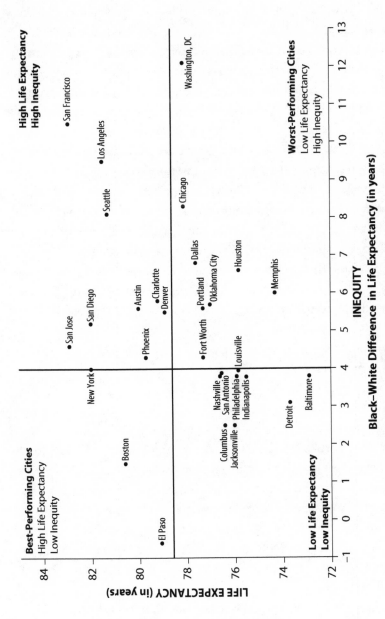

Figure 3.4. Life Expectancy and Racial Inequity in Life Expectancy. *Notes:* Life expectancy at birth in years; 5-year averages (2013–2017). Quadrants are separated by lines representing the US outcomes (for both life expectancy and the Black:white difference in life expectancy).

City Spotlight: Chicago

Many readers will come to this chapter focused on a particular city. Here we highlight Chicago as an example of how city residents, leaders, or other stakeholders could assess these data for their own cities of interest. Overall, Chicago fares poorly relative to the national averages for all-cause mortality rates, life expectancy, and premature mortality (figure 3.5). Moreover, Chicago has more racial inequities in these outcomes than the United States as a whole, as well as more than most of the other large cities. Black residents of Chicago have a 55% higher mortality rate than white residents (compared to a 23% higher rate for Blacks compared to whites nationally). Similarly, Chicago's gaps in Black and white life expectancies and premature mortality are more than twice as large as those for the whole country. Only a small handful of large cities fare worse in these equity measures. Chicago has its work cut out for it. The root causes of such disparities, including levels of racial segregation and poverty, are explored in chapter 6, and specific examples of how the city is addressing inequities in life expectancy are provided in chapter 9.

Conclusions

Clearly, mortality in the United States depends on the color of your skin and the city in which you live. Across the United States, a white baby can expect to live 4 years longer than a Black baby. And if you are lucky enough to be born in certain cities, such as San Francisco or San Jose, you can expect to live 10 years longer than someone born in Baltimore. Even more striking is the difference in survival by race *and* city. A white baby born in Washington, DC, can expect to live to age 86; a Black baby born in several other big US cities cannot expect to live to age 72. Remember, this huge difference is between babies born in two of our country's largest cities, with all of their considerable resources (health care and otherwise).

Looking beyond life expectancy, we found that mortality disparities reveal that an additional 190 Black people in the United States died *every day* as a result of a mortality rate higher than their white counter-

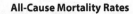

All-Cause Mortality Rates

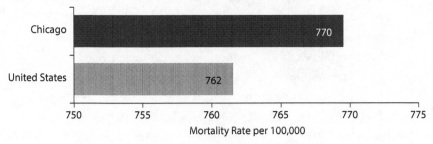

Life Expectancy

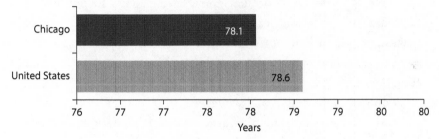

Premature Mortality

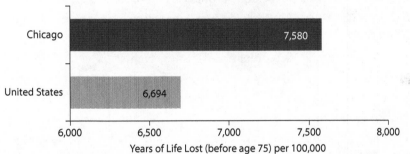

Figure 3.5. City Spotlight: Comparison of Summary Mortality Measures in Chicago and the United States. *Notes:* Mortality rates are age-adjusted. All data are 5-year averages (2013–2017).

parts. These are hidden deaths, easily overlooked or ignored without the necessary data to locate them. Delving deeper into the data, we showed even more prominent inequities in premature mortality. At the national level, the number of years of life lost (before age 75) for Blacks is 59% higher than that for whites. These lost years place a huge burden (personal, financial, and otherwise) on one particular group of urban residents. And to be sure, the costs grow and compound over time—as Camara Jones, former president of the American Public Health Association, observed, racism "saps the strength of the whole society" (p. 231).[29] Premature mortality and excess mortality stress family bonds and community ties, with many negative corollary effects.

Despite the magnitude of these racial and geographic disparities, examined separately, they still tell only part of the story. Not only do mortality outcomes vary by race and by city, but racial inequities within these outcomes also vary by city. Most importantly, the data show that city-level racial inequities are not universal. Although some cities had huge disparities (such as a 12-year difference in life expectancy between Blacks and whites living in Washington, DC), one city (El Paso) actually had a lower mortality rate (and higher life expectancy) for Blacks compared to whites. Other cities, such as Boston, showed similar mortality outcomes for Blacks and whites.

These findings provide more evidence that racial disparities are largely driven by social, not genetic or biological, factors.[30,31] As outlined in chapter 2, these social factors include the political and structural characteristics of places, such as levels of racial discrimination and public policies related to health, education, and housing. Together, these societal factors influence more "downstream" determinants of health, such as living conditions, health behaviors, and psychosocial factors. Thus, cities with poor mortality rates or large racial inequities will first need to consider how their policies and structures across sectors may be influencing these outcomes.

We are not the first to document that the mortality experiences of Americans vary by race.[32-34] Similarly, our results showing geographic variation in health outcomes complement a large and growing body of work documenting such differences at the regional, state, county, and local levels.[5,11,17,24,35] However, the comprehensive city-level information provided here on three different but complementary measures of mortality, as well as inequities within, enables us to identify which cities need the most support and which are performing relatively well.

To move forward, urban leaders and health advocates across the country still need more information. The reasons why people die are varied. Consequently, the strategies to address poor health or health inequities must be developed and implemented accordingly. To further our understanding of mortality inequities, chapter 4 will examine city-level mortality rates (and disparities within) for the leading causes of death. Following that, we investigate additional priority causes of death, such as HIV and opioid-related deaths, where existing evidence indicates large or growing inequities (chapter 5). Chapter 6 assesses the patterns seen across all mortality outcomes and explores potential ecological explanations. Together, these data can empower cities and other public health stakeholders to more strategically pursue specific policy and programmatic changes to improve health equity for their residents. This, in turn, can enable the United States to move toward its goal of eliminating health inequities, as set out in the Healthy People initiative.

References

1. Harkness AG. Age at Marriage and at Death in the Roman Empire. *Transactions of the American Philological Association (1869–1896)*. 1896;27:35–72.

2. Woods R. Ancient and Early Modern Mortality: Experience and Understanding. *Economic History Review*. 2007;60(2):373–399.

3. Haines MR. Ethnic Differences in Demographic Behavior in the United States: Has There Been Convergence? *Historical Methods*. 2003;36(4):157–195.

4. *Healthy People: The Surgeon General's Report on Health Promotion and Disease Prevention*. United States Public Health Service; 1979.

5. Arias E, Escobedo L, Kennedy J, Fu C, Cisewski J. U.S. Small-Area Life Expectancy Estimates Project: Methodology and Results Summary. *Vital Health Statistics*. 2018;2(181).

6. Centers for Disease Control and Prevention, National Center for Health Statistics. About Multiple Cause of Death, 1999–2018. http://wonder.cdc.gov /mcd-icd10.html.

7. Murphy S, Xu J, Kochanek K, Arias E. *Mortality in the United States, 2017*. Hyattsville, MD: National Center for Health Statistics. 2018.

8. Khazan O. Americans Are Dying Even Younger: Drug Overdoses and Suicides Are Causing American Life Expectancy to Drop. *Atlantic*. November 29, 2018.

9. Kochanek KD MS, Xu JQ, Arias E. *Mortality in the United States, 2016*. Hyattsville, MD: National Center for Health Statistics; 2017.

10. Lartey J. "It's Totally Unfair": Chicago, Where the Rich Live 30 Years Longer Than the Poor. *Guardian*. June 23, 2019.

11. Hunt BR, Tran G, Whitman S. Life Expectancy Varies in Local Communities in Chicago: Racial and Spatial Disparities and Correlates. *Journal of Racial and Ethnic Health Disparities*. 2015;2(4):425–433.

12. GBD 2016 Mortality Collaborators. Global, Regional, and National under-5 Mortality, Adult Mortality, Age-Specific Mortality, and Life Expectancy, 1970–2016: A Systematic Analysis for the Global Burden of Disease Study 2016. *Lancet.* 2017;390(10100):1084–1150.

13. Centers for Disease Control and Prevention. Premature Mortality in the United States: Public Health Issues in the Use of Years of Potential Life Lost. *Morbidity and Mortality Weekly Report.* 1986;35(Suppl 2):1S–11S.

14. Gardner JW, Sanborn JS. Years of Potential Life Lost (YPLL)—What Does It Measure? *Epidemiology.* 1990;1(4):322–329.

15. Xu J, Murphy SL, Kochanek KD, Bastian B, Arias E. Deaths: Final Data for 2016. *National Vital Statistics Reports.* 2018;67(5):1–76.

16. Buchanich JM, Doerfler SM, Lann MF, Marsh GM, Burke DS. Improvement in Racial Disparities in Years of Life Lost in the USA since 1990. *PLOS One.* 2018;13(4):1–12.

17. Mokdad AH, Ballestros K, Echko M, et al. The State of U.S. Health, 1990–2016: Burden of Diseases, Injuries, and Risk Factors among U.S. States. *Journal of the American Medical Association.* 2018;319(14):1444–1472.

18. Hedegaard H, Miniño AM, Warner M. Drug Overdose Deaths in the United States, 1999–2017. *NCHS Data Brief.* 2018;329.

19. Grove R, Hetzel, AM. *Vital Statistics Rates in the United States, 1940–1960.* Washington, DC: National Center for Health Statistics; 1968.

20. Harper S, MacLehose RF, Kaufman JS. Trends in the Black-White Life Expectancy Gap among U.S. States, 1990–2009. *Health Affairs.* 2014;33(8):1375–1382.

21. Cunningham TJ, Croft JB, Liu Y, Lu H, Eke PI, Giles WH. Vital Signs: Racial Disparities in Age-Specific Mortality among Blacks or African Americans—United States, 1999–2015. *Morbidity and Mortality Weekly Report.* 2017;66(17):444–456.

22. Woolf SH, Schoomaker H. Life Expectancy and Mortality Rates in the United States, 1959–2017. *Journal of the American Medical Association.* 2019;322(20):1996–2016.

23. University of Wisconsin Population Health Institute. County Health Rankings. 2020. www.countyhealthrankings.org.

24. Dwyer-Lindgren L, Bertozzi-Villa A, Stubbs RW, et al. Inequalities in Life Expectancy among US Counties, 1980 to 2014: Temporal Trends and Key Drivers. *JAMA Internal Medicine.* 2017;177(7):1003–1011.

25. Whitman S, Shah AM, Benjamins MR, eds. *Urban Health: Combating Disparities with Local Data.* New York: Oxford University Press; 2011.

26. US Census Bureau. American Fact Finder. 2020. https://data.census.gov /cedsci/.

27. US Conference of Mayors. *Metro Economies: Past and Future Employment Levels: Transportantion and the Cost of Congestion, Population Forecast.* Washington, DC; 2018.

28. World Bank. Life Expectancy at Birth. 2019. https://data.worldbank.org/indicator/SP.DYN.LE00.IN.

29. Jones CP. Toward the Science and Practice of Anti-racism: Launching a National Campaign against Racism. *Ethnicity and Disease*. 2018;28(Suppl 1):231–234.

30. Goodman AH. Why Genes Don't Count (for Racial Differences in Health). *American Journal of Public Health*. 2000;90(11):1699–1702.

31. Templeton AR. Biological Races in Humans. *Studies in History and Philosophy of Biological and Biomedical Sciences*. 2013;44(3):262–271.

32. Orsi JM, Margellos-Anast H, Whitman S. Black–White Health Disparities in the United States and Chicago: A 15-Year Progress Analysis. *American Journal of Public Health*. 2010;100(2):349–356.

33. Satcher D, Fryer GE, McCann J, Troutman A. What If We Were Equal? A Comparison of the Black-White Mortality Gap in 1960 and 2000. *Health Affairs*. 2005;24(2):459–464.

34. Hummer RA. Black-White Differences in Health and Mortality: A Review and Conceptual Model. *Sociological Quarterly*. 1996;37(1):105–125.

35. Fenelon A, Boudreaux M. Life and Death in the American City: Men's Life Expectancy in 25 Major American Cities from 1990 to 2015. *Demography*. 2019;56(6):2349–2375.

FOUR

Inequities in the 10 Leading Causes of Death

ABIGAIL SILVA, NAZIA SAIYED, FERNANDO G. DE MAIO,
AND MAUREEN R. BENJAMINS

A S DOCUMENTED IN CHAPTER 3, the overall mortality experience and nature of racial inequities clearly differ across US cities. But overall indicators like life expectancy and premature mortality only tell part of the story. Another essential way to understand mortality patterns in a population is to rank the causes of death in order of frequency to identify those that are of most public health importance. The leading causes of death are considered a primary indicator of a population's overall health status and quality of life.[1] In the United States, the 10 leading causes of death in 2017 accounted for 74% of all deaths and included heart disease, cancer, accidents (unintentional injuries), chronic lower respiratory disease (CLRD), stroke (cerebrovascular disease), Alzheimer's disease, diabetes, influenza and pneumonia, kidney disease, and suicide.[2,3] What might city-level data on racial inequities in these outcomes reveal about the nature of health inequities in the country? Here we conduct an examination of cause-specific mortality and related inequities at the city level to identify geographic areas, specific outcomes, or population groups of particular concern for targeted interventions.

Any potential city-level initiatives need to be developed and implemented within a framework that incorporates the wide range of individual, social, and structural factors that contribute to these outcomes (see chapter 2). At the most proximal level, common modifiable factors such as tobacco use, inadequate physical activity, alcohol consumption, and an unhealthy diet contribute substantially to the leading causes of death.[4-8] Social and structural factors, though more distal, are clearly important contributors since they influence individual behaviors. For instance, many of these leading causes of death (e.g., heart disease, some cancers, diabetes, stroke, kidney disease, and CLRD) are considered amenable to health care, meaning that they are potentially preventable with the provision of timely and effective health care.[9] Furthermore, policies related to issues such as health care coverage, tobacco control, motor vehicle safety, and gun control have been shown to affect both overall and cause-specific mortality.[10-15] Finally, policies in other sectors, including those related to housing and education, help create social conditions that produce racialized patterns in health inequity.[16] Through these multiple avenues, cities can utilize evidence-based policies and interventions to address inequities in outcomes.[17] Toward the end of this chapter, we use Chicago as a case study to illustrate how a city may employ the cause-specific mortality data and proposed framework to begin tackling its Black:white mortality inequities.

Nationally, Black and white mortality experiences differ.[18] Black Americans have historically been at a *disadvantage* for most, but not all, of the leading causes of death. In terms of deaths resulting from heart disease, cancer, stroke, diabetes, and kidney disease, the Black rate is consistently higher than the white rate.[18-23] These causes contribute substantially to the racial inequity observed in all-cause mortality and life expectancy.[24,25] For mortality due to influenza and pneumonia, the racial inequity is considerably less pronounced.[22,23,26] On the other hand, Black Americans have a demonstrated *advantage* over white Americans in mortality related to suicide, accidents, CLRD, and Alzheimer's disease.[22,27,28] However, these patterns are not consistent across all of the large cities. To understand how cities compare for both mortality rates and racial equity, we conclude the chapter with a discussion of the best- and worst-performing cities.

Examining Cause-Specific Mortality at the City Level

In this chapter, we show the 2013–2017 average annual age-adjusted mortality rates for the top 10 leading causes of death for the 29 largest US cities (see the appendix for more details on the data sources, measures, and analyses). We calculate rate ratios to compare the (non-Hispanic) Black and (non-Hispanic) white mortality rates. We also calculate the number of excess deaths due to differences in mortality rates. Looking at the number of excess deaths (primarily for Blacks), as well as the percentage of these excess deaths from specific conditions, gives cities valuable motivation, and insight, as they determine how and where to allocate their increasingly constrained resources.

Here we present the findings in two general sections: causes of death where (at the national level) Black Americans have a mortality *disadvantage*, and causes of death where they have a mortality *advantage*.

Black Mortality Disadvantage

Black Americans have a higher mortality rate than white Americans for 6 of the 10 leading causes of death: heart disease, cancer, stroke, diabetes, kidney disease, and influenza and pneumonia (figure 4.1). These causes constitute 57% of all deaths nationally. We first focus on the top two causes of death (heart disease and cancer), followed by the others in order of frequency (stroke, diabetes, kidney disease, and influenza and pneumonia).

Heart Disease and Cancer

Heart disease and cancer were responsible for approximately half of all US deaths (23% and 22%, respectively) in 2013–2017. Heart disease alone accounted for over one-quarter of the disparity found in life expectancy between Black and white populations.[24] The age-adjusted mortality rate per 100,000 population for the United States was 175 for heart disease and 165 for cancer (table 4.1). Clearly, the mortality rates for these two causes are considerably higher than all other specific causes of death (e.g., the mortality rate for the third-leading cause of death—CLRD—is

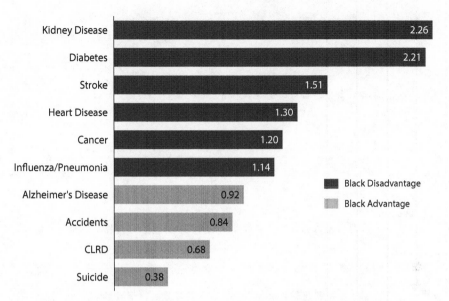

Figure 4.1. Black:White Mortality Rate Ratios for the Leading Causes of Death in the United States. *Notes:* Rate ratios calculated using age-adjusted 5-year average (2013–2017) mortality rates. CLRD = chronic lower respiratory disease.

43 per 100,000 population). As with all-cause mortality, there is considerable variation in cause-specific mortality rates at the city level. Detroit and Baltimore had the highest heart disease and cancer mortality rates, while San Jose and San Francisco had the lowest rates. The magnitude of the difference between cities was quite stark. For instance, Detroit had a heart disease mortality rate that was more than double that of San Jose (295 vs. 115 per 100,000, respectively). The difference in the cancer mortality rate ranged from 134 in San Jose to 215 in Baltimore.

Nationally, heart disease mortality was approximately 6% higher than cancer mortality. In some cities (such as Detroit and New York), heart disease mortality was more than 30% higher than the rate for cancer mortality. However, for 11 of the 29 cities examined, cancer was the leading cause of death. In Boston and San Francisco, for example, the cancer mortality rate was approximately 20%–25% higher than the heart disease mortality rate.

Table 4.2 displays the Black:white mortality rate ratios, which indicate the relative inequity in rates by race for the United States as a whole

Table 4.1. Mortality Rates for the 10 Leading Causes of Death in the United States and the 29 Largest Cities

	Heart Disease	Cancer	CLRD	Accidents	Stroke	Alzheimer's Disease	Diabetes	Influenza/ Pneumonia	Kidney Disease	Suicide
United States	175	165	43	43	39	29	21	15	14	13
Austin, TX	138	144	31	52	42	31	17	11	14	13
Baltimore, MD	251	215	37	42	56	14	31	22	18	8
Boston, MA	125	156	27	40	27	17	20	13	15	5
Charlotte, NC	140	155	33	33	43	17	20	15	21	10
Chicago, IL	196	177	29	34	43	40	24	18	19	7
Columbus, OH	189	177	52	55	47	21	28	20	18	11
Dallas, TX	186	166	36	40	53	26	19	14	21	10
Denver, CO	146	158	48	51	36	38	20	13	11	16
Detroit, MI	295	186	34	54	44	31	28	20	23	8
El Paso, TX	155	147	33	34	37	18	36	9	17	11
Fort Worth, TX	181	176	50	33	54	40	29	13	18	11
Houston, TX	204	191	32	48	51	37	26	16	24	12
Indianapolis, IN	192	192	64	54	42	30	25	13	23	15
Jacksonville, FL	183	179	50	62	46	29	25	17	15	15
Los Angeles, CA	168	144	27	24	35	16	24	22	12	8
Louisville, KY	175	187	53	59	36	34	23	17	22	16
Memphis, TN	224	200	37	52	57	34	32	20	18	9
Nashville, TN	200	182	49	62	48	41	24	17	11	14
New York, NY	191	144	20	23	21	11	24	25	11	6
Oklahoma City, OK	195	161	59	56	41	36	28	12	5	16
Philadelphia, PA	214	196	37	62	43	12	23	15	12	10
Phoenix, AZ	141	142	48	51	32	39	28	10	21	15
Portland, OR	164	194	44	50	48	39	27	12	3	18
San Antonio, TX	207	173	38	45	52	38	31	12	18	13
San Diego, CA	136	149	28	31	36	36	20	11	3	13
San Francisco, CA	115	139	21	32	33	30	13	12	8	12
San Jose, CA	115	134	23	27	33	7	27	12	8	10
Seattle, WA	130	148	25	40	31	36	19	10	4	8
Washington, DC	206	170	23	45	36	20	20	13	9	6

Notes: Age-adjusted 5-year average (2013–2017) mortality rates are expressed per 100,000 population. Bold numbers represent city rates that are higher than the US rate, and gray numbers represent city rates that are equal to or lower than the US rate. CLRD = chronic lower respiratory disease.

and for each of the largest cities. These rate ratios reveal that the US Black mortality rates for heart disease and cancer were 30% and 20% higher than the white rates, respectively. This Black:white inequity in heart disease and cancer mortality was present in virtually every city as demonstrated by the rate ratios that are greater than 1 and statistically significant. There are, however, some notable exceptions to these trends. First, El Paso showed no racial inequity for these two main causes of death. This may help to explain the earlier finding in which only El Paso had a higher white than Black all-cause mortality rate (chapter 3, figure 3.1). Second, two cities had inequities within either heart disease or cancer, but not for both. Columbus and Boston had no mortality inequities in terms of heart disease but did show inequities in cancer. Interestingly, their inequities in cancer were among one of the smallest among the cities. Third, the magnitude of the inequities among the cities varied substantially. As an example, for the 26 cities with a racial inequity in heart disease mortality, the Black rate was between 8% (Baltimore) and 144% (Washington, DC) higher than the white rate. Similarly, among the 28 cities that had a cancer mortality disparity, the Black rate was between 5% (Jacksonville and Louisville) and 92% (Washington, DC) higher than the white rate. Exposing this intercity variability (and ultimately understanding the causes of that variability) is necessary to drive efforts aimed at eliminating health inequities.

As a result of these inequities, 32,883 (potentially preventable) annual excess US Black deaths were attributed to these two causes of death alone (table 4.3). Inequities in heart disease and cancer mortality accounted for 47% of all excess Black deaths in the country. In other words, achieving equity in these two conditions, at the national level, would reduce excess US Black deaths by almost half. Across the cities examined, racial differences in heart disease and cancer mortality contributed 29% (Baltimore) to 70% (Detroit) of all excess Black deaths.

Stroke
Mortality due to stroke, also known as cerebrovascular disease, has been steadily decreasing over the past several decades in the United States, thanks in large part to improvements in modifiable risk factors and more

Table 4.2. Black:White Mortality Rate Ratios for the 10 Leading Causes of Death

| | Black Mortality Disadvantage | | | | | | Black Mortality Advantage | | | |
	Heart Disease	Cancer	Stroke	Diabetes	Kidney	Influenza/ Pneumonia	CLRD	Accidents	Alzheimer's Disease	Suicide
United States	1.30	1.20	1.51	2.21	2.26	1.14	0.68	0.84	0.92	0.38
Austin, TX	1.63	1.43	1.81	3.09	2.88	0.90	0.83	1.01	1.05	0.49
Baltimore, MD	1.08	1.08	1.25	1.79	1.94	0.89	0.67	0.87	0.85	0.44
Boston, MA	0.90	1.06	1.53	2.48	2.24	0.65	0.64	0.78	0.92	0.76
Charlotte, NC	1.49	1.35	1.70	2.95	3.88	1.26	0.82	0.97	1.36	0.43
Chicago, IL	1.40	1.46	1.77	2.18	2.42	1.18	1.22	1.59	1.18	0.46
Columbus, OH	1.03	1.07	1.23	1.94	2.03	1.07	0.63	0.83	0.75	0.55
Dallas, TX	1.61	1.46	1.76	2.50	2.79	1.41	0.99	1.16	1.17	0.31
Denver, CO	1.45	1.43	1.49	2.28	2.14	1.40	0.84	0.97	0.79	0.70
Detroit, MI	1.25	1.29	1.81	1.51	2.39	1.10	0.62	0.53	1.07	0.52
El Paso, TX	0.92	0.91	1.18	1.55	1.14	0.78	0.68	1.16	0.57	0.35
Fort Worth, TX	1.29	1.28	1.56	2.36	2.44	1.15	0.75	0.96	0.92	0.23
Houston, TX	1.55	1.30	1.69	2.58	2.41	1.41	0.88	1.01	0.95	0.43
Indianapolis, IN	1.13	1.10	1.37	2.14	1.83	0.92	0.55	0.77	1.14	0.44
Jacksonville, FL	1.15	1.05	1.42	2.13	2.43	1.17	0.58	0.57	0.80	0.27
Los Angeles, CA	1.87	1.56	2.20	3.27	2.84	1.47	1.54	1.49	1.14	0.68
Louisville, KY	1.09	1.05	1.21	1.62	1.97	1.07	0.76	0.65	0.63	0.43
Memphis, TN	1.42	1.57	1.89	2.90	2.89	1.05	0.69	0.67	0.96	0.36
Nashville, TN	1.38	1.19	1.41	2.32	1.77	1.07	0.65	0.71	0.94	0.32
New York, NY	1.21	1.18	1.66	3.17	1.88	1.19	1.02	0.91	1.08	0.54
Oklahoma City, OK	1.40	1.30	1.68	2.59	2.60	1.36	0.70	0.97	1.00	0.46
Philadelphia, PA	1.24	1.20	1.38	1.79	1.79	0.90	0.85	0.65	1.22	0.40
Phoenix, AZ	1.37	1.17	1.62	2.39	2.27	1.15	0.69	1.15	1.05	0.52
Portland, OR	1.25	1.31	1.55	3.05	3.04	1.53	1.05	1.21	0.63	0.62
San Antonio, TX	1.20	1.15	1.56	2.28	2.43	1.04	0.73	1.10	0.75	0.42
San Diego, CA	1.66	1.21	1.51	3.77	1.83	1.12	1.12	1.17	0.85	0.47
San Francisco, CA	1.55	1.65	1.93	3.86	3.33	1.37	1.88	2.44	1.40	0.61
San Jose, CA	1.35	1.29	1.71	2.80	1.11	1.57	0.85	1.57	2.52	0.51
Seattle, WA	1.47	1.45	1.74	3.91	4.14	1.17	1.30	1.84	0.88	0.71
Washington, DC	2.44	1.92	1.69	6.82	5.92	1.58	1.69	2.39	1.03	0.74

Notes: Age-adjusted 5-year average (2013–2017) mortality rates were used to calculate the rate ratios. Bold numbers denote statistically significant rate ratios (p < 0.05). CLRD = chronic lower respiratory disease.

Table 4.3. Annual Excess Black Deaths due to Unequal Mortality Rates between Races

	Black Mortality Disadvantage						Black Mortality Advantage			
	Heart Disease	Cancer	Stroke	Diabetes	Kidney	Influenza/ Pneumonia	CLRD	Accidents	Alzheimer's Disease	Suicide
United States	**20,228**	**12,655**	**6,703**	**7,365**	**5,205**	**895**	**-4,346**	**-2,339**	**-689**	**-4,007**
Austin, TX	**50**	**37**	**16**	**13**	9	0	-1	3	1	-6
Baltimore, MD	**101**	**74**	**51**	**65**	**43**	-8	**-63**	**-19**	-8	**-31**
Boston, MA	-17	**15**	**18**	**28**	**20**	-7	**-16**	**-13**	-2	-2
Charlotte, NC	**127**	**118**	**49**	**47**	**58**	7	-4	0	**14**	**-20**
Chicago, IL	**679**	**688**	**236**	**167**	**153**	**31**	**67**	**162**	**31**	**-52**
Columbus, OH	23	**30**	**19**	**36**	**24**	3	**-34**	**-15**	-9	**-12**
Dallas, TX	**302**	**209**	**91**	**50**	**62**	**16**	5	**29**	**13**	**-40**
Denver, CO	**41**	**42**	**10**	**12**	6	3	-5	-1	-5	-4
Detroit, MI	**373**	**280**	**125**	**57**	**90**	13	**-117**	**-219**	10	**-37**
El Paso, TX	0	-2	1	2	1	0	-3	2	-2	-3
Fort Worth, TX	**72**	**63**	**30**	**32**	**21**	3	**-15**	-1	-2	**-19**
Houston, TX	**489**	**274**	**137**	**113**	**100**	**29**	**-12**	8	-5	**-55**
Indianapolis, IN	**59**	**43**	**32**	**47**	**35**	-1	**-64**	**-31**	7	**-27**
Jacksonville, FL	**67**	**26**	**37**	**44**	**33**	6	**-44**	**-79**	-5	**-36**
Los Angeles, CA	**587**	**336**	**133**	**130**	**67**	**39**	**66**	**53**	**20**	**-18**
Louisville, KY	**40**	**18**	**15**	**20**	**26**	2	**-18**	**-35**	**-15**	**-18**
Memphis, TN	**274**	**314**	**116**	**103**	**57**	5	**-37**	**-77**	-4	**-38**
Nashville, TN	**98**	**51**	**26**	**32**	10	4	**-21**	**-28**	-4	**-22**
New York, NY	**784**	**547**	**214**	**468**	**73**	**87**	19	**-26**	12	**-76**
Oklahoma City, OK	**60**	**35**	**20**	**26**	10	4	**-11**	4	0	-9
Philadelphia, PA	**320**	**259**	**95**	**87**	**78**	-9	**-35**	**-170**	**14**	**-58**
Phoenix, AZ	**42**	**19**	**13**	**19**	2	1	-8	9	0	-8
Portland, OR	**15**	**19**	7	**14**	4	2	-8	6	-4	-3
San Antonio, TX	**40**	**28**	**24**	**21**	**15**	1	**-11**	5	-8	**-13**
San Diego, CA	**71**	**29**	**12**	**27**	1	2	4	7	-4	-8
San Francisco, CA	**44**	**58**	**16**	**16**	9	2	**13**	**29**	**9**	-3
San Jose, CA	**14**	**12**	5	8	0	2	0	6	2	-2
Seattle, WA	**29**	**29**	9	**17**	6	0	5	**17**	-2	-2
Washington, DC	**575**	**377**	**62**	**96**	**42**	**20**	**44**	**128**	0	-9

Notes: Excess deaths represent the average number of excess Black deaths annually due to their higher mortality rate compared to the white rate (2013–2017). Cities labeled "Black Mortality Advantage" have negative Black excess deaths (due to a higher white mortality rate). Bold numbers denote statistically significant Black-white disparities (p < 0.05). CLRD = chronic lower respiratory disease.

effective treatments.[29,30] While stroke was the third-leading cause of death in 1960,[31] it now ranks fifth and accounts for 5% of all deaths. For 2013–2017, the US stroke mortality rate was 39 per 100,000 population and ranged from a low of 21 (New York) to a high of 57 (Memphis) per 100,000 population across the cities (table 4.1). A total of 17 cities had a stroke mortality rate that was higher than the national rate.

When comparing the outcomes among race groups, we see that the Black stroke mortality rate was 51% higher than the white rate (table 4.2). Significant and wide-ranging inequities in stroke mortality were present in all but one (El Paso) of the largest US cities. As an example, Louisville experienced a Black stroke mortality rate that was 21% higher than the white rate, while Los Angeles had a Black rate that was 120% higher than the white rate. Within almost all the cities, the Black:white inequity was larger for stroke than for the two leading causes of death (heart disease and cancer).

Nationally, the Black:white inequity in stroke mortality resulted in 6,703 excess Black deaths (table 4.3). This represents 10% of all excess Black deaths, though, at the city level, this proportion was as low as 3% (Washington, DC) and as high as 32% (Boston). Compare this finding with an earlier one in which heart disease and cancer mortality accounted for 29% of excess Black deaths in Baltimore. The implication here is that in order to ameliorate racial inequities in mortality, Boston might consider prioritizing efforts aimed at reducing mortality due to stroke, while Baltimore might be better off tackling heart disease and cancer.

Diabetes and Kidney Disease

More than 100 million Americans have diabetes or prediabetes, and an estimated 37 million have chronic kidney disease.[32,33] Although the burden of morbidity is high, diabetes and kidney disease account for only 3% and 2% of all US deaths, respectively. The mortality rate for diabetes was 21 per 100,000 population in the United States and ranged from a low of 13 (San Francisco) to a high of 36 (El Paso). Within the largest cities, 19 experienced a diabetes mortality rate higher than that of the nation (table 4.1). The mortality rate for kidney disease in the United States was 14 per 100,000 population. Mortality due to kidney disease varied considerably across cities, with Houston experiencing a rate (24) eight times the rate of San Diego (3) or Phoenix (3). Sixteen cities had a rate that was higher than the national rate.

While the mortality rates for these two causes were considerably lower than for heart disease, cancer, or stroke, the magnitude of the racial inequity was much larger. Nationally, the Black mortality rates for diabetes and kidney disease were more than twice as high as the white rates (table 4.2). The disparity due to these two causes resulted in 12,570 excess Black deaths annually, which represents 18% of all excess Black deaths in the country (table 4.3).

Diabetes is the only leading cause of death showing racial inequities in all cities. Even in the city with the least disparity for this outcome, Detroit, the Black diabetes mortality rate was 51% higher than the white rate. The most extreme inequity was seen in the US capital, where the Black rate exceeded the white rate by an astounding 582%.

In terms of kidney disease, all cities except San Jose and El Paso exhibited racial inequities in mortality. Among the cities with inequities, almost all had Black rates *at least double* the white rates. Nashville had the smallest disparity (Black:white mortality rate ratio = 1.77), while the US capital had the largest (Black:white mortality rate ratio = 5.92). For 18 of the largest cities, the Black:white kidney disease mortality inequity was larger than the disparity for diabetes (or any of the other leading causes of death).

Influenza and Pneumonia
Although influenza and pneumonia are vaccine preventable and amenable to health care (i.e., treatment),[9,34-36] together they represent the eighth-leading cause of death and account for 2% of all US deaths. The US mortality rate due to these conditions was 15 per 100,000 population (table 4.1). Among the 29 cities compared, the rate was as low as 9 deaths per 100,000 population in El Paso and as high as 25 in New York. Eleven cities had a rate higher than the US rate.

At the national level, the Black mortality rate for influenza and pneumonia was 14% higher than the white rate (table 4.2). The Black:white differences in mortality experiences varied more widely across the largest

US cities than any causes of death previously discussed in which Black Americans experienced a mortality disadvantage over their white counterparts. More specifically, the Black mortality rate was higher than the white rate in 12 cities, while 16 cities experienced no racial inequities. In one city, Boston, the Black rate was actually lower than the white rate (Black:white mortality rate ratio=0.65). Among the cities with a Black:white disparity, the Black rate was 18% (Chicago) to 58% (Washington, DC) higher than the white rate. Given the low rates of mortality due to this cause and the relatively small inequities, influenza and pneumonia are not primary contributors to the number of excess Black deaths across cities.

Black Mortality Advantage

For the remaining leading causes of death, the national Black mortality rate was lower than the white rate. Black Americans have a mortality advantage compared to white Americans for CLRD, accidents, Alzheimer's disease, and suicide. Together, these four causes accounted for 16% of all US deaths from 2013 to 2017.

Chronic Lower Respiratory Disease

CLRD includes diseases such as chronic obstructive pulmonary disease, asthma, emphysema, and chronic bronchitis and is the third-leading cause of death in the United States, totaling 6% of all deaths. The national mortality rate due to CLRD was 43 per 100,000 population (table 4.1). Like the other leading causes, this rate varied widely across cities. As an example, New York had a rate as low as 20 per 100,000, while Indianapolis has a rate as high as 64. Ten of the largest cities had a rate that was higher than the US rate.

The national Black mortality rate for CLRD was 32% lower than the white rate (table 4.2). For 17 of the big cities, a Black mortality advantage was apparent. Among the cities with a Black advantage, the Black rate was 12% (Houston) to 45% (Indianapolis) lower than the white rate. However, Seattle, San Francisco, Chicago, Los Angeles, and the US capital had a Black rate that was 22% to 88% higher than the white rate. The Black and white mortality rates were statistically equivalent for seven cities.

The Black advantage in mortality due to CLRD meant that there were 4,346 excess white deaths per year from this cause (table 4.3). The Black mortality advantage in Detroit accounted for 117 excess white deaths, while the Black mortality disadvantage in Chicago accounted for 67 excess Black deaths.

Accidents

Accidental deaths, including those related to motor vehicle accidents and falls, were the fourth-leading cause of death, representing 5% of all US deaths. The national mortality rate for accidental deaths was 43 per 100,000 population (table 4.1). There was more than a twofold difference across the cities, with a rate as low as 23 in New York and a rate as high as 62 in three cities. Sixteen cities had a mortality rate that was higher than the US rate.

Nationally, the Black rate for accidental deaths was 16% lower than the white rate (table 4.2). The nature and extent of the inequity varied across the cities. The Black advantage in accidental deaths was present in 11 of the largest cities. In Detroit, the Black rate was 47% lower than the white rate, while it was 9% lower in New York. Conversely, eight cities had a Black rate that was significantly higher than the white rate. Among these cities, the Black mortality rate was 15% (Phoenix) to 144% (San Francisco) higher than the white rate. Ten cities showed no significant racial differences in accident-related mortality.

Across the country, the Black advantage in mortality due to accidents translated into 2,339 excess white deaths per year that would be prevented if whites died of accidents at the same rate as Blacks (table 4.3). The Black mortality advantage in Detroit alone accounted for 219 excess white deaths. Note, however, that eight cities still showed excess Black deaths. For example, the Black mortality disadvantage in Chicago accounted for 162 excess Black deaths each year.

Alzheimer's Disease

Alzheimer's disease is a progressive brain disorder that impacts cognitive and functional abilities, including the ability to swallow and breathe.[37] The number of deaths due to Alzheimer's disease has increased, in part, because of growth in the aging population.[38] The US mortality rate due to Alzheimer's disease was 29 per 100,000 population (table 4.1). It is the sixth-leading cause of death and is responsible for 4% of all deaths. The mortality experience varied considerably across the largest cities. For instance, Nashville's mortality rate was 45 per 100,000 population, which is more than six times the rate for San Jose (7). Of the largest cities, 18 had a rate that was higher than the US rate.

At the national level, the Black mortality rate for Alzheimer's disease was 8% lower than the white rate (table 4.2). However, of the big cities, 7 had a significant Black mortality advantage and 7 others had a Black mortality disadvantage. Among the cities with a Black mortality advantage, the Black rate was 20% (Jacksonville) to 43% (El Paso) lower than the white rate. Cities with a Black disadvantage in mortality due to Alzheimer's disease experienced a Black rate 14% (Los Angeles) to 152% (San Jose) higher than the white rate. The remaining cities had comparable mortality rates for their Black and white populations. Given the relatively low rates of mortality due to Alzheimer's disease and the relatively small disparity, this cause of death was not a major contributor to racial inequities in excess deaths nationally or across cities.

Suicide

The US mortality rate due to suicide has been steadily increasing over the past two decades.[39] The most common methods of suicide include by hanging/strangulation/suffocation, by a firearm, and by poisoning.[40] These three methods alone account for 92% of suicide deaths.[40] In the United States, suicide is the 10th-leading cause of death, with a 2013–2017 average annual age-adjusted rate of 13 per 100,000 population (table 4.1). As with all other causes, the rate varied substantially across the 29 largest cities. As an example, Boston had a rate as low as 5, while Portland had a rate of 18. Eight of the largest cities had a higher suicide rate than the country.

The Black advantage for suicide mortality was striking, with the US Black mortality rate being 62% lower than the white rate (table 4.2). This level of racial inequity was much wider than that found for the other leading causes of death where a Black advantage exists. In addition, 27 cities had a significant disparity; of these, the Black rate was 26% (Washington, DC) to 77% (Fort Worth) lower than the white rate. Only Boston and Seattle showed similar mortality rates between races.

At the national level, if the white rate equaled the Black rate, 4,007 excess white deaths that occur yearly as a result of suicide could be eliminated (table 4.3). Across cities, the Black mortality advantage for suicide contributed anywhere from 2 (San Jose) to 76 (New York) excess white deaths annually.

Further Insight into Excess Black Deaths

The mortality experiences for Black and white Americans varied widely across the largest US cities, and thus so did the level of excess deaths. Figure 4.2 and table 4.3 show excess Black deaths resulting from the

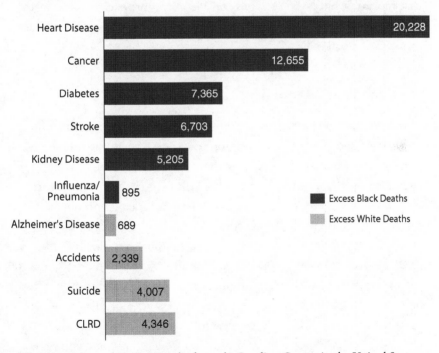

Figure 4.2. Annual Excess Deaths from the Leading Causes in the United States. *Notes:* Excess deaths represent the average number of excess deaths in a group annually due to racial differences in mortality rates, 2013–2017. CLRD = chronic lower respiratory disease.

Black mortality disadvantage and the excess white deaths attributable to the Black mortality advantage. Two things are apparent. First, when considering all leading causes of death, the total number of *excess white deaths* (n = 11,381) does not come close to offsetting the total number of *excess Black deaths* (n = 53,051). Second, the level of excess Black deaths varies dramatically across cities. Consider the number of excess Black deaths attributed to heart disease. In Chicago, New York, Los Angeles, and Washington, DC, the number of annual excess Black deaths ranged from 575 to 784. In contrast, San Jose, Portland, and Seattle each had less than 30 excess Black deaths each year due to heart disease. It is important to note, however, that the number of excess Black deaths is a function of the size of the Black population in addition to the racial inequity in rates. Take New York and Portland: these cities have similar Black:white rate ratios (1.21 and 1.25, respectively) for heart disease mortality, but New York has considerably more excess Black deaths owing to the fact that its Black population is approximately 50 times larger than Portland's.

Best- and Worst-Performing Cities

In this chapter, we have provided huge amounts of data regarding mortality rates and levels of inequity for 10 causes of death for the largest US cities. To help summarize how these cities fared across the various causes of death, we can plot their rankings for cause-specific mortality rates and racial equity (figure 4.3). Here our focus is on the leading causes exhibiting a Black mortality disadvantage. These six causes—heart disease, cancer, stroke, diabetes, influenza/pneumonia, and kidney disease—are responsible for over half of all deaths in the United States each year. The cities fell into four quadrants based on their ranking (top half vs. bottom half) in terms of cause-specific mortality rates and Black:white rate ratios. The best-performing cities, those ranking in the top half of the cities for both mortality (i.e., lower rates) and equity (i.e., smaller Black:white rate ratios), included El Paso, Boston, Phoenix, and New York. Four cities fell squarely in the "worst performing" quadrant. Those ranked in the bottom half of cities for both mortality (i.e., higher

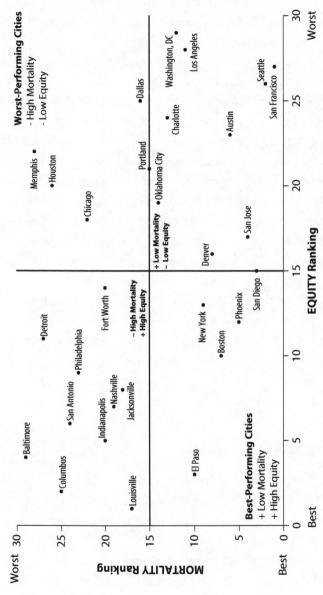

Figure 4.3. Ranking Mortality and Equity within the Six Leading Causes of Death with a Black Mortality Disadvantage. *Notes:* The six causes include heart disease, cancer, stroke, diabetes, kidney disease, and influenza and pneumonia. Mortality ranking is based on a city's age-adjusted 5-year average (2013–2017) mortality rate. Equity ranking is based on the Black:white mortality rate ratios. Quadrants are separated by lines representing the average ranking (out of 29 cities) for each outcome.

rates) and equity (i.e., larger Black:white rate ratios) included Dallas, Memphis, Houston, and our home city, Chicago. The vast majority of cities, however, ranked poorly in either cause-specific mortality or equity. An evaluation of city-level characteristics that might help us explain these patterns is presented in chapter 6.

Moving forward, an examination of the leading causes of death for these cities can highlight potential focus areas for intervention. For instance, although Boston ranked well in cause-specific mortality and racial equity in those outcomes, its mortality rate for kidney disease was 11% higher than the national rate. Additionally, the leading cause of death in Boston was cancer, not heart disease. These pieces of information offer Boston an opportunity to further improve the overall health of its residents by targeting their unique health issues. Cities can use existing frameworks and models to design and implement new initiatives, such as those aimed at improving kidney care[41] or cancer control.[42–44] As another example, Los Angeles did well in cause-specific mortality overall but poorly in terms of equity for each of the 10 leading causes. Thus, for that city, it would not be sufficient to improve overall city rates for these causes since such general efforts would likely maintain (or even exacerbate) racial inequities. Instead, initiatives there should be led in conjunction with Black communities (and relevant community organizations and institutions) to remedy policies and systems that have created and maintained the racial inequities over time.

City Spotlight: Chicago

In chapter 3, we found that Chicago performed poorly regarding both mortality-related outcomes and racial equity (figure 3.4), having a higher all-cause mortality rate and lower life expectancy than the nation as a whole. Chicago's level of inequity was also higher, with Black residents experiencing a 55% higher mortality rate than their white counterparts, resulting in 3,341 excess Black deaths annually. As noted above, a closer examination of cause-specific mortality is needed to provide insight into potential focus areas for the city.

Among the leading causes of death, Chicago had higher mortality rates than the nation for heart disease, cancer, and stroke. The mortality rates from these three causes were 40%–70% higher for Blacks than whites. The inequities seen in these three causes alone account for almost half of the excess Black deaths. The primary risk factors for heart disease, cancer, and stroke are largely modifiable, and evidence-based interventions are available for implementation.[45–48] Thus, in addition to policies aimed at eliminating structural barriers to health (like poverty and residential segregation), Chicagoans could benefit from the implementation of evidence-based policies and programs targeting risk factors related to diet (e.g., taxation of unhealthy foods), lifestyle (e.g., incentives for using public transportation or bikes), and tobacco use (e.g., cessation interventions, increasing tobacco-restricted areas).[49–52] For high-risk communities, ensuring access to cancer and cardiovascular health screening and general health care is also critical for improving outcomes and addressing racial inequities.[49,53,54] As discussed in chapter 7, elected officials and other leaders must engage the community, particularly its Black residents, in developing, implementing, and sustaining any health improvement efforts.

Conclusion

This chapter revealed huge variations in the direction and extent of geographic and racial disparities in the leading causes of death across America's largest cities. For the number one cause of death, heart disease, the worst-performing city (Detroit) had double the mortality rate of the best-performing cities (San Francisco and San Jose). Some causes, like kidney disease, showed even more dramatic geographic variation, with a eightfold difference in the rates between the worst- and best-performing cities (Houston and Phoenix, respectively). When racial inequities were examined, Black residents fared worse than whites for most causes of death, but the magnitude of the disparity varied considerably.

Cause-specific mortality data at the city level allow us to (1) compare results across the largest cities and (2) provide cities with data specific to their jurisdiction. The data shown here can help nationally focused groups (including philanthropies, health care providers and insurers, advocates, and researchers) identify which cities need the most attention and support, as well as those leading the way. At the local level, the data can enable cities to target activities toward their biggest issues, supported by existing evidence-based policies and programs. Cities may also find the information useful in identifying potential partner cities facing the same challenges (to perhaps pool information and resources) or that have achieved better outcomes (to serve as a model). Finally, these types of data allow us to set goals and establish a baseline for the hard work still ahead to attain equity in our largest urban areas.

Looking at similar data for other causes provides additional insight into racial inequities in mortality. The following chapter addresses selected causes of death that have significant Black disadvantages, such as HIV and homicide, as well as a critical emerging cause that has remarkable variation in racial inequities, opioid-related deaths. Combined, these two chapters provide cities with detailed information to help support funding and programming decision-making.

References

1. Mokdad AH, Ballestros K, Echko M, et al. The State of US Health, 1990–2016: Burden of Diseases, Injuries, and Risk Factors among US States. *Journal of the American Medical Association.* 2018;319(14):1444–1472.

2. Murphy SL, Xu J, Kochanek KD, Arias E. Mortality in the United States, 2017. *NCHS Data Brief.* 2018(328):1–8.

3. Heron M. Deaths: Leading Causes for 2016. *National Vital Statistics Reports.* 2018;67(6):1–77.

4. Carlson SA, Adams EK, Yang Z, Fulton JE. Percentage of Deaths Associated with Inadequate Physical Activity in the United States. *Preventing Chronic Disease.* 2018;15:E38.

5. Lariscy JT, Hummer RA, Rogers RG. Cigarette Smoking and All-Cause and Cause-Specific Adult Mortality in the United States. *Demography.* 2018;55(5):1855–1885.

6. Long G, Watkinson C, Brage S, et al. Mortality Benefits of Population-Wide Adherence to National Physical Activity Guidelines: A Prospective Cohort Study. *European Journal of Epidemiology.* 2015;30(1):71–79.

7. Ma J, Siegel RL, Jacobs EJ, Jemal A. Smoking-Attributable Mortality by State in 2014, U.S. *American Journal of Preventive Medicine.* 2018;54(5):661–670.

8. Liese AD, Krebs-Smith SM, Subar AF, et al. The Dietary Patterns Methods Project: Synthesis of Findings across Cohorts and Relevance to Dietary Guidance. *Journal of Nutrition*. 2015;145(3):393–402.

9. Nolte E, McKee M. Measuring the Health of Nations: Analysis of Mortality Amenable to Health Care. *BMJ*. 2003;327(7424):1129.

10. Sommers BD. State Medicaid Expansions and Mortality, Revisited: A Cost-Benefit Analysis. *American Journal of Health Economics*. 2017;3(3):392–421.

11. Jones B, Dellinger A, Wallace D. Achievements in Public Health, 1900–1999. Motor Vehicle Safety; a 20th Century Public Health Achievement. *Morbidity and Mortality Weekly Report*. 1999;48(18):369–374.

12. Miller S, Altekruse S, Johnson N, Wherry LR. *Medicaid and Mortality: New Evidence from Linked Survey and Administrative Data*. National Bureau of Economic Research; 2019. 0898-2937.

13. Kaufman EJ, Morrison CN, Branas CC, Wiebe DJ. State Firearm Laws and Interstate Firearm Deaths from Homicide and Suicide in the United States: A Cross-Sectional Analysis of Data by County. *JAMA Internal Medicine*. 2018;178(5):692–700.

14. Friedman LS, Hedeker D, Richter ED. Long-Term Effects of Repealing the National Maximum Speed Limit in the United States. *American Journal of Public Health*. 2009;99(9):1626–1631.

15. Paoletti L, Jardin B, Carpenter MJ, Cummings KM, Silvestri GA. Current Status of Tobacco Policy and Control. *Journal of Thoracic Imaging*. 2012;27(4):213–219.

16. Raphael D. Health Inequities in the United States: Prospects and Solutions. *Journal of Public Health Policy*. 2000;21(4):394–427.

17. Williams DR, Cooper LA. Reducing Racial Inequities in Health: Using What We Already Know to Take Action. *International Journal of Environmental Research and Public Health*. 2019;16(4):606.

18. Chang MH, Moonesinghe R, Athar HM, Truman BI. Trends in Disparity by Sex and Race/Ethnicity for the Leading Causes of Death in the United States—1999–2010. *Journal of Public Health Management and Practice*. 2016;22(Suppl 1):S13–S24.

19. Van Dyke M, Greer S, Odom E, et al. Heart Disease Death Rates among Blacks and Whites Aged ≥35 Years—United States, 1968–2015. *MMWR Surveillance Summaries*. 2018;67(5):1.

20. O'Keefe EB, Meltzer JP, Bethea TN. Health Disparities and Cancer: Racial Disparities in Cancer Mortality in the United States, 2000–2010. *Frontiers in Public Health*. 2015;3(51).

21. Hunt BR, Whitman S, Henry CA. Age-Adjusted Diabetes Mortality Rates Vary in Local Communities in a Metropolitan Area: Racial and Spatial Disparities and Correlates. *Diabetes Care*. 2014;37(5):1279–1286.

22. Xu J, Murphy SL, Kochanek KD, Bastian B, Arias E. Deaths: Final Data for 2016. *National Vital Statistics Reports*. 2018;67(5):1–76.

23. Centers for Disease Control and Prevention (CDC). Deaths: Final Data for 2017. June 24, 2019. https://www.cdc.gov/nchs/data/nvsr/nvsr68/nvsr68_09 -508.pdf.

24. Kochanek KD, Arias E, Anderson RN. How Did Cause of Death Contribute to Racial Differences in Life Expectancy in the United States in 2010? *NCHS Data Brief.* 2013(125):1–8.

25. Wong MD, Shapiro MF, Boscardin WJ, Ettner SL. Contribution of Major Diseases to Disparities in Mortality. *New England Journal of Medicine.* 2002;347(20):1585–1592.

26. American Lung Association. Trends in Pneumonia and Influenza Morbidity and Mortality. November 1, 2015. https://www.lung.org/getmedia /98f088b5-3fd7-4c43-a490-ba8f4747bd4d/pi-trend-report.pdf.pdf.

27. Curtin SC, Hedegaard H. Suicide Rates for Females and Males by Race and Ethnicity: United States, 1999 and 2017. *NCHS Reports.* 2019.

28. Kramarow EA, Tejada-Vera B. Dementia Mortality in the United States, 2000–2017. *National Vital Statistics Reports.* 2019;68(2):1–29.

29. Yang Q, Tong X, Schieb L, et al. Vital Signs: Recent Trends in Stroke Death Rates—United States, 2000–2015. *MMWR Morbidity and Mortality Weekly Report.* 2017;66(35):933.

30. Jemal A, Ward E, Hao Y, Thun M. Trends in the Leading Causes of Death in the United States, 1970–2002. *Journal of the American Medical Association.* 2005;294(10):1255–1259.

31. National Center for Health Statistics. *Vital Statistics of the United States 1960: Volume II—Mortality, Part A.* Washington, DC: National Center for Health Statistics; 1963. https://www.cdc.gov/nchs/data/vsus/VSUS_1960_2A.pdf.

32. Centers for Disease Control and Prevention (CDC). Chronic Kidney Disease in the United States, 2019. March 11, 2019. https://www.cdc.gov /kidneydisease/pdf/2019_National-Chronic-Kidney-Disease-Fact-Sheet.pdf.

33. Centers for Disease Control and Prevention (CDC). New CDC Report: More Than 100 Million Americans Have Diabetes or Prediabetes. July 18, 2017. https://www.cdc.gov/diabetes/pdfs/data/statistics/national-diabetes-statistics -report.pdf.

34. Arriola C, Garg S, Anderson EJ, et al. Influenza Vaccination Modifies Disease Severity among Community-Dwelling Adults Hospitalized with Influenza. *Clinical Infectious Diseases.* 2017;65(8):1289–1297.

35. Flannery B, Reynolds SB, Blanton L, et al. Influenza Vaccine Effectiveness against Pediatric Deaths: 2010–2014. *Pediatrics.* 2017;139(5).

36. Tanzella G, Motos A, Battaglini D, Meli A, Torres A. Optimal Approaches to Preventing Severe Community-Acquired Pneumonia. *Expert Review of Respiratory Medicine.* 2019.

37. Ballard C, Gauthier S, Corbett A, Brayne C, Aarsland D, Jones E. Alzheimer's Disease. *Lancet.* 2011;377(9770):1019–1031.

38. Taylor CA, Greenlund SF, McGuire LC, Lu H, Croft JB. Deaths from Alzheimer's Disease—United States, 1999–2014. *MMWR Morbidity and Mortality Weekly Report.* 2017;66(20):521.

39. Hedegaard H, Curtin SC, Warner M. Suicide Mortality in the United States, 1999–2017. *NCHS Data Brief.* 2018.

40. Stone DM, Simon TR, Fowler KA, et al. Vital Signs: Trends in State Suicide Rates—United States, 1999–2016 and Circumstances Contributing to Suicide—27 States, 2015. *Morbidity and Mortality Weekly Report.* 2018;67(22):617.

41. Mendu ML, Waikar SS, Rao SK. Kidney Disease Population Health Management in the Era of Accountable Care: A Conceptual Framework for Optimizing Care across the CKD Spectrum. *American Journal of Kidney Diseases.* 2017;70(1):122–131.

42. Seeff LC, Major A, Townsend JS, et al. Comprehensive Cancer Control Programs and Coalitions: Partnering to Launch Successful Colorectal Cancer Screening Initiatives. *Cancer Causes and Control.* 2010;21(12):2023–2031.

43. Sighoko D, Murphy AM, Irizarry B, Rauscher G, Ferrans C, Ansell D. Changes in the Racial Disparity in Breast Cancer Mortality in the Ten US Cities with the Largest African American Populations from 1999 to 2013: The Reduction in Breast Cancer Mortality Disparity in Chicago. *Cancer Causes Control.* 2017;28(6):563–568.

44. Grubbs SS, Polite BN, Carney J Jr, et al. Eliminating Racial Disparities in Colorectal Cancer in the Real World: It Took a Village. *Journal of Clinical Oncology.* 2013;31(16):1928–1930.

45. Sabatino SA, Lawrence B, Elder R, et al. Effectiveness of Interventions to Increase Screening for Breast, Cervical, and Colorectal Cancers: Nine Updated Systematic Reviews for the Guide to Community Preventive Services. *American Journal of Preventive Medicine.* 2012;43(1):97–118.

46. US Department of Health and Human Services. Healthy People 2020 Evidence-Based Resource Tool. 2019. https://www.healthypeople.gov/2020/tools -resources/Evidence-Based-Resources.

47. Emmons KM, Colditz GA. Realizing the Potential of Cancer Prevention—the Role of Implementation Science. *New England Journal of Medicine.* 2017;376(10):986–990.

48. Zaza S, Briss PA, Harris KW. *The Guide to Community Preventive Services: What Works to Promote Health?* Oxford: Oxford University Press; 2005.

49. Pearson TA. Public Policy Approaches to the Prevention of Heart Disease and Stroke. *Circulation.* 2011;124(23):2560–2571.

50. Block JP, Subramanian SV. Moving Beyond "Food Deserts": Reorienting United States Policies to Reduce Disparities in Diet Quality. *PLOS Med.* 2015;12(12):e1001914.

51. Warren M, Beck S, Rayburn J. The State of Obesity 2018: Better Policies for a Healthier America. *Washington (DC): Trust for America's Health and the Robert Wood Johnson Foundation.* 2018:1–68.

52. Rhoades RR, Beebe LA, Boeckman LM, Williams MB. Communities of Excellence in Tobacco Control: Changes in Local Policy and Key Outcomes. *American Journal of Preventive Medicine.* 2015;48(1):S21–S28.

53. Mensah GA. Eliminating Disparities in Cardiovascular Health: Six Strategic Imperatives and a Framework for Action. *Circulation.* 2005;111(10):1332–1336.

54. Buchmueller TC, Levinson ZM, Levy HG, Wolfe BL. Effect of the Affordable Care Act on Racial and Ethnic Disparities in Health Insurance Coverage. *American Journal of Public Health.* 2016;106(8):1416–1421.

FIVE

Inequities in Selected Causes of Death

HIV, Homicide, and Opioid

ABIGAIL SILVA, NAZIA SAIYED, AND MAUREEN R. BENJAMINS

M ORTALITY STATISTICS provide valuable insight into the health of our urban populations. Chapters 3 and 4 illustrate the considerable variation in mortality rates and racial inequities across US cities for both all-cause mortality and mortality due to the leading causes of death. Beyond these, however, other priority causes of death also demand our attention owing to the magnitude of the racial inequities observed within the causes or to recent increases in mortality rates—increases that have contributed to an alarming decrease in life expectancy across the United States since 2015. These outcomes include deaths due to HIV, homicide, and opioids.

The unequal burden of mortality shouldered by one group in the United States is most clearly demonstrated in the cases of HIV and homicide. Consider that although Black Americans make up only 13% of the nation's population, they account for 43% of HIV diagnoses.[1] From 2010 to 2016, HIV incidence and mortality have slowly decreased.[2–4] Public health and medical advances have provided an increasingly complete arsenal of tools to combat HIV, including evidence-based behavioral interventions, as well as effective screening, pre-exposure prophylaxis, and treatment.[5,6] However, stark racial inequities in HIV diagnoses and mortality persist.[7,8] The Black community has also been greatly impacted by another epidemic, gun violence. National- and state-level data show that the Black homicide rate is substantially higher than that of the white population.[7,9] Homicide deaths, the majority of which involve firearms, are a significant contributor to the Black:white gap in life expectancy and potential years of life lost.[10,11] While gun violence is a complex societal problem, a growing base of evidence-informed solutions exists, including recommended policies related to the purchase, possession, and transfer of firearms.[12–14]

An additional pressing public health threat is the opioid overdose epidemic.[15] During the past 15 years (2001–2016), the number of opioid-related deaths increased by 345%.[16] In 2018, approximately 128 people died per day as a result of this epidemic in the United States.[17] Opioid-related mortality rates increased similarly in both Black and white populations between 1980 and 2000, but since then, white rates have increased more rapidly, driven largely by prescription painkillers.[18] Like the causes discussed above, there are promising public health interventions that can help mitigate this epidemic.[19,20]

Examining Mortality at the City Level

Historically, urban centers have been disproportionately affected by HIV, gun violence, and drug overdoses, and thus these are issues of serious concern for city leaders and residents.[21–23] Unfortunately, mortality rates related to these causes are not readily available at the city level.[8,24,25] Local data on race-specific mortality are even more scant despite evidence showing that the Black population has among the highest mortality rates for HIV, homicide, and opioids.[9,26,27] We need to close this knowledge gap. Government officials, public health professionals, and health care providers must have timely access to such data, particularly local data, in order to monitor such epidemics and target the urgently needed interventions required to improve total population health and ameliorate racial inequities.[28]

To better understand city-level patterns in mortality rates for these three causes of death (HIV, homicide, and opioids), we provide new data on mortality rates and racial inequities within them for each of the country's 29 largest cities. We used the same data sources and a similar methodology for calculating rates and measures of disparities as seen in chapters 3 and 4. The details are described in the appendix. Rates and measures of inequity are provided for the city, as well as for the non-Hispanic Black and non-Hispanic white populations. Note that rates based on fewer than 20 deaths were suppressed, as they are considered statistically unreliable for presentation.[7] Therefore, race-specific rates for all three causes are not displayed for El Paso and San Jose. Similarly, the race-specific rates for HIV- and homicide-related mortality are not presented for Washington, DC. A small number of other cities also lack race-specific rates owing to too few deaths.

HIV

The United States has made remarkable gains related to HIV-related mortality since HIV/AIDS was first identified in the early 1980s. From this time, the number of HIV deaths in the United States climbed sharply, until it peaked in 1995 with 50,628 deaths.[29] With the introduction of highly active antiretroviral therapy, HIV deaths declined substantially between 1995 and 1998.[29,30] Since then, HIV deaths have slowly but steadily continued to decline.[3] While HIV mortality rates have decreased for both Blacks and whites in the United States, the Black rate has remained markedly higher than the white rate since at least 1990.[3] In 2017, HIV was among the top 10 causes of death for those aged 25–44 years, largely driven by deaths in the Black population.[7]

For the period 2013–2017, the HIV mortality rate was 2 per 100,000 population. As a comparison, recall that the mortality rate for the leading cause of death (heart disease) was 175 per 100,000, while the rate for the 10th-leading cause of death (suicide) was 13. Clearly, HIV ranks well below the top 10 causes of death across the US population. However, that is not to minimize the burden HIV deaths present, particularly since we have evidence-based prevention methods and effective treatment that could conceivably eliminate HIV mortality in this country.

Of the largest cities, the HIV mortality rate ranged from a low of 1 per 100,000 (San Jose) to a high of 15 (Baltimore) (table 5.1). Twenty cities had an HIV mortality rate above the US rate.

Although HIV does not rank as a major killer in the United States, race-specific HIV death data reveal vast inequities. Nationally, the average annual Black HIV mortality rate was almost 10 times as high as the white rate (table 5.1). The 22 cities with a sufficient number of race-

Table 5.1. HIV and Homicide Mortality Rates and Black:White Rate Ratios in the United States and the 29 Largest Cities

	HIV Mortality Rate	HIV B:W Rate Ratio	Homicide Mortality Rate	Homicide B:W Rate Ratio
United States	2	9.9	6	8.2
Austin, TX	2	7.3	3	3.9
Baltimore, MD	**15**	4.2	37	11.3
Boston, MA	3	3.2	5	...
Charlotte, NC	**4**	6.1	**8**	7.8
Chicago, IL	**4**	4.9	**18**	26.4
Columbus, OH	2	3.3	**11**	7.1
Dallas, TX	**6**	2.7	10	7.1
Denver, CO	3	...	6	9.3
Detroit, MI	5	...	37	3.2
El Paso, TX	2	...	3	...
Fort Worth, TX	3	4.3	**7**	3.9
Houston, TX	**8**	4.7	**14**	6.5
Indianapolis, IN	2	2.6	**16**	6.7
Jacksonville, FL	**7**	8.5	**13**	4.7
Los Angeles, CA	3	4.2	**7**	17.4
Louisville, KY	2	5.4	**12**	6.4
Memphis, TN	**9**	...	**25**	7.3
Nashville, TN	3	4.1	10	6.5
New York, NY	5	7.6	4	9.9
Oklahoma City, OK	3	2.0	**11**	6.3
Philadelphia, PA	5	5.2	**17**	8.7
Phoenix, AZ	2	3.1	**8**	5.4
Portland, OR	3	...	4	8.3
San Antonio, TX	**4**	2.3	**9**	6.0
San Diego, CA	2	2.9	3	7.5
San Francisco, CA	**6**	2.4	4	19.5
San Jose, CA	1	...	4	...
Seattle, WA	2	4.3	3	24.1
Washington, DC	**11**	...	15	...

Notes: Age-adjusted 5-year average (2013-2017) mortality rates per 100,000 population. Bold numbers represent city rates that are higher than the US rate, and gray numbers represent city rates that are equal to or lower than the US rate. All rate ratios displayed here were statistically significant (p < 0.05). Rate ratios were suppressed (...) when either race had <20 deaths.

specific HIV deaths to analyze displayed significant and wide-ranging inequities in HIV mortality. As an example, Oklahoma City experienced a Black HIV mortality rate that was 100% higher than the white rate, while Jacksonville's Black rate was 750% higher than the white rate. It should also be noted that none of these 22 cities had a greater Black:white disparity than the one found at the national level, which suggests that even larger inequities may exist in smaller cities or rural populations.[31-34]

Homicide

Published mortality data for 2017 show that homicide was the 20th-leading cause of death in the United States, contributing to less than 1% of all deaths.[7] But, as with HIV, while homicide is not a major driver of overall mortality rates, it is a telling indicator of the state of health inequities in the United States because it is the seventh-leading cause of death for Blacks. Homicide accounted for 3% of all deaths in 2017 among Blacks, primarily among men.[7] It is a major contributor to the Black:white inequity in life expectancy, as these deaths tend to occur in the younger age groups.[11,35-37] Three in four homicides involve a gun.[38] Recently, deaths due to guns have increased following a 15-year period of stability.[39] The gun violence epidemic is a grave public health concern that threatens to impact the life expectancy of the US population.[37,40]

In 2013–2017, the US mortality rate for homicide deaths was 6 per 100,000 population (table 5.1). More than a 10-fold difference was experienced across the cities, with a low rate of approximately 3 per 100,000 in Austin, El Paso, San Diego, and Seattle and a rate as high as 37 in Detroit and Baltimore. Nineteen cities had a mortality rate higher than the US rate. For all but two cities (New York and San Francisco), the mortality rate for homicide was higher than for HIV. These 27 cities experienced a homicide rate that was approximately 30% (Portland) to 700% higher (Indianapolis) than the HIV rate.

Nationally, the Black rate for homicide deaths was 8.2 times the white rate (table 5.1). The nature and extent of the inequities varied across the cities. A total of 25 cities had a sufficient number of race-specific homicide-related deaths that would allow us to assess inequities. In

Detroit, the Black rate was 3.2 times the white rate, while it was an extraordinary 26.4 times the white rate in Chicago. Additionally, Baltimore, Los Angeles, San Francisco, and Seattle had Black rates that were more than 10 times higher than white rates.

Opioid

According to the Centers for Disease Control and Prevention, between 1990 and 2017, 700,000 people died of a drug overdose. More than half involved an opioid.[41] Opioids include prescription opioids, illegal opioids such as heroin, and illicitly manufactured fentanyl. From 2006 to 2014, overdose deaths increased about 3% per year, but between 2014 and 2016 the annual rate of growth increased sharply to 18%.[20] This recent upsurge has been primarily driven by deaths from synthetic

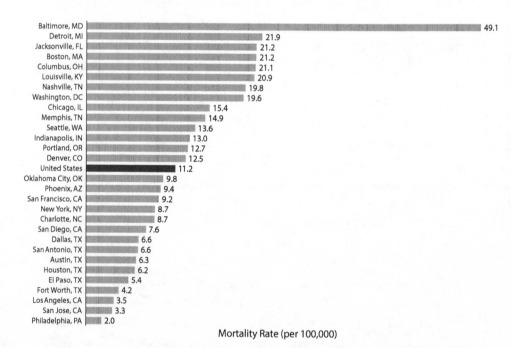

Mortality Rate (per 100,000)

Figure 5.1. Opioid-Related Mortality Rates in the United States and the 29 Largest Cities. *Note:* Age-adjusted 5-year average (2013–2017) mortality rates per 100,000 population.

opioids, such as fentanyl.[41] In 2016 alone, the opioid epidemic was responsible for 1.7 million years of life lost in this country.[16]

The age-adjusted opioid-related mortality rate for the United States from 2013 to 2017 was 11 per 100,000 population (figure 5.1). The rates ranged from 2 per 100,000 (Philadelphia) to 49 (Baltimore), representing more than a 24-fold difference between these cities. For this cause, 14 of the big cities studied here had higher opioid-related mortality rates than the nation. In 18 of the big cities, the opioid overdose mortality rate actually surpassed that for HIV and homicide.

Figure 5.2 displays the Black:white mortality rate ratios to show the relative inequity in opioid mortality rates by race. Unlike for HIV and

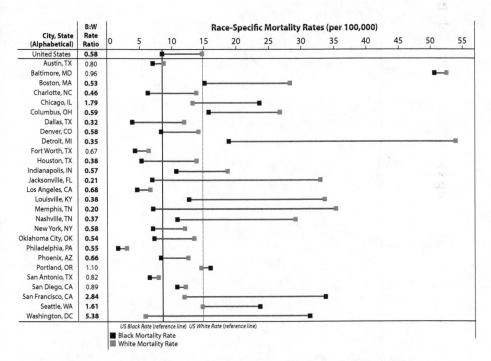

Figure 5.2. Race-Specific Opioid-Related Mortality Rates and Black:White Ratios in the United States and the 27 Largest Cities. *Notes:* Age-adjusted 5-year average (2013–2017) mortality rates per 100,000 population. Bold numbers denote statistically significant rate ratios (p < 0.05). Rates and rate ratios were suppressed for El Paso and San Jose owing to <20 deaths for one or both race groups.

homicide, Blacks exhibit a mortality advantage in opioid-related mortality at the national level. Specifically, the US Black opioid-related mortality rate was 42% lower than the white rate. A total of 27 cities had a sufficient number of race-specific opioid deaths to permit an assessment of disparities. Of these, a Black advantage was apparent in 17 cities, whereby the Black rate was 32% (Los Angeles) to 80% (Memphis) *below* the white rate. On the other hand, Black residents in four cities (Chicago, San Francisco, Seattle, and Washington, DC) fared worse than their white counterparts, experiencing rates 61% (Seattle) to 438% (Washington DC) *higher* than whites. Six cities had statistically equivalent Black and white rates.

Best- and Worst-Performing Cities

Baltimore stands out as having the highest mortality rate for all three causes of death considered here (HIV, homicide, and opioid). Perhaps this is not surprising, as research shows that economic conditions are implicated in these outcomes and Baltimore is one of the poorest and most unequal among the largest cities (tables A.1 and A.2).[42–44] Other cities with poor mortality outcomes across the three selected causes include Washington, DC, Jacksonville, and Memphis. The rates for these three cities were consistently among the 10 highest over the course of 2013–2017. At the other end of the spectrum, San Jose and El Paso had some of the lowest mortality rates attributable to HIV, homicide, or opioids. Despite these patterns, it is evident that many of the large cities struggled with just one (or two) of these causes of death. San Francisco, for example, had an HIV mortality rate more than three times the national average and had one of the worst rates among the cities included here; however, its homicide mortality rate was lower than the national rate and that of most other large cities. Similarly, Philadelphia performed poorly for HIV and homicide mortality but appears to have been spared by the opioid crisis. In fact, it had the lowest opioid mortality rate of the largest cities.

In terms of racial inequities, Black Americans in the urban centers of the United States had a substantial disadvantage in mortality due to HIV and homicide but tended to have an advantage in mortality due to opioids. Jacksonville, New York, and Austin had the highest Black:white rate ratios for HIV, while Chicago, Seattle, and San Francisco had the highest Black:white rate ratios for homicide. Opioid-related mortality displayed a more complicated pattern. Memphis and Washington, DC, illustrate the complex nature of the opioid mortality inequity. While in Memphis the Black rate was 80% *lower* than the white rate, in the nation's capital the Black rate was 438% *higher* than the white rate. Six cities had no inequities in opioid mortality. These cross-sectional results likely reflect the changing trends seen in the Black and white populations nationally and by geography.[18,45] Only Chicago, San Francisco, and Seattle consistently showed a Black mortality disadvantage across all three causes.

City Spotlight: Chicago

Chicago was worse than the nation as whole (and most other large cities) in terms of the three causes of deaths evaluated in this chapter (figure 5.3). Its mortality rates related to opioids, HIV, and homicide were 36%, 100%, and 200% higher than the US rates, respectively. Among the largest cities, Chicago ranked 10th for opioid-related mortality and 14th for HIV-related mortality. In homicides, the city fared considerably worse, with the fourth-highest mortality rate of the largest cities. Although it was not ranked worst of the large cities, Chicago attracts considerable local and national attention from public health researchers and the media for its levels of violence.[46–51] To address the issue, Chicago has numerous long-time violence prevention efforts and recently developed new initiatives (led by academic, health care, and government stakeholders) to tackle this public health crisis.[52–55] The data here provide critical baseline information that can help the city monitor its progress in reducing its staggering homicide mortality rates.

Chicago also performed poorly in terms of racial equity within these outcomes. It was one of three cities showing a Black disadvantage in all three causes of death (figure 5.3). Recall that in chapter 3 we found that Blacks Chicagoans lived, on average, 8.3 years less than their white counterparts. Although the overall mortality rates due to HIV, homicide,

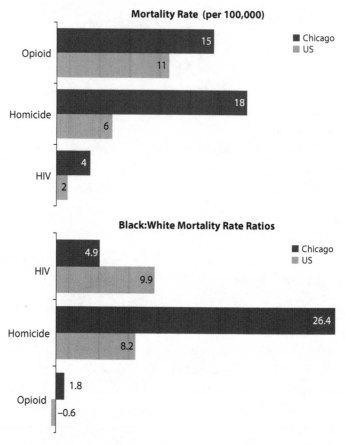

Mortality Rate (per 100,000)

Chicago / US

Opioid — Chicago: 15, US: 11
Homicide — Chicago: 18, US: 6
HIV — Chicago: 4, US: 2

Black:White Mortality Rate Ratios

Chicago / US

HIV — Chicago: 4.9, US: 9.9
Homicide — Chicago: 26.4, US: 8.2
Opioid — Chicago: 1.8, US: −0.6

Figure 5.3. City Spotlight: Mortality Rates and Black:White Rate Ratios in Chicago and the United States for Select Causes. *Notes:* Age-adjusted 5-year average (2013–2017) mortality rates per 100,000 population. All rate ratios displayed here were statistically significant (p < 0.05).

and opioids were considerably lower than those of the leading causes of death examined in chapter 4, the related Black:white inequity is likely a significant contributor to the racial gap in life expectancy since these causes tend to impact younger populations as noted previously.[11,16,35] Addressing the inequities should entail focusing resources in communities that are disproportionately affected by all three epidemics (HIV, gun violence, and opioids). Chicago could thereby make considerable gains in closing its unacceptably wide racial gap in life expectancy.

Conclusion

As found in the previous two chapters, the priority causes of death we examined here—HIV, homicide, and opioids—showed substantial geographic and racial disparities across the largest US cities. But here we observed an additional twist: both the range of mortality rates and the racial inequities in rates were generally much greater compared to the disparities found within the *leading* causes of death. For example, here the worst-performing large city (Baltimore, for HIV, homicide, and opioids) had mortality rates 12–23 times higher than the rates in the best-performing cities for each outcome (San Jose for HIV, San Diego or El Paso for homicide, and Philadelphia for opioids). The racial inequities within HIV and homicide mortality were striking. *All* the cities for which race-specific rates could be calculated exhibited Black:white rate ratios greater than 2. This means that for both HIV mortality and homicides, the Black rate was *at least double* the white rate across the largest US cities. Turning to racial inequities within opioid mortality, the data we found highlighted a need to focus *locally* on that epidemic. Public health officials and health care providers responsible for addressing the opioid issue need data to ensure that they are identifying and reaching the communities most at risk. Given that in 4 cities the Black rate was higher while in 17 cities the white rate was higher, it is clear that city-level policies and environments strongly influence this increasingly grave health problem and that cities must tailor their solutions to their particular circumstances. Compared to most of the leading causes of death, the three causes examined in this chapter tend to disproportionately impact younger age groups.[56,57] Therefore, they require immediate attention if we want to reduce premature mortality, improve life expectancy, and achieve racial equity in those outcomes across our largest cities.[16,40,57]

Fortunately, as noted earlier in this chapter, evidence-informed interventions for each of these three health issues are available. The availability of city-level rates and measures of inequities can help motivate and mobilize our policy makers, community leaders, and stakeholders to address pressing health issues, with an eye toward achieving health equity.

This is particularly true for causes of death like HIV for which effective preventive measures exist. For instance, pre-exposure prophylaxis (PrEP), a daily pill to help decrease the risk of HIV infection, is a highly effective prevention strategy that can be used to treat high-risk HIV-negative individuals.[58] HIV screening tests can be utilized to identify individuals who are infected.[59] Individuals who test positive have recourse to antiviral therapy, thereby reducing morbidity and mortality.[60] However, we must be vigilant to ensure that there is equitable access to these strategies.[61]

An examination of city-level data is a critical step toward improving the health of our population and ensuring racial equity in health. To that end, we have presented a huge amount of data in part II of this book. Readers may ask why we see such different patterns for mortality and equity outcomes across these cities. The next steps for improving population health entail understanding and subsequently addressing the root causes of excess mortality and mortality disparities. The chapter that follows will help identify city-level characteristics that are linked to the variation in mortality experiences seen here, including racial inequities. The theoretical framework presented in chapter 2 will serve as a guide as we grapple with the causes producing such patterns of inequity in outcomes, finding economic inequality and racial segregation to be fundamental drivers of Black:white mortality disparities. The final section of the book will lay out concrete approaches for how cities might employ their local data to empower their leaders and communities to invest in local solutions.

References

1. Centers for Disease Control and Prevention (CDC). HIV in the United States and Dependent Areas. October 30, 2019. https://www.cdc.gov/hiv /statistics/overview/ataglance.html.

2. Centers for Disease Control and Prevention (CDC). Estimated HIV Incidence and Prevalence in the United States (2010–2016). July 5, 2019. https://www.cdc.gov/hiv/pdf/library/slidesets/cdc-hiv-incidence-prevalence-2010 -2016.pdf.

3. Centers for Disease Control and Prevention (CDC). HIV Mortality 2017. https://www.cdc.gov/hiv/pdf/library/slidesets/cdc-hiv-surveillance-mortality -2017.pdf.

4. Centers for Disease Control and Prevention (CDC). Epidemiology of HIV Infection 2018 (Preliminary). https://www.cdc.gov/hiv/pdf/library/slidesets/cdc-hiv-surveillance-epidemiology-2018.pdf.

5. Kelly JA. Ten Things We Need to Do to Achieve the Goals of the End the HIV Epidemic Plan for America. *Journal of Acquired Immune Deficiency Syndrome*. 2019;82(Suppl 2):S94–S98.

6. Gandelman A, Dolcini MM. The Influence of Social Determinants on Evidence-Based Behavioral Interventions—Considerations for Implementation in Community Settings. *Translational Behavioral Medicine*. 2012;2(2):137–148.

7. Centers for Disease Control and Prevention (CDC). Deaths: Final Data for 2017. June 24, 2019. https://www.cdc.gov/nchs/data/nvsr/nvsr68/nvsr68_09-508.pdf.

8. Hess KL, Johnson SD, Hu X, et al. Diagnoses of HIV Infection in the United States and Dependent Areas, 2017. November 2018. https://stacks.cdc.gov/view/cdc/60911.

9. Riddell CA, Harper S, Cerdá M, Kaufman JS. Comparison of Rates of Firearm and Nonfirearm Homicide and Suicide in Black and White Non-Hispanic Men, by U.S. State. *Annals of Internal Medicine*. 2018;168(10):712–720.

10. Rosenberg M, Ranapurwala SI, Townes A, Bengtson AM. Do Black Lives Matter in Public Health Research and Training? *PLOS One*. 2017;12(10):e0185957.

11. Roberts MT, Reither EN, Lim S. Contributors to Wisconsin's Persistent Black-White Gap in Life Expectancy. *BMC Public Health*. 2019;19(1):891.

12. Crifasi CK, McCourt AD, Booty MD, Webster DW. Policies to Prevent Illegal Acquisition of Firearms: Impacts on Diversions of Guns for Criminal Use, Violence, and Suicide. *Current Epidemiology Reports*. 2019;6(2):238–247.

13. Rudolph KE, Stuart EA, Vernick JS, Webster DW. Association between Connecticut's Permit-to-Purchase Handgun Law and Homicides. *American Journal of Public Health*. 2015;105(8):e49–54.

14. American Psychological Association. *Gun Violence: Prediction, Prevention, and Policy: APA Panel of Experts Report*. American Psychological Association; 2013.

15. Scholl L, Seth P, Kariisa M, Wilson N, Baldwin G. Drug and Opioid-Involved Overdose Deaths—United States, 2013–2017. *MMWR Morbidity and Mortality Weekly Report*. 2018;67(5152):1419–1427.

16. Gomes T, Tadrous M, Mamdani MM, Paterson JM, Juurlink DN. The Burden of Opioid-Related Mortality in the United States. *JAMA Network Open*. 2018;1(2):e180217-e180217.

17. Wilson N. Drug and Opioid-Involved Overdose Deaths—United States, 2017–2018. *MMWR Morbidity and Mortality Weekly Report*. 2020;69.

18. Alexander MJ, Kiang MV, Barbieri M. Trends in Black and White Opioid Mortality in the United States, 1979–2015. *Epidemiology*. 2018;29(5):707–715.

19. Bardwell G, Kerr T, McNeil R. The Opioid Overdose Epidemic and the Urgent Need for Effective Public Health Interventions That Address Men Who Use Drugs Alone. *American Journal of Men's Health.* 2019;13(3):1557988319859113.

20. Salmond S, Allread V. A Population Health Approach to America's Opioid Epidemic. *Orthopaedic Nursing.* 2019;38(2):95–108.

21. Hall HI, Espinoza L, Benbow N, Hu YW. Epidemiology of HIV Infection in Large Urban Areas in the United States. *PLOS One.* 2010;5(9):e12756.

22. Ingram DD, Chen L-H. Age-Adjusted Homicide Rates, by Urbanization of County of Residence—United States, 2004 and 2013. Centers for Disease Control and Prevention; 2015.

23. Hedegaard H, Miniño AM, Warner M. Urban–Rural Differences in Drug Overdose Death Rates, by Sex, Age, and Type of Drugs Involved, 2017. *NCHS Data Brief.* 2019;345.

24. Kegler SR, Dahlberg LL, Mercy JA. Firearm Homicides and Suicides in Major Metropolitan Areas—United States, 2012–2013 and 2015–2016. *Morbidity and Mortality Weekly Report.* 2018;67(44):1233–1237.

25. Seth P, Scholl L, Rudd RA, Bacon S. Overdose Deaths Involving Opioids, Cocaine, and Psychostimulants—United States, 2015–2016. *Morbidity and Mortality Weekly Report.* 2018;67(12):349.

26. Lippold KM, Jones CM, Olsen EOM, Giroir BP. Racial/Ethnic and Age Group Differences in Opioid and Synthetic Opioid–Involved Overdose Deaths among Adults Aged ≥18 Years in Metropolitan Areas—United States, 2015–2017. *Morbidity and Mortality Weekly Report.* 2019;68(43):967.

27. Allgood KL, Hunt B, Rucker MG. Black:White Disparities in HIV Mortality in the United States: 1990–2009. *Journal of Racial and Ethnic Health Disparities.* 2016;3(1):168–175.

28. Davis CS, Green TC, Zaller ND. Addressing the Overdose Epidemic Requires Timely Access to Data to Guide Interventions. *Drug and Alcohol Review.* 2016;35(4):383–386.

29. Centers for Disease Control and Prevention (CDC). HIV Surveillance—United States, 1981–2008. *MMWR Morbidity and Mortality Weekly Report.* 2011;60(21):689.

30. Fauci AS. The AIDS Epidemic—Considerations for the 21st Century. *New England Journal of Medicine.* 1999;341(14):1046–1050.

31. Singh GK, Siahpush M. Widening Rural-Urban Disparities in All-Cause Mortality and Mortality from Major Causes of Death in the USA, 1969–2009. *Journal of Urban Health.* 2014;91(2):272–292.

32. Weissman S, Duffus WA, Iyer M, Chakraborty H, Samantapudi AV, Albrecht H. Rural-Urban Differences in HIV Viral Loads and Progression to AIDS among New HIV Cases. *Southern Medical Journal.* 2015;108(3):180–188.

33. Reif S, Pence BW, Hall I, Hu X, Whetten K, Wilson E. HIV Diagnoses, Prevalence and Outcomes in Nine Southern States. *Journal of Community Health.* 2015;40(4):642–651.

34. Vaughan AS, Rosenberg E, Shouse RL, Sullivan PS. Connecting Race and Place: A County-Level Analysis of White, Black, and Hispanic HIV Prevalence, Poverty, and Level of Urbanization. *American Journal of Public Health*. 2014;104(7):e77-e84.

35. Kochanek KD, Arias E, Anderson RN. How Did Cause of Death Contribute to Racial Differences in Life Expectancy in the United States in 2010? *NCHS Data Brief*. 2013(125):1–8.

36. Cunningham TJ, Croft JB, Liu Y, Lu H, Eke PI, Giles WH. Vital Signs: Racial Disparities in Age-Specific Mortality among Blacks or African Americans—United States, 1999–2015. *MMWR Morbidity and Mortality Weekly Report*. 2017;66(17):444–456.

37. Howard G, Peace F, Howard VJ. The Contributions of Selected Diseases to Disparities in Death Rates and Years of Life Lost for Racial/Ethnic Minorities in the United States, 1999–2010. *Preventing Chronic Disease*. 2014;11:E129.

38. Jack SPD, Petrosky E, Lyons BH, et al. Surveillance for Violent Deaths—National Violent Death Reporting System, 27 States, 2015. *MMWR Surveillance Summaries*. 2018;67(11):1–32.

39. Goldstick JE, Zeoli A, Mair C, Cunningham RM. US Firearm-Related Mortality: National, State, and Population Trends, 1999–2017. *Health Affairs (Millwood)*. 2019;38(10):1646–1652.

40. Redelings M, Lieb L, Sorvillo F. Years off Your Life? The Effects of Homicide on Life Expectancy by Neighborhood and Race/Ethnicity in Los Angeles County. *Journal of Urban Health*. 2010;87(4):670–676.

41. Centers for Disease Control and Prevention (CDC). Opioid Basics: Understanding the Epidemic. December 19, 2018. https://www.cdc.gov/drugoverdose/epidemic/index.html.

42. Friedman J, Kim D, Schneberk T, et al. Assessment of Racial/Ethnic and Income Disparities in the Prescription of Opioids and Other Controlled Medications in California. *JAMA Internal Medicine*. 2019;179(4):469–476.

43. Kennedy BP, Kawachi I, Prothrow-Stith D, Lochner K, Gupta V. Social Capital, Income Inequality, and Firearm Violent Crime. *Social Science and Medicine*. 1998;47(1):7–17.

44. Pellowski JA, Kalichman SC, Matthews KA, Adler N. A Pandemic of the Poor: Social Disadvantage and the U.S. HIV Epidemic. *Am Psychol*. 2013;68(4):197–209.

45. Kiang MV, Basu S, Chen J, Alexander MJ. Assessment of Changes in the Geographical Distribution of Opioid-Related Mortality across the United States by Opioid Type, 1999–2016. *JAMA Network Open*. 2019;2(2):e190040–e190040.

46. Fitzpatrick V, Castro M, Jacobs J, et al. Nonfatal Firearm Violence Trends on the Westside of Chicago between 2005 and 2016. *Journal of Community Health*. 2019;44(5):866–873.

47. Kieltyka J, Kucybala K, Crandall M. Ecologic Factors Relating to Firearm Injuries and Gun Violence in Chicago. *Journal of Forensic and Legal Medicine*. 2016;37:87–90.

48. Matoba N, Reina M, Prachand N, Davis MM, Collins JW. Neighborhood Gun Violence and Birth Outcomes in Chicago. *Maternal and Child Health Journal*. 2019;23(9):1251–1259.

49. Whitman S, Benbow N, Good G. The Epidemiology of Homicide in Chicago. *J Natl Med Assoc*. 1996;88(12):781–787.

50. Fessenden F, Park H. Chicago's Murder Problem. *New York Times*. May 27, 2016.

51. Sun-Times Wire. 1 Killed, 9 Wounded in Thanksgiving Shootings. *Chicago Sun-Times*. November 29, 2019.

52. Yang B. GIS Crime Mapping to Support Evidence-Based Solutions Provided by Community-Based Organizations. *Sustainability*. 2019;11(18):4889.

53. Butts JA, Roman CG, Bostwick L, Porter JR. Cure Violence: A Public Health Model to Reduce Gun Violence. *Annual Review of Public Health*. 2015;36:39–53.

54. Webster DW, Whitehill JM, Vernick JS, Curriero FC. Effects of Baltimore's Safe Streets Program on Gun Violence: A Replication of Chicago's Ceasefire Program. *Journal of Urban Health*. 2013;90(1):27–40.

55. Office of Senator Dick Durbin. Chicago Heal Initiative: Hospital Engagement, Action, and Leadership. 2018. https://www.durbin.senate.gov/imo/media/doc/Chicago%20HEAL%20Initiative%20FINAL.pdf.

56. Miniño A. Mortality among Teenagers Aged 12–19 Years: United States, 1999–2006. *NCHS Data Brief*. 2010(37):1–8.

57. Marcus JL, Chao CR, Leyden WA, et al. Narrowing the Gap in Life Expectancy between HIV-Infected and HIV-Uninfected Individuals with Access to Care. *Journal of Acquired Immune Deficiency Syndrome*. 2016;73(1):39–46.

58. Fonner VA, Dalglish SL, Kennedy CE, et al. Effectiveness and Safety of Oral HIV Preexposure Prophylaxis for All Populations. *AIDS*. 2016;30(12):1973–1983.

59. Branson BM, Handsfield HH, Lampe MA, et al. Revised Recommendations for HIV Testing of Adults, Adolescents, and Pregnant Women in Health-Care Settings. *Morbidity and Mortality Weekly Report: Recommendations and Reports*. 2006;55(14):1-CE-4.

60. Palella FJ Jr, Delaney KM, Moorman AC, et al. Declining Morbidity and Mortality among Patients with Advanced Human Immunodeficiency Virus Infection. HIV Outpatient Study Investigators. *New England Journal of Medicine*. 1998;338(13):853–860.

61. Grossman CI, Purcell DW, Rotheram-Borus MJ, Veniegas R. Opportunities for HIV Combination Prevention to Reduce Racial and Ethnic Health Disparities. *American Psychologist*. 2013;68(4):237–246.

PART III EPIDEMIOLOGICAL PATTERNS AND SOCIOLOGICAL EXPLANATIONS

We know that health is determined by—not influenced by—*determined* by social conditions. That is why social, economic, political, educational inequalities *produce* health inequalities.

—Linda Rae Murray, MD, MPH
Presidential Address at the American
Public Health Association Annual
Meeting, 2011

We have made the case that city-level data are of paramount importance. We have examined stark differences in the epidemiology of mortality, life expectancy, and premature death. We have quantified the magnitude of racial inequities in these outcomes and how these inequities vary from city to city. We have also explored patterns in the leading causes of death, contrasting "Black Mortality Advantage" and "Black Mortality Disadvantage" causes, plus selected other priority causes.

We now know that mortality rates and racial inequities in mortality vary extensively across our nation's largest urban areas. But why? In part III, we test some of the relationships discussed in chapter 2 and empirically examine "upstream" causes of mortality. We provide a simple but powerful ecological analysis to assess correlations between city-level characteristics and mortality patterns. Our results highlight the relationships among poverty, income inequality, residential segregation, and mortality patterns across and within large US cities. The answers, as we will see, are not always clear-cut. There is no one factor that can explain all of the variability in mortality rates and racial inequities in mortality by city, and thus no "magic solution" to the problems described in chapters 3–5. Yet this only reinforces the urgency of our message—to make real progress on health equity, we must strive to better understand mortality patterns and their roots in social conditions. Health advocates need this knowledge to create and implement more effective solutions, solutions that are multifaceted and take different forms in different cities.

SIX

Understanding Mortality Patterns and Inequities across US Cities

FERNANDO G. DE MAIO, MAUREEN R. BENJAMINS,
ABIGAIL SILVA, AND NAZIA SAIYED

HOW CAN WE MAKE sense of the data we have seen so far? Are there city-level characteristics that can help us understand the patterns we observed in chapters 3–5? If we recall figures 3.4 and 4.3, do the four quadrants in those figures reflect different kinds of cities, with different social and demographic characteristics? Are there essential differences between cities that do relatively well on both overall rates and racial equity, cities that do well in one dimension but not the other, and cities that rank poorly in both dimensions? In this chapter, we draw on the theoretical literature on health inequities reviewed in chapter 2, as well as previous studies, which together suggest a few critical structural and social determinants of health. These factors may help us better understand why some cities do well in some respects but not others.

But first, a word of caution: pinpointing a single causal factor as the *only* and *perfect* solution to the problem of unequal cities is impossible. The causes of geographic and racial health inequities, as we saw in chapter 2, are very complex and thus cannot be reduced to a single variable in a statistical analysis. Mortality data reflect a lifetime of exposure to widely different conditions; the data reflect generations' worth of history. So it is not a surprise that there is no simple and definitive explanation to what makes US cities unequal in their mortality profiles.

This is not to say, however, that we cannot identify a set of issues that matter or help us understand why mortality rates show distinct patterns across the largest cities in the United States. In particular, our review of the health inequities literature and theories highlights income inequality and structural racism as root causes of health inequities. Both issues challenge the way many people think about the causes of poor health, shifting our attention "upstream" and away from the behaviors of individuals.[1-5] In chapter 2, we discussed theoretical models that drew our attention to these deeper, structural issues. Those models highlight the harmful effects of living in a society with large economic differences between the poorest and the richest.[6-8] They also attest to the health effects of discriminatory practices embedded within not only the health care system but also society in general that disproportionately limit opportunities for people of color in the United States.[9-12]

Most people can readily appreciate the link between socioeconomic conditions and mortality patterns. Just as a social gradient in health exists across the population—the richer a person is, the longer their life expectancy tends to be—we might expect to find a social gradient at the city level. That is, there might be an association between a city's wealth (this is typically measured by a city's median household income) and life expectancy, premature mortality, and years of life lost in that city. Are our healthiest cities, those with the highest levels of life expectancy and lowest levels of premature mortality, our richest cities? Or might our healthiest cities be those with the highest levels of educational attainment, lowest levels of poverty, or other basic markers of socioeconomic status?

The research literature on health inequities finds considerable nuance for understanding these potential explanations. While income and poverty are well-known social determinants of health at the individual and household levels, previous studies suggest that explaining patterns across cities will require us to broaden our thinking beyond variables like household income, poverty, and education.[13-15] As discussed in chapter 2, there are other city-level characteristics that likely matter, including income inequality and racial segregation.

In this chapter, we explore the ecological associations between city-level characteristics and mortality outcomes. We begin with the cornerstone variables—poverty, median household income, and educational attainment—but go beyond, to look at racial composition of cities and, most importantly, more sophisticated variables quantifying segregation and income inequality. We end the chapter, as we have concluded the previous chapters, by spotlighting our home city of Chicago—zooming in to explore the complex patterns among economic inequality, racial segregation, and mortality *within* the city as illustrated by patterns across its 77 communities.[16]

What Are Essential Characteristics of Unequal Cities?

So far in the book we have documented inequality between and within the largest US cities by examining mortality rates. We have quantified and organized cities by their mortality outcomes, as well as by levels of mortality inequality. We have examined striking patterns in Black:white inequities in all-cause mortality, life expectancy, and premature mortality, as well as in mortality rates for specific causes of death, from heart disease to homicide. We now turn to a different way of thinking about "unequal cities"—how they differ in social and demographic characteristics. Guided by theory discussed in chapter 2, previously published work, and existing city-level data, we selected a core group of variables to quantify basic socioeconomic conditions, racial segregation, and income inequality in our cities.

To gauge the effect of basic socioeconomic conditions of a city, we used three important variables: percent poverty, median household income, and percent with a high school diploma. To account for racial segregation, we used two measures of demographic composition (percent non-Hispanic Black and percent non-Hispanic white; hereafter Black and white, respectively), as well as the index of concentration at the extremes (ICE) and the index of isolation (IOI; Black and white). For income inequality, we used two measures: the Gini coefficient and the ICE, which, as chapter 2 showed, can quantify racial segregation, economic inequality, and, importantly, the presence of both.[17,18] These measures are described in more detail below.

Poverty

Many might assume that poverty is the most important driver of health inequities; the damaging health effects of living below the poverty line are well documented for individuals and their families.[6,19] Yet while an *individual* living below the poverty line may face more limited opportunities to make healthy choices, the link between a *city's* level of poverty and its mortality profile or—most importantly for us—its level of racial inequity in mortality is *not* well documented. Our investigation therefore takes this critical cornerstone variable as our starting point. We obtained data on the percentage of a city's population that lives below the poverty line ("poverty status in the past 12 months") from the 2009–2013 American Community Survey.

Median Household Income

Given the large body of evidence confirming the general relationship between socioeconomic status and health (the ubiquitous "social gradient in health"), any investigation of city-level health inequities must also incorporate income.[6,20,21] To measure average income across a city, researchers often use median household income. We obtained median household income ("income in the past 12 months," in 2013 inflation-adjusted dollars) from the 2009–2013 American Community Survey.

Educational Attainment

A third socioeconomic variable considered was educational attainment, which most researchers recognize as an important social determinant of health.[1,6] For our city-level analysis, we defined educational attainment as the percentage of residents aged 18 years or older with at least a high school diploma. We also obtained these data ("percent high school graduate or higher") from the 2009–2013 American Community Survey.

Racial Segregation

As we saw in chapter 2, theories of health inequities increasingly point toward structural racism as a critical determinant of health.[11,22-25] Earlier research based on the psychosocial model focused on the health effects of perceived discrimination. A newer wave of research has taken a place-based approach to study the health effects of structural racism— the ways in which historical and contemporary racial inequities are perpetuated by social, economic, and political systems.[9,26,27] Although not perfect, one approach for incorporating this concept into statistical analyses is to use measures of racial segregation. Our analysis utilized several measures to assess the racial makeup and distribution across a city. The first two were simple measures of racial composition: the percentages of a city's population that are composed of Black and white residents. We obtained these data from the 2009–2013 American Community Survey. While important starting points, these measures alone are insufficient to understand racial segregation. To deepen our analysis, we also employ two more advanced measures: the IOI and the ICE.

The IOI is perhaps the most commonly used measure in research on racial segregation.[28-30] It measures "the extent to which minority members are exposed only to one another" (p. 288).[31] The IOI quantifies the percentage of same-group population in the census tract where the average member of a racial/ethnic group lives. It has a lower bound of zero (which would occur when a very small group is widely dispersed in a city) and a higher bound of 100 (a situation of hypersegregation, where group members are entirely isolated from other racial/ethnic groups in a city).[32] The IOI can be measured for Black and white populations separately, creating IOI(Black) and IOI(white) variables. These data were obtained from Brown University's Diversity and Disparities Project website.

Previously described in this book, the ICE also allows us to examine segregation by race. In this measure of segregation, ICE(race), the extremes are defined by the proportion of Black and white residents in a city. An ICE(race) of −1 would indicate that the city is composed solely of Black residents, and an ICE(race) of +1 would indicate that the city is composed solely of white residents. An ICE(race) value of 0 would suggest a city composed equally of Blacks and whites, or with large proportions of other groups.[16,33] We calculated ICE(race) values using 2013–2017 American Community Survey data. More details about the ICE variables are available in the appendix.

Income Inequality

Theoretical grounds might support the claim that a city's level of income inequality—not just its overall income or poverty level—is associated with the health of its residents. Previous work examining all-cause mortality in US cities suggests that the effect of income inequality may be even more significant than the effect of overall income, as measured by median household income.[15] Research also indicates that the picture may be more complex when we consider cause-specific patterns of mortality. Previously published results from the Sinai Urban Health Institute have shown a possible association between city-level income inequality and Black:white inequities in heart disease mortality[13] and lung cancer mortality,[34] but less of an association (or none at all) for diabetes and prostate cancer mortality.[14,30]

In our analysis, we used two different measures of income inequality. One is the Gini coefficient, a well-known measure of income inequality often used in economics and public health.[35–39] The Gini coefficient is a flexible and powerful way to quantify income inequality. It ranges from 0 (complete equality, where all households in a city earn the same income) to 1 (complete inequality, where all the income in a city is earned by one household). We obtained Gini values from the American Fact-Finder website, based on 2013 American Community Survey data.

Our second measure of income inequality is ICE(income), used by the Robert Wood Johnson Foundation–funded City Health Dashboard and many researchers interested in health inequities.[16,17] For a given city, it compares the number of households in the bottom 20% of national household income ("deprived") to the number of households in the top 20% of national household income ("privileged"). The result is a number that describes the mix of household incomes in a city, ranging from −1 (all households are in the deprived category) to +1 (all households are in the privileged category), with 0 signifying that both income groups are present in equal numbers, or that the city is composed of households that fall within the 20th–80th percentiles. We calculated ICE(income) values with 2013 American Community Survey data.

Lastly, our ICE(combined) variable quantified the joint effect of racial segregation and income inequality in a city. For a given city, it compares the number of Black residents in the bottom 20% of national household income ("deprived") to the number of white residents with incomes that fall in the top 20% of national household income ("privileged"). The result is a number that describes the extremes of deprivation and affluence in a city, ranging from −1 (all residents are Black and poor) to +1 (all residents are white and rich), with 0 signifying that both race and income groups are present in equal numbers, or that the city is composed of residents of any race/ethnicity whose income falls within the 20th–80th percentiles of the national income distribution. We calculated ICE(combined) values with 2013 American Community Survey data. More details on these variables are available in the appendix.

Our analysis was guided by a very clear objective: to understand, in broad terms, which city-level attributes might explain patterns in city mortality rates and inequities in mortality. We examined total rates (for all people in a city, regardless of their race or ethnicity), race-specific rates (for Black and white populations), and—most importantly—the Black:white mortality rate difference, following the example of previous studies from the Sinai Urban Health Institute. We chose the rate difference rather than the rate ratio for these analyses because it can be a particularly powerful indicator of the public health importance of the inequity in question. In addition to our core measures of poverty, median household income, educational attainment, racial segregation, and income inequality, we also considered population size, since there are considerable differences in population size across the 30 largest cities. The extent to which population size explains between-city variability in mortality inequities, however, is an open question.

Looking for Patterns

We used a simple but powerful analytical approach. Specifically, we examined correlations between city-level factors and mortality outcomes using Spearman's rank-order coefficient (or Spearman's correlation for short). This statistic measures the strength and direction of the association between two variables, which are ranked, and produces a coefficient (ρ) that can range from -1 to 1. A correlation of $\rho = -1$ indicates a perfect negative correlation (as one variable goes up, the other goes down), and a correlation of $\rho = 1$ indicates a perfect positive correlation (both variables go up and down together).

This type of analysis is called "ecological analysis." It is particularly useful for understanding patterns between places and for identifying possible determinants of disease distribution, in this case Black:white differences in life expectancy, mortality, or years of life lost. But ecological analysis has well-known limitations: (1) from ecological associations we cannot infer individual associations, and (2) from correlations we cannot prove causation. The first of these limitations, often described as the "ecological fallacy," has deeply concerned social researchers for decades.[40-42] The central problem is that inferences cannot be drawn about the relationships between variables at one level (say, among individuals) from the relationships between variables at a group, or ecologic, level (in our case, the city level). However, since our primary aim here was to understand how city-level characteristics may be associated with a city's mortality patterns, it was an appropriate method of analysis, as long as our findings are not used to make inferences about individual-level relationships. The second limitation (related to causation) is also important to acknowledge. It is well known that correlation does not prove causation; other kinds of data and analyses are better suited for that. Our aim here was not to substantiate any particular causal pattern but, far more simply, to document associations between city-level socioeconomic characteristics and mortality patterns to gain better understanding of inequality in US cities.

How Are Our Cities Different?

We begin by exploring the descriptive summaries of our independent variables (see table 6.1). Although all 30 cities included here are "large" cities, they differ in population size. As seen in table 6.1, the mean population size across the cities is approximately 1.3 million, but that number is distorted by the three largest cities (New York, Los Angeles, and Chicago). (See table A.1 in the appendix for selected city-level sociodemographic characteristics.) The median value for population size, or the value at which half the cities have larger populations and half have smaller, is just over 780,000 (not shown). The three smallest cities in the analysis have populations of less than 600,000 (Las Vegas, Oklahoma City, and Portland).

Our cities also vary substantially in their poverty levels. Across the 30 cities, we see a 20% poverty rate (itself higher than the 15% rate for the country overall). Yet this hides important differences between the best-off cities (San Jose, 12%; San Francisco, 14%; and Seattle, 14%; see table A.1) and the worst-off cities (Philadelphia, 27%; Memphis, 27%; and Detroit, 39%). This mirrors differences we see across cities in terms of median household income. Across the United States, median household income stands at $53,046. In these large cities, the median household income is just over $50,000, ranging from the mid $20,000s (Detroit) to the low $80,000s (San Jose).

Differences are also apparent in our third indicator of basic socioeconomic condition: the percentage of residents aged 18 years or older with at least a high school diploma. Nationally, 86% of adults have graduated from high school, while across our 30 cities this number stands at 83%. We see a range from 74% (Dallas) to 93% (Seattle). As might be expected, our 30 cities differ markedly from one another.

Also not surprisingly, the largest cities show wide variability in racial composition. While Blacks constitute 12% of the total US population, this percentage is almost double in our 30 cities. Yet this masks wide variation between cities. The percentage of Black residents ranges from 3% (El Paso and San Jose) to 81% (Detroit) (see table A.2 for data

Table 6.1. Descriptive Characteristics for the 30 Largest US Cities and the United States

| | Socioeconomic | | | | Racial Segregation | | | | | Income Inequality | | |
	Population	% Poverty	Median Household Income	% High School Diploma	% NH Black	% NH White	ICE (Race)	IOI (Black)	IOI (White)	Gini	ICE (Income)	Combined ICE (Race + Income)
Mean	1,309,888	21	$50,000	83	23	42	0.17	43.3	59.0	0.50	−0.06	0.03
Standard deviation	1,523,483	5	$11,527	5	20	16	0.29	25.4	13.0	0.03	0.14	0.12
Minimum	590,995	12	$26,325	74	3	8	−0.69	4.6	21.8	0.46	−0.42	−0.37
Maximum	8,268,999	39	$81,829	93	81	72	0.65	91.5	78.2	0.55	0.26	0.22
United States	311,536,594	15	$53,046	86	12	63	—	46	74	0.48	—	—

Notes: NH = Non-Hispanic; ICE = index of concentration at the extremes; IOI = index of isolation.

on individual cities). Across the cities, an average of 42% of the population is white. This, too, ranges dramatically, from a low of 8% (Detroit) to a high of 72% (Portland).

Looking at our indicators of racial segregation, we see similar wide-ranging differences between cities. IOI(Black) has a mean value of 42.4—meaning that an average Black person lives in an area with 42.4% Black residents. This is lowest in San Jose (4.6) and highest in Detroit (91.5). IOI(white) has a mean of 59.0, with a minimum of 21.8 (Detroit) and a maximum of 78.2 (Louisville). Both IOI measures illustrate the well-known segregation that afflicts US cities. Our second measure of segregation, ICE(race), paints a similar picture. It has a mean value of 0.18 (on a scale ranging from −1, where all residents would be Black, to +1, where all residents of a city would be white), with a minimum of −0.69 (Detroit) and a maximum of 0.65 (Portland).

Lastly, we see large between-city variation in both variables that measure income inequality. Across the United States as a whole, we have a Gini coefficient of 0.48 (on a scale ranging from 0 to 1, with higher values indicating higher levels of inequality). Across our cities, the mean is 0.50, with a minimum of 0.46 (in five cities: Columbus, Nashville, Oklahoma, San Antonio, and San Jose) and a maximum of 0.55 (in two cities: Dallas and New York). This is mirrored with variability in the ICE(income) variable, which has a mean value of 0.18 (on a scale ranging from −1 to +1, with lower values reflecting the concentration of poverty and higher values reflecting the concentration of affluence), with a minimum value of −0.42 (Detroit) and a maximum value of 0.26 (San Jose).

Lastly, our combined measure of economic inequality and racial segregation, ICE(combined), has a mean value of 0.03 (recall that this measure ranges from −1, where all residents would be Black and poor, to +1, where all residents would be rich and white). Across our cities, ICE(combined) ranges from a minimum of −0.37 (Detroit) to a maximum of 0.22 (in San Francisco and Seattle).

These descriptive data illustrate an important point: our cities are not a homogenous group. We saw in chapters 3–5 how much they vary in their overall mortality rates and in their levels of equity. In this chapter, we have glimpsed how the cities differ in their socioeconomic and demographic characteristics. In the section below, we examine the ecological associations between city-level characteristics and mortality outcomes.

Ecological Correlates of All-Cause Mortality, Life Expectancy, and Years of Life Lost

First, we examined the outcomes from chapter 3—all-cause mortality, life expectancy, and years of life lost—looking at the total city rate, the Black rate, the white rate, and the Black:white rate difference (see table 6.2). Note that data for Las Vegas are not shown (see Appendix).

The results revealed several important patterns. These emerged when we considered the size of the correlation, its direction (positive or negative), and its significance. How one interprets the size of correlation coefficients depends on context (and sample size), but in general the higher the absolute value of the coefficient, the greater the association between the two variables. The direction tells about the flow of the relationship: as one variable goes up, what happens to the other? The significance of the correlation tells us whether we can reject the idea that there is no association between variables (but with the now standard caveat that one should be mindful of the limitations associated with placing too much emphasis on statistical significance).

To begin, we observed that population size is not strongly related to mortality, being significantly correlated with neither total- or race-specific summary measures. Note that none of the mortality rate differences were associated with population size. In other words, the differences in levels of racial inequity *between* cities cannot be explained by the sizes of the cities themselves.

The data showed significant correlations between poverty and total all-cause mortality ($\rho = 0.53$, $p < 0.05$), implying that as a city's level of poverty increases, all-cause mortality rates also rise. Similar correlations were found between poverty and total life expectancy ($\rho = -0.53$, $p < 0.05$) and total years of life lost ($\rho = 0.57$, $p < 0.05$). Poverty was significantly and negatively correlated with white rates for life expectancy and years of life lost, but not with the Black:white rate difference

Table 6.2. Associations between City-Level Characteristics and Summary Measures of Mortality

		Socioeconomic			Racial Segregation						Income Inequality		
	Population	% Poverty	Median Household Income	% High School Diploma	% NH Black	% NH White	ICE (Race)	IOI (Black)	IOI (White)	Gini	ICE (Income)	Combined ICE (Race + Income)
All-Cause Mortality													
Total	−0.26	**0.53**	**−0.80**	−0.12	**0.60**	−0.07	−0.37	**0.58**	0.11	−0.07	**−0.79**	−0.84
Black	−0.24	0.10	−0.34	−0.08	0.23	0.06	0.02	0.20	0.05	0.15	−0.26	−0.29
White	−0.32	0.26	**−0.66**	−0.05	0.21	0.17	0.02	0.21	0.21	**−0.41**	**−0.68**	**−0.61**
B:W difference	0.13	−0.21	**0.44**	0.09	−0.03	−0.11	−0.03	−0.14	−0.20	0.36	**0.54**	**0.40**
Life Expectancy													
Total	0.27	**−0.53**	**0.81**	0.13	**−0.62**	0.06	**0.37**	**−0.60**	−0.12	0.07	**0.80**	**0.85**
Black	0.20	−0.22	**0.38**	0.15	−0.30	0.06	0.14	−0.26	0.06	−0.22	0.30	0.34
White	0.21	**−0.40**	**0.75**	0.18	−0.29	−0.02	0.14	−0.30	−0.08	0.33	**0.77**	**0.71**
B:W difference	0.08	−0.23	**0.44**	0.10	−0.01	−0.02	0.05	−0.09	−0.11	**0.42**	**0.54**	**0.40**
Years of Life Lost													
Total	−0.24	**0.57**	**−0.82**	0.14	**0.67**	−0.08	**−0.42**	**0.67**	0.13	−0.01	**−0.82**	**−0.87**
Black	−0.19	0.28	**−0.47**	−0.17	0.34	−0.09	−0.18	0.36	−0.05	0.22	**−0.42**	**−0.44**
White	−0.20	**0.45**	**−0.81**	−0.21	0.35	−0.02	−0.19	0.36	0.09	−0.27	**0.82**	**−0.75**
B:W difference	−0.05	−0.08	0.30	0.07	−0.03	0.00	0.06	−0.11	−0.05	0.32	0.39	0.32

Notes: Associations described with Spearman rank-order coefficients. Bold numbers indicate $p < 0.05$. NH = Non-Hispanic; ICE = index of concentration at the extremes; IOI = index of isolation; B:W = Black:white.

in all-cause mortality, life expectancy, or years of life lost. This suggests that it is not necessarily poorer cities that have larger inequities in mortality. Poverty was certainly associated with overall levels of health, as measured by all-cause mortality, life expectancy, and years of life lost. But a city's level of poverty does not help us understand variability in racial equity across cities.

Continuing to move to the right within table 6.2, we saw correlations between median household income and our summary measures of mortality. Here we found many more significant associations—suggesting more explanatory power for median household income than poverty. This is important because although median household income and poverty both describe a city's basic socioeconomic status, they focus on very different characteristics of that socioeconomic status. The poverty rate is a reflection of the low end of the socioeconomic distribution, while median household income is a better reflection of the middle part of the distribution. Median household income was strongly correlated with total all-cause mortality ($\rho = -0.80$, $p < 0.05$) and, interestingly, the Black:white rate difference in all-cause mortality ($\rho = 0.44$, $p < 0.05$). The latter finding suggests that richer cities have *larger* racial inequities in all-cause mortality than cities with lower median income levels.

Interestingly, the percentage of residents with a high school diploma was not correlated with any of the mortality outcomes in table 6.2. In other words, city-level educational attainment was not associated with all-cause mortality rates, life expectancy, or years of life lost.

The racial distribution of a city's population was only marginally related to mortality and mortality inequities. We found that the percentage of a city's population that is Black was associated with total all-cause mortality ($\rho = 0.60$, $p < 0.05$), total life expectancy ($\rho = -0.62$, $p < 0.05$), and total years of life lost ($\rho = 0.67$, $p < 0.05$). However, the percentage of a city's population that is Black was not correlated with Black:white differences in these summary mortality measures. The percentage of a city's population that is white is also not associated with any of these measures.

The most interesting results, however, appear further still to the right in table 6.2. We will consider two sets of results: those examining racial segregation using the IOI and ICE(race), and those examining income inequality using the Gini coefficient and ICE(income).

At first glance, there appears to be little explanatory power with the IOI. But we did detect significant correlations between IOI(Black) and total all-cause mortality ($\rho = 0.58$, $p < 0.05$), total life expectancy ($\rho = -0.60$, $p < 0.05$), and total years of life lost ($\rho = 0.67$, $p < 0.05$). In other words, as the segregation of Black people increased, total all-cause mortality increased, life expectancy decreased, and total years of life lost increased. In contrast, IOI(white) was not associated with any of these mortality outcomes. This is an important finding, suggesting that segregation is associated with poorer health for Blacks but not whites. It may be that psychosocial stressors are particularly heightened in segregated Black communities. It is also true that segregated Black communities have less of the structural amenities that other communities benefit from.[43] Segregation additionally limits Black peoples' access to the health care system. Recall all the "upstream" issues discussed in chapter 2. All are heightened—powered—by segregation. We also found that neither IOI(Black) nor IOI(white) was associated with any of the mortality or life expectancy rate differences. That is, at this level of analysis, and for these particular outcomes, segregation did not show a clear-cut association with inequities in mortality. Similarly, ICE(race) displayed relatively little explanatory power for city-level differences in inequities.

When we examined income inequality, some strong patterns emerged. As discussed earlier in the chapter, we utilized two measures of income inequality: the Gini coefficient and ICE(income). As might be expected given that they both measure income inequality (albeit in different ways), the results obtained were generally, but not perfectly, aligned.

Looking at the Gini coefficient first, we found no association with total or race-specific rates except for white all-cause mortality ($\rho = 0.41$, $p < 0.005$), and we did find correlations with Black:white differences in all-cause mortality ($\rho = 0.38$, $p < 0.005$), life expectancy ($\rho = 0.41$, $p < 0.005$), and years of life lost ($\rho = 0.32$, $p < 0.005$). In all three cases, cities with higher levels of income inequality showed larger Black:white differences in mortality.

This is further supported by the correlations with our second measure of income inequality, ICE(income). To begin, we saw strong correlations with all-cause mortality ($\rho=-0.79$, $p<0.05$), white all-cause mortality ($\rho=-0.68$, $p<0.05$), and the Black:white rate difference in all-cause mortality ($\rho=0.54$, $p<0.05$). These correlations are mirrored in table 6.2 when we considered life expectancy and years of life lost; ICE(income) was correlated with Black:white differences in life expectancy ($\rho=0.54$, $p<0.05$) and Black:white differences in years of life lost ($\rho=0.39$, $p<0.05$). Again, cities with higher levels of income inequality had larger racial inequities in mortality.

When interpreting correlation coefficients, it is often helpful to examine the data visually. Figure 6.1 more clearly illustrates the correlation between ICE(income) and total all-cause mortality. At higher levels of inequality, as ICE(income) increased, we saw lower levels of all-cause

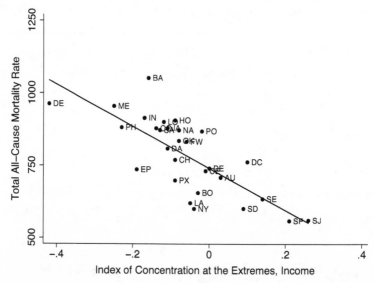

Figure 6.1. Relationship between Income Inequality (ICE(income)) and All-Cause Mortality (per 100,000). *Notes:* $\rho=-0.79$, $p<0.05$. City names have been abbreviated: Austin (AU), Baltimore (BA), Boston (BO), Charlotte (CE), Chicago (CH), Columbus (CO), Dallas (DA), Denver (DN), Detroit (DE), El Paso (EP), Fort Worth (FW), Houston (HO), Indianapolis (IN), Jacksonville (JA), Los Angeles (LA), Louisville (LO), Memphis (ME), Nashville (NA), New York (NY), Oklahoma City (OK), Philadelphia (PH), Phoenix (PX), Portland (PO), San Antonio (SA), San Diego (SD), San Francisco (SF), San Jose (SJ), Seattle (SE), Washington, DC (DC).

mortality. In other words, as a city's economic makeup leans toward the economically privileged part of the spectrum, overall mortality rates go down, mirroring the correlation between median household income and all-cause mortality. In figure 6.1, there is a strong linear relationship between inequality and mortality. Detroit had the lowest ICE(income) value, suggesting concentration of poverty, while San Francisco and San Jose were on the opposite end of the spectrum, with a concentration of affluence.

However, the data also provided support for a harmful effect of income inequality—measured as either the Gini coefficient or ICE(income)—when we focused on inequities. In figure 6.2, we see the spread of cities by level of ICE(income) and the Black:white rate difference in all-cause mortality. Here cities with higher concentrations of affluence in contrast to poverty tend to have *larger* Black:white rate differences. Similarly, in figure 6.3, we plot the spread of cities by the Gini coefficient and Black:white differences in life expectancy.

The patterning in figure 6.2 and 6.3 was not as "tight" as it was in figure 6.1—reflective of smaller correlation coefficients between the city

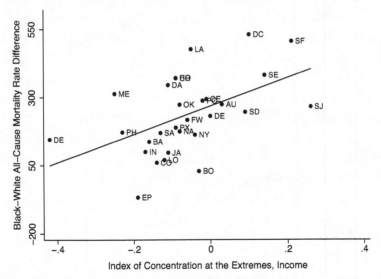

Figure 6.2. Relationship between Income Inequality (Gini Coefficient) and the Black:White Rate Difference in Total All-Cause Mortality (per 100,000). *Note:* $\rho = 0.54$, $p < 0.05$.

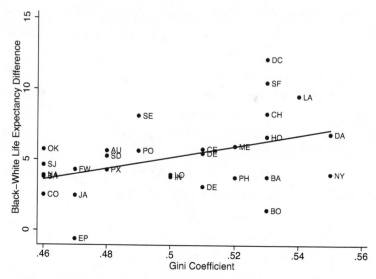

Figure 6.3. Relationship between Income Inequality (Gini Coefficient) and the Black:White Rate Difference in Life Expectancy (in Years). *Note:* $\rho=0.42$, $p<0.05$.

characteristics and the equity outcomes. Yet the patterns were still pronounced, with larger racial rate differences in the more unequal cities, as measured by ICE(income) or the Gini coefficient. Los Angeles, San Francisco, and Washington, DC, were all examples of this. Boston was an interesting exception, with high levels of income inequality but low Black:white rate differences for all-cause mortality (figure 6.2) and life expectancy (figure 6.3). ICE(combined) generally had similar or, at times, smaller coefficients with our summary mortality measures than ICE(income) did.

These results point toward a relationship between income inequality and health inequities (defined as Black:white rate differences for all-cause mortality, life expectancy, and years of life lost). This is consistent with the psychosocial theoretical tradition (discussed in chapter 2), which found income inequality to be a fundamental determinant of health. In that tradition, exposure to higher levels of inequality activates a range of bodily systems linked to stress responses—eventually leading to avoidable morbidity and premature mortality.[6,7,20,21] This is also consistent with the sociopolitical tradition. From that perspective, higher levels of inequality are associated with a range of structural issues in cities; income inequality, in this way, is a proxy measure that captures a wide range of characteristics, from the quality of education systems to the state of public hospitals to a city's transportation system.[21]

Across these results, we also found very mixed evidence of city-level correlations between racial segregation and overall mortality inequities. Contrary to what we might have expected, the IOI and the ICE(race) variables displayed little explanatory power in these analyses. At first glance, this may appear to contradict the evidence we reviewed in chapter 2 and the growing literature on the health effects of structural racism and residential segregation.[44–48] But we think that these results are not necessarily inconsistent with that literature; instead, we believe that the findings reflect an important methodological issue: the level at which we measure and correlate concepts. Throughout this book we have argued for the value of a city-level analysis; we believe that it is imperative to collect and analyze data at the city level to understand health inequities. Yet what we have here is an important twist—to understand variability *between* and *within* cities, we ultimately need analyses that compare cities across cities and also analyses that take a more local turn, examining communities within cities as well. We will return to this idea later in this chapter, under our Chicago spotlight, to examine the association between the ICE and premature mortality across Chicago's 77 community areas.[16]

Ecological Correlates of the Leading Causes of Death: Black Mortality Disadvantage and Black Mortality Advantage

To better understand the associations between our city-level characteristics and health inequities, it would be useful to go beyond our summary measures of population health to examine correlations with levels of mortality by cause of death. We organize the analysis using the same categorization used in chapter 4, distinguishing between causes of death that have a Black Mortality Disadvantage (heart disease, cancer, stroke, diabetes, kidney disease, and influenza/pneumonia; see table 6.3) and outcomes with a Black Mortality Advantage (accidents, chronic lower respiratory disease, Alzheimer's, and suicide; see table 6.4).

Table 6.3. Associations between City-Level Socioeconomic Characteristics and "Black Mortality Disadvantage" Causes of Death—Heart Disease, Cancer, Stroke, Diabetes, Kidney Disease, and Influenza/Pneumonia

	Socioeconomic				Racial Segregation					Income Inequality		
	Population	% Poverty	Median Household Income	% High School Diploma	% NH Black	% NH White	ICE (Race)	IOI (Black)	IOI (White)	Gini	ICE (Income)	Combined ICE (Race + Income)
Heart Disease												
Total	0.00	**0.64**	**-0.72**	-0.34	**0.70**	**-0.38**	**-0.66**	**0.69**	-0.12	0.15	**-0.71**	**-0.80**
Black	0.09	**0.41**	**-0.42**	**-0.42**	**0.46**	-0.35	**-0.44**	**0.42**	-0.26	0.24	-0.35	**-0.44**
White	-0.02	**0.50**	**-0.81**	**-0.47**	0.29	-0.22	-0.30	0.36	-0.09	-0.18	**-0.82**	**-0.72**
B:W difference	0.15	-0.05	0.25	-0.06	0.08	-0.18	-0.09	-0.06	-0.26	0.26	**0.37**	0.24
Cancer												
Total	-0.28	0.44	**-0.65**	0.01	**0.63**	0.02	-0.35	**0.62**	0.25	0.06	**-0.65**	**-0.74**
Black	-0.12	0.07	-0.15	-0.04	0.20	0.06	0.00	0.16	0.07	0.28	-0.10	-0.15
White	-0.20	0.15	**-0.48**	-0.05	0.09	0.18	0.06	0.12	0.26	-0.28	**-0.51**	**-0.44**
B:W difference	0.04	-0.08	0.33	0.05	0.10	-0.14	-0.09	-0.01	-0.20	**0.39**	0.42	0.28
Stroke												
Total	-0.10	0.43	**-0.57**	-0.18	**0.42**	-0.25	**-0.42**	0.32	-0.19	-0.11	**-0.55**	**-0.66**
Black	0.04	0.11	-0.20	-0.15	0.06	-0.05	-0.04	-0.07	-0.17	-0.15	-0.16	-0.22
White	-0.21	0.09	**-0.43**	0.01	0.09	0.18	0.07	0.02	0.14	**-0.41**	**-0.42**	**-0.43**
B:W difference	0.23	0.04	0.12	-0.22	-0.08	-0.27	-0.10	-0.19	**-0.44**	0.09	0.17	0.12

Diabetes

Total	-0.10	0.36	**-0.55**	-0.35	0.03	-0.34	-0.28	0.03	-0.28	**-0.44**	**-0.60**	**-0.49**
Black	-0.17	**-0.45**	0.27	0.27	**-0.41**	**0.43**	**0.55**	**-0.44**	0.29	**-0.54**	0.26	0.34
White	-0.36	0.06	**-0.41**	0.00	-0.07	0.27	0.25	-0.06	0.27	**-0.60**	**-0.44**	-0.33
B:W difference	-0.08	**-0.56**	**0.60**	0.34	**-0.39**	0.29	**0.42**	**-0.47**	0.14	-0.24	**0.61**	**0.60**

Kidney Disease

Total	0.06	**0.56**	**-0.70**	-0.32	**0.59**	-0.23	**-0.48**	**0.53**	-0.12	0.20	**-0.69**	**-0.77**
Black	0.09	0.24	-0.35	-0.06	0.36	0.11	-0.12	0.32	0.09	0.10	**-0.37**	**-0.46**
White	0.07	**0.41**	**-0.61**	-0.27	0.33	-0.04	-0.24	0.31	0.03	-0.02	**-0.64**	**-0.65**
B:W difference	0.07	0.13	-0.21	-0.04	0.28	0.08	-0.09	0.25	0.01	0.14	-0.22	-0.32

Influenza and Pneumonia

Total	0.17	**0.48**	**-0.41**	-0.27	**0.69**	-0.24	**-0.55**	**0.78**	-0.04	**0.44**	**-0.41**	**-0.61**
Black	0.07	0.16	-0.22	-0.17	**0.37**	-0.15	-0.27	**0.50**	-0.06	0.26	-0.18	-0.34
White	0.11	0.42	**-0.46**	-0.26	**0.56**	-0.16	**-0.41**	**0.68**	-0.02	0.28	**-0.48**	**-0.60**
B:W difference	0.11	-0.31	**0.42**	-0.01	-0.17	-0.04	0.09	-0.15	-0.14	0.24	**0.49**	**0.37**

Notes: Associations described with Spearman rank-order coefficients. Bold numbers indicate p < 0.05. NH = Non-Hispanic; ICE = index of concentration at the extremes; IOI = index of isolation; B:W = Black:White.

Table 6.4. Associations between City-Level Characteristics and the "Black Mortality Advantage" Causes of Death

	Socioeconomic				Racial Segregation					Income Inequality		
	Population	% Poverty	Median Household Income	% High School Diploma	% NH Black	% NH White	ICE (Race)	IOI (Black)	IOI (White)	Gini	ICE (Income)	Combined ICE (Race + Income)
Accidents												
Total	-0.37	0.23	**-0.53**	0.24	0.33	**0.39**	0.11	0.32	**0.49**	**-0.35**	**-0.52**	**-0.50**
Black	-0.21	-0.31	0.19	0.33	**-0.39**	0.29	**0.45**	**-0.43**	0.17	-0.30	0.21	0.34
White	-0.30	0.219	**-0.62**	0.09	0.23	0.27	0.11	0.23	0.34	**-0.37**	**-0.62**	**-0.52**
B:W difference	0.19	-0.37	**0.63**	0.05	**-0.53**	-0.11	0.19	**-0.59**	-0.27	0.13	**0.65**	**0.68**
CLRD												
Total	-0.36	0.15	**-0.55**	0.07	0.16	**0.43**	0.24	0.11	**0.42**	**-0.50**	**-0.54**	**-0.47**
Black	-0.16	-0.09	-0.17	-0.07	-0.33	0.33	**0.47**	-0.34	0.17	-0.21	-0.13	0.07
White	-0.36	0.18	**-0.61**	-0.08	0.01	0.27	0.21	-0.02	0.23	**-0.58**	**-0.61**	**-0.47**
B:W difference	0.30	-0.24	**0.61**	0.06	-0.19	-0.16	-0.01	-0.19	-0.18	**0.55**	**0.65**	**0.58**
Alzheimer's Disease												
Total	0.30	-0.10	-0.09	0.07	-0.21	0.15	0.26	**-0.39**	-0.03	-0.31	-0.04	0.10
Black	-0.05	-0.23	0.14	0.05	-0.15	0.20	0.30	-0.34	-0.03	-0.09	0.23	0.24
White	-0.32	-0.19	0.01	0.18	-0.21	0.32	**0.42**	-0.34	0.19	-0.26	0.06	0.19
B:W difference	**0.46**	0.10	0.15	-0.27	0.22	-0.26	-0.32	0.13	-0.30	**0.43**	0.18	0.01
Suicide												
Total	-0.35	-0.33	-0.06	0.35	-0.38	**0.65**	**0.72**	**-0.41**	**0.51**	**-0.55**	-0.02	0.14
Black	-0.23	-0.30	0.08	0.27	**-0.53**	**0.41**	**0.69**	**-0.60**	0.28	-0.36	0.15	**0.41**
White	-0.19	-0.13	-0.32	0.01	**-0.38**	0.23	**0.37**	**-0.40**	0.14	**-0.54**	-0.31	-0.11
B:W difference	0.06	-0.03	**0.44**	0.17	0.15	0.00	-0.06	0.16	0.08	**0.51**	**0.46**	0.37

Notes: Associations described with Spearman rank-order coefficients. Bold numbers indicate p < 0.05. NH = Non-Hispanic; ICE = index of concentration at the extremes; IOI = index of isolation; B:W = Black:White; CLRD = chronic lower respiratory disease.

Looking first at the Black Mortality Disadvantage results, once again population size holds little explanatory power and is not correlated with any of the Black:white rate differences. Poverty is also relatively weakly associated with the mortality outcomes, though it is positively and significantly correlated with mortality from a few causes, including total heart disease mortality ($\rho=0.64$, $p<0.05$) and total kidney disease mortality ($\rho=0.56$, $p<0.05$). The most interesting poverty results, however, concerned diabetes mortality. Here we saw a positive (but not statistically significant) correlation with overall mortality ($\rho=0.36$) but a negative correlation with the Black diabetes mortality rate ($\rho=-0.45$, $p<0.05$) and a *negative* correlation with the Black:white difference ($\rho=-0.56$, $p<0.05$). Contrary to what might have been expected, as poverty increased, the Black:white difference in diabetes mortality rate decreased. This was echoed in a negative correlation between percent Black and the Black:white difference in diabetes mortality ($\rho=-0.39$, $p<0.05$).

Median household income was an important correlate of many of the Black Mortality Disadvantage outcomes, including the Black:white difference in diabetes mortality ($\rho=0.60$, $p<0.05$) and Black:white difference in influenza/pneumonia mortality ($\rho=0.42$, $p<0.05$). In both cases, the positive correlation implies that as income increases, Black:white differences increase (contrary to what we saw above with diabetes mortality). However, median household income was not associated with the Black:white difference in the three leading causes of death, heart disease, cancer, and stroke.

The racial segregation variables produced few significant correlations across the Black Mortality Disadvantage outcomes. Of note, IOI(Black) was significantly correlated with city mortality rates from heart disease ($\rho=0.69$, $p<0.05$), cancer ($\rho=0.62$, $p<0.05$), kidney disease ($\rho=0.53$, $p<0.05$), and influenza/pneumonia ($\rho=0.78$, $p<0.05$). IOI(Black) was significantly correlated with *only one* of the Black:white rate differences (diabetes, $\rho=-0.47$, $p<0.05$). ICE(race) generally did not hold much statistical power in these results, with the exception of the rate difference in diabetes mortality ($\rho=0.42$, $p<0.05$).

Our most important correlations, again, appeared with our measures of income inequality. Here the correlations with Black Mortality

Disadvantage outcomes generally supported the patterns we saw earlier with the summary mortality measures. ICE(income) showed the most explanatory power, being significantly associated with Black:white rate differences in four of the six outcomes, including the two leading causes of death. In particular, ICE(income) was correlated with Black:white rate differences in mortality due to heart disease ($\rho=0.37$, $p<0.05$), cancer ($\rho=0.42$, $p<0.05$), diabetes ($\rho=0.61$, $p<0.05$), and influenza/pneumonia ($\rho=0.49$, $p<0.05$). The Gini coefficient displayed less consistent and weaker correlations with these outcomes, with the only significant correlation with a measure of racial equity occurring with the Black:white cancer mortality rate difference ($\rho=0.39$, $p<0.05$; see figure 6.4). In this case, the relatively more equal cities of Columbus, San Antonio, and Nashville stood in contrast to the more unequal cities with larger cancer rate differences, including Los Angeles, San Francisco, and Washington, DC.

Turning our attention to the Black Mortality Advantage outcomes (accidents, CLRD, Alzheimer's, and suicide), we found additionally in-

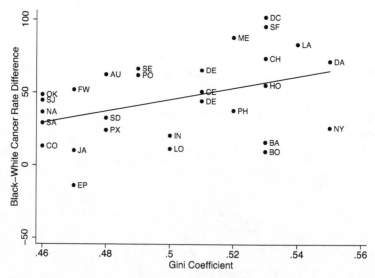

Figure 6.4. Relationship between Income Inequality (Gini Coefficient) and the Black:White Rate Difference in Cancer Mortality (per 100,000). *Note:* $\rho=0.39$, $p<0.05$.

teresting results. For the first time, population size showed explanatory power—but with a significant association with only one of the four rate differences: Alzheimer's ($\rho = 0.46$, p < 0.05). In this case, larger cities had a larger Black:white difference in Alzheimer's mortality. Across the four Black Mortality Advantage outcomes, population size had a negative relationship with white mortality rates (with correlations bordering statistical significance for three of the four outcomes), generating a hypothesis that inequities may be created by differentially greater benefit for white populations in larger cities. Neither poverty or educational attainment was correlated with any of the four Black Mortality Advantage rate differences.

Looking at our segregation variables, again we observed relatively little explanatory power. Percent Black and IOI(Black) were correlated with only one of four rate differences (accidents; $\rho = -0.53$, p < 0.05 for percent Black and $\rho = -0.59$, p < 0.05 for IOI(Black)). ICE(race) was not correlated with any of the Black Mortality Advantage rate differences.

Mirroring the previous results from our correlations with summary measures and with Black Mortality Disadvantage outcomes, we saw significant correlations between income inequality and Black Mortality Advantage outcomes. The Gini coefficient was significantly correlated with three of the four rate differences, including Alzheimer's mortality ($\rho = 0.43$, p < 0.05; see figure 6.5). Here San Jose was an outlier, with a relatively low Gini coefficient and a relatively high Black:white gap in Alzheimer's mortality rate. Reflecting the Black Mortality *Advantage*, most cities showed a negative rate difference on the graph (indicating a lower mortality rate for Blacks over whites). However, at higher levels of Gini, we saw that the cities clustered *above* the value of 0 on the Y-axis (a positive rate difference brings us back to the territory of Black Mortality Disadvantage). This is congruent with correlations found between ICE(income) and accidents ($\rho = 0.65$, p < 0.05), CLRD ($\rho = 0.65$, p < 0.05), and suicide ($\rho = 0.46$, p < 0.05). Again, cities with more unequal distributions of income tended to have larger rate differences between Blacks and whites for these causes of death.

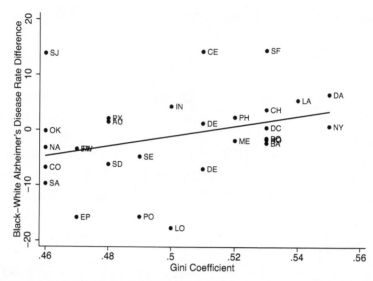

Figure 6.5. Relationship between Income Inequality (Gini Coefficient) and the Black:White Rate Difference in Alzheimer's Disease Mortality (per 100,000). *Note:* $\rho = 0.43$, $p < 0.05$.

Ecological Correlates of the Selected Priority Causes

We now turn our attention to the additional priority causes first explored in chapter 5: homicide, HIV, and opioids. Again, population size was not associated with homicide or HIV-related mortality, but it was associated with opioid-related deaths, whether we examined the total rate, the Black rate, or the white rate. For opioid mortality, larger cities tended to have *lower* mortality rates. However, population size did not explain the Black:white difference in opioid-related mortality ($\rho = 0.17$, not significant; see table 6.5).

Poverty had a strong positive relationship with total homicide mortality ($\rho = 0.59$, $p < 0.05$) but none of the other outcomes. Median household income showed explanatory power with homicide (significantly so with total, Black, and white rates) and the Black:white rate difference for opioid mortality ($\rho = 0.57$, $p < 0.05$), the latter correlation implying that richer cities had larger Black:white differences in opioid-related mortality rates. Percent high school diploma showed relatively little explanatory power and was not associated with racial equity in rates.

Table 6.5. Associations between City Level Socioeconomic Characteristics and Mortality due to Homicide, HIV, and Opioids

	Socioeconomic				Racial Segregation					Income Inequality		
	Population	% Poverty	Median Household Income	% High School Diploma	% NH Black	% NH White	ICE (Race)	IOI (Black)	IOI (White)	Gini	ICE (Income)	Combined ICE (Race +Income)
Homicide												
Total	-0.03	**0.59**	**-0.67**	-0.20	**0.80**	-0.21	**-0.60**	**0.81**	0.02	0.25	**-0.67**	**-0.83**
Black	-0.10	0.35	**-0.47**	-0.09	**0.53**	-0.06	-0.29	**0.60**	0.04	0.28	**-0.45**	**-0.52**
White	-0.19	0.33	**-0.72**	-0.22	0.22	-0.02	-0.09	0.22	0.00	-0.35	**-0.71**	**-0.64**
B:W difference	-0.08	0.29	**-0.37**	-0.03	**0.49**	-0.03	-0.26	**0.56**	0.08	**0.37**	-0.35	**-0.42**
HIV												
Total	0.09	0.34	-0.23	-0.22	**0.56**	**-0.44**	**-0.69**	**0.63**	-0.25	**0.62**	-0.21	**-0.39**
Black	-0.15	-0.26	0.20	0.21	-0.17	0.00	0.11	-0.19	0.00	-0.17	0.22	0.29
White	0.08	-0.11	0.11	0.04	-0.24	-0.09	-0.03	-0.09	-0.05	0.20	0.02	0.14
B:W difference	-0.12	-0.28	0.22	0.22	-0.15	0.02	0.13	-0.19	0.00	-0.17	0.26	0.31
Opioid-Related												
Total	**-0.52**	0.07	-0.18	**0.39**	**0.46**	0.31	0.02	**0.57**	**0.42**	0.04	-0.22	-0.33
Black	**-0.46**	-0.18	0.19	**0.50**	0.19	0.32	0.19	0.26	0.32	0.09	0.18	0.11
White	**-0.48**	0.14	-0.36	0.24	**0.38**	0.28	0.05	**0.44**	0.36	-0.03	-0.35	**-0.39**
B:W difference	0.17	**-0.37**	**0.57**	0.18	**-0.38**	-0.03	0.16	**-0.39**	-0.10	0.06	**0.55**	**0.55**

Notes: Associations described with Spearman rank-order coefficients. Bold numbers indicate p<0.05. NH=Non-Hispanic; ICE=index of concentration at the extremes; IOI=index of isolation; B:W=Black:White.

Looking at the measures of racial segregation, we found very mixed results. For example, percent Black was positively correlated with the Black:white rate difference in homicide mortality ($\rho = 0.49$, p < 0.05) but negatively correlated with the rate difference in opioid-related mortality ($\rho = -0.38$, p < 0.05). IOI(Black) was positively correlated with total rates for homicide, HIV, and opioid-related mortality as well as the Black:white difference in homicide.

Finally, looking at the measures of income inequality, mixed results again emerged. The Gini coefficient was associated with the Black:white difference in homicide mortality ($\rho = 0.37$, p < 0.05) but not with differences with HIV or opioid-related mortality, while ICE(income) was negatively correlated with homicide outcomes (total: $\rho = -0.67$, p < 0.05; Black: $\rho = -0.45$, p < 0.05; white: $\rho = -0.71$, p < 0.05) and, marginally, with the Black:white rate difference (total: $\rho = -0.35$, p = 0.06).

Summing Up: What Have We Learned about Mortality Inequities across US Cities?

Looking across these results, there are several issues worth highlighting:

1. Health inequities, assessed by Black:white mortality rate difference, are not a product of population size. The problem of inequities is not limited to only the largest of our large cities.
2. Poverty—one of the most traditional and important predictors of health at the individual level—is not a particularly powerful correlate of city-level health inequities as defined by Black:white mortality rate differences.
3. There is, however, some evidence that median household income—the second of our traditional socioeconomic measures—is correlated with larger Black:white rate differences.
4. Across these analyses, income inequality is correlated with mortality, but this relationship varies considerably by cause of death and by income inequality measure. The associations were strongest with all-cause mortality, life expectancy, years of life

lost, and some specific causes, including cancer and heart disease. The correlations between income inequality and the other causes of death studied here were small or inconsistent.

5. Across these analyses (and contrary to our initial expectations), racial segregation was generally less correlated with our mortality indicators than income inequality.

A word of caution is warranted on these last two points. We believe that what we are seeing here partly reflects the different geographical levels at which we can measure and analyze data. We have made the case in this book for the value of city-level data. However, we are also cognizant that some processes occur at levels larger than a city (e.g., state and federal health policy) and some issues manifest at levels smaller than a city (e.g., community-level segregation). To explore this in more depth, we turn to our Chicago spotlight, where we have seen the evidence of the correlation among income inequality, residential segregation, and premature mortality firsthand.

City Spotlight: Chicago

Examining the Index of Concentration at the Extremes and Premature Mortality in Chicago's 77 Community Areas

In 2018, a group of researchers (including one of the authors of this chapter, as well as authors from chapter 9) examined economic inequality and racial segregation as predictors of premature mortality among Chicago's 77 officially designated community areas.[16] This followed on the heels of similar studies using data from New York City and Boston.[17,49] In this case, premature mortality was defined as deaths that occurred before age 65. Looking across Chicago's 77 communities, we found a range from 94 premature deaths per 100,000 population to 699 deaths per 100,000 population. These striking differences between community areas are illustrated in figure 6.6.

Looking further into the data, we found that ICE(combined) was strongly associated with premature mortality rates at the community level. Most importantly, when we looked across Chicago communities,

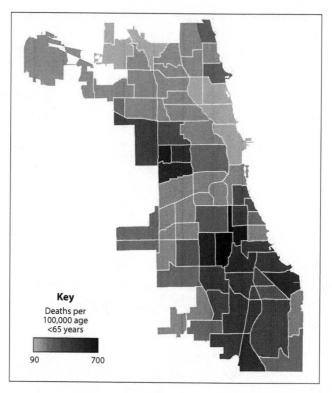

Key

Deaths per
100,000 age
<65 years

90   700

Figure 6.6. Premature Mortality Rates (2011–2015; per 100,000 Population
Age <65 Years) by Chicago Community Area. *Source:* Lange-Maia BS, De Maio F,
Avery EF, et al. Association of Community-Level Inequities and Premature Mortality:
Chicago, 2011–2015. *Journal of Epidemiology and Community Health.*
2018;72(12):1099–1103. Used with permission.

ICE(combined) was more strongly correlated with premature mortality ($\rho=-0.86$, $p<0.01$) than ICE(income) ($\rho=-0.76$, $p<0.01$) or
ICE(race) ($\rho=-0.83$, $p<0.01$) by themselves (see figure 6.7).

These results are important for a few reasons. First, they reaffirm
the importance of examining both *between-* and *within-*city variability.
Without doing so, it is easy to overlook the finer details of how health
is socially patterned in US cities. This echoes recent calls from the Sinai
Urban Health Institute and others for the need for local data.[50,51] Second, our between-city correlations, as well as our Chicago spotlight,
reinforce the idea that some processes occur, and therefore have to be
measured, across large geographic levels, while others require us to

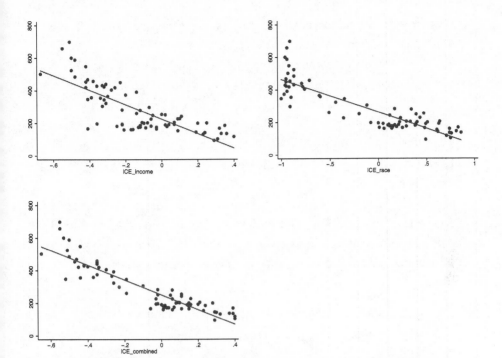

Figure 6.7. Association between the Index of Concentration at the Extremes and Premature Mortality among Chicago's 77 Communities. *Notes:* 2011–2015 data. Premature mortality defined as deaths per 100,000 population age <65 years. *Source:* Lange-Maia BS, De Maio F, Avery EF, et al. Association of Community-Level Inequities and Premature Mortality: Chicago, 2011–2015. *Journal of Epidemiology and Community Health.* 2018;72(12):1099–1103. Used with permission.

zoom in to smaller geographic levels. The concept of income inequality, for example, must be measured at relatively high levels of geography, levels large enough to contain substantial variance. It would be methodologically incorrect, for example, to calculate a Gini coefficient for a very small area like a neighborhood block or, arguably, a Chicago community. In this case, we are pointed toward a city-level unit of analysis, not a community-level definition.

However, while we have reason to believe that income inequality is best measured at the level of a city, we may also have reason to believe that racial segregation is best measured at a more local, community level. Looking at our city-level data, Chicago has an ICE(race) score of 0.03—

very close to the midpoint of the scale, suggesting a balance of white and Black residents. And at that level of geography, if we look at the city overall without acknowledging the internal patterning, we would conclude that Chicago is not a segregated city. However, if we focus in more closely and examine segregation *within* the city of Chicago, the results are very different. In the Chicago spotlight, we saw a previous analysis of community-level data from Chicago where the median ICE(race) value was 0.11—but the range was from −1.0 (a hypersegregated Black community) to 0.86 (a segregated white community).[16] It is only with this variance that we can detect the relationship between segregation and health outcomes. In this way, we need both city-level data to compare across cities and community-level data within cities to fully understand the relationships that make our cities so unequal.

Beyond Sociodemographic Characteristics: The Importance of Local Policies

So far in this chapter we have explored important demographic and socioeconomic characteristics of cities. But, of course, the differences that set cities apart from one another cannot always be reduced to attributes such as levels of educational attainment or income inequality. An important part of what differentiates cities is their approach to public policy. Recall that in chapter 2 all three of our "big picture" models—the BARHII model from the San Francisco Bay Area, the model of the WHO Commission on the Social Determinants of Health, and the more academic model from David Coburn illustrating the political roots of the income inequality hypothesis—incorporated "policy" as a fundamental piece of their causal chains leading to health outcomes.

To ground this idea in data, in this section we explore the importance of city-level policies through an innovative healthy policy scorecard developed by the de Beaumont Foundation and Kaiser Permanente. This scorecard assesses each city's implementation of policies that help their residents lead healthier lives, including evidence-based policies such as inclusionary zoning regulations that boost affordable housing stock, stringent anti-tobacco policies, and universal access to

Table 6.6. Health Policy Awards by City

City	Overall	Affordable Housing	Alcohol Sales Control	Complete Streets	Earned Sick Leave	Food Safety	Healthy Food Procurement	Universal Pre-K	Smoke-Free Indoor Air	Tobacco 21
Austin, TX	Bronze			Gold	Gold			Bronze	Silver	
Baltimore, MD	Bronze	Bronze		Gold	Bronze		Bronze	Bronze	Silver	Gold
Boston, MA	Gold	Silver	Gold	Silver	Bronze	Gold	Gold	Gold	Silver	
Charlotte, NC	Bronze			Silver		Gold		Gold	Silver	
Chicago, IL	Gold	Gold	Gold	Gold	Silver		Silver	Silver	Gold	Gold
Columbus, OH				Gold		Gold			Gold	Gold
Dallas, TX				Gold				Bronze	Gold	
Denver, CO	Bronze	Bronze	Gold	Silver				Bronze	Gold	
Detroit, MI				Gold				Silver	Gold	
El Paso, TX								Bronze	Silver	
Fort Worth, TX				Gold				Bronze	Silver	
Houston, TX	Bronze			Gold			Bronze	Bronze	Gold	
Indianapolis, IN				Gold					Bronze	
Jacksonville, FL				Silver				Bronze		
Los Angeles, CA	Gold	Gold		Gold	Gold	Gold	Gold	Bronze	Silver	Gold
Louisville, KY	Bronze		Silver			Gold	Silver	Silver	Gold	
Memphis, TN		Silver	Gold					Bronze		
Nashville, TN		Silver						Gold		
New York, NY	Gold	Gold		Gold	Silver	Gold	Gold	Gold	Gold	Gold
Oklahoma City, OK								Bronze	Bronze	
Philadelphia, PA	Silver			Gold	Silver		Gold	Silver	Silver	
Phoenix, AZ		Bronze		Gold	Bronze				Gold	
Portland, OR	Bronze				Bronze	Silver			Gold	
San Antonio, TX	Silver	Silver	Silver	Silver	Gold	Silver		Gold	Gold	Gold
San Diego, CA	Silver	Silver	Silver	Gold	Silver	Gold	Gold	Bronze	Silver	Gold
San Francisco, CA	Silver	Bronze	Silver	Gold	Bronze	Silver	Gold	Bronze	Gold	Gold
San Jose, CA	Gold	Silver		Bronze	Silver	Gold	Bronze	Silver	Gold	Gold
Seattle, WA	Silver	Silver				Gold		Silver	Gold	Gold
Washington, DC	Silver	Silver	Gold	Gold	Bronze	Gold	Gold	Bronze	Bronze	Gold

Note: Adapted from www.cityhealth.org.

prekindergarten. The scorecard gives cities a medal (gold, silver, bronze, or no award) based on their implementation of the specific policies (see table 6.6).

Across our sample, five cities were awarded gold medals (New York, Los Angeles, Chicago, and San Jose), six were awarded silver (Philadelphia, San Antonio, San Diego, San Francisco, Seattle, and Washington), and seven were awarded bronze (Houston, Austin, Charlotte, Denver, Baltimore, Portland, and Louisville) in 2017. The remaining cities did not receive any medal, indicating that they lagged behind the others in proposing, implementing, or evaluating these needed policies.

Is there a link between different award levels and mortality profiles? Do the cities with more progressive policy portfolios have better mortality rates or smaller health inequities? To explore this, we conducted a simple descriptive analysis (see figure 6.8).

It is clear that the policy awards have some relationship to overall levels of health. Figure 6.8 shows a boxplot of all-cause mortality by policy award level. The line in the middle of the box represents the me-

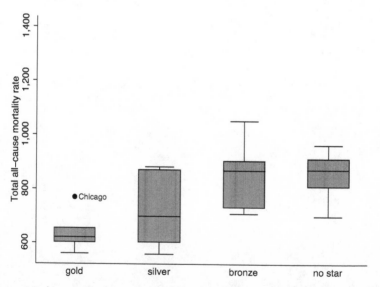

Figure 6.8. Association between Health Policy Award Level and Total All-Cause Mortality Rate.

dian value for that group, and the bottom and top limits of the box represent the 25th and 75th percentiles, respectively. Outliers, cities that are unlike the rest of their group, are isolated and labeled. Overall, the "gold" cities have lower all-cause mortality rates than do "silver" cities, and they are, overall, lower than "bronze" cities and cities with no award. Our home city of Chicago is an outlier in the "gold" group, with higher all-cause mortality rates than the rest. Yet if we look at Black:white mortality rates separately, a different pattern emerges—one that reminds us of the critical challenges that remain, even in "gold" cities. In figure 6.9, we examine Black and white all-cause mortality rates separately. The pattern is clear: there are mortality inequalities at every level of policy ranking, even among the cities that were awarded gold medals for having the best health-related policies.

Conclusion

In this chapter, we have grappled with a huge amount of data to explore a relatively simple objective: to understand, in broad terms, which city-

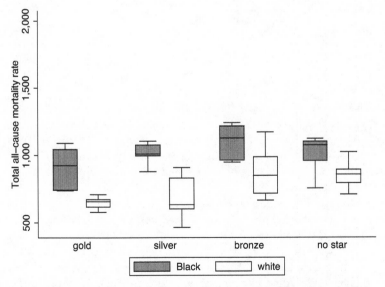

Figure 6.9. Association between Health Policy Award Level and Total All-Cause Black and White Mortality Rates.

level attributes may help us understand variation in a city's mortality profile. We looked at total rates, Black- and white-specific rates, and the inequities in mortality as measured by rate differences across a city. We knew that no single, easy answer was likely to emerge. The roots of health inequities in the United States are simply too complex and multifaceted to be attributed to any one variable.

Understanding mortality patterns and inequities across the United States requires us to move beyond easy narratives that point the finger at poverty in isolation from other issues. We have seen here that city-level poverty is a remarkably weak correlate of mortality rates. Yet median household income does show some associations with racial inequities in rates. We saw, for example, that richer cities have *larger* Black:white inequities in all-cause mortality. And we saw that cities with higher levels of income inequality have larger Black:white inequities in all-cause mortality, life expectancy, and years of life lost. These are results that should alarm us all. They are indicative of an economic system that prizes economic growth above all, even above the health of our neighbors.

Part IV of this book will focus on the potential for change, motivated by a social justice framework (chapter 7), and evidenced by the work of the Sinai Urban Health Institute (chapter 8) and West Side United (chapter 9).

References

1. Bay Area Regional Health Inequities Initiative. *Applying Social Determinants of Health Indicators to Advance Health Equity: A Guide for Local Health Department Epidemiologists and Public Health Professionals.* Oakland, CA; 2015.

2. World Health Organization. *Closing the Gap in a Generation: Health Equity through Action on the Social Determinants of Health.* Geneva: World Health Organization; 2008.

3. Coburn D. Beyond the Income Inequality Hypothesis: Class, Neo-liberalism, and Health Inequalities. *Social Science and Medicine.* 2004;58(1):41–56.

4. Coburn D. Income Inequality, Welfare, Class and Health: A Comment on Pickett and Wilkinson, 2015. *Social Science and Medicine.* 2015;146:228–232.

5. Williams DR, Lawrence JA, Davis BA, Vu C. Understanding How Discrimination Can Affect Health. *Health Services Research.* 2019;54(Suppl 2): 1374–1388.

6. Marmot M. *The Health Gap*. New York: Bloomsbury; 2015.

7. Wilkinson RG, Pickett K. *The Inner Level*. London: Penguin; 2018.

8. De Maio F. Advancing the Income Inequality Hypothesis. *Critical Public Health*. 2012;22(1):39–46.

9. Bailey ZD, Krieger N, Agenor M, Graves J, Linos N, Bassett MT. Structural Racism and Health Inequities in the USA: Evidence and Interventions. *Lancet*. 2017;389(10077):1453–1463.

10. Jones CP. Levels of Racism: A Theoretic Framework and a Gardener's Tale. *American Journal of Public Health*. 2000;90(8):1212–1215.

11. Krieger N. Living and Dying at the Crossroads: Racism, Embodiment, and Why Theory Is Essential for a Public Health of Consequence. *American Journal of Public Health*. 2016;106(5):832–833.

12. Williams DR, Lawrence JA, Davis BA. Racism and Health: Evidence and Needed Research. *Annual Review of Public Health*. 2019;40:105–125.

13. Benjamins MR, Hirschtick JL, Hunt BR, Hughes MM, Hunter B. Racial Disparities in Heart Disease Mortality in the 50 Largest U.S. Cities. *Journal of Racial and Ethnic Health Disparities*. 2016.

14. Benjamins MR, Hunt BR, Raleigh SM, Hirschtick JL, Hughes MM. Racial Disparities in Prostate Cancer Mortality in the 50 Largest US Cities. *Cancer Epidemiology*. 2016;44:125–131.

15. Ross NA, Wolfson MC, Dunn JR, Berthelot JM, Kaplan GA, Lynch JW. Relation between Income Inequality and Mortality in Canada and in the United States: Cross Sectional Assessment Using Census Data and Vital Statistics. *British Medical Journal*. 2000;320(7239):898–902.

16. Lange-Maia BS, De Maio F, Avery EF, et al. Association of Community-Level Inequities and Premature Mortality: Chicago, 2011–2015. *Journal of Epidemiology and Community Health*. 2018;72(12):1099–1103.

17. Krieger N, Waterman PD, Spasojevic J, Li W, Maduro G, Van Wye G. Public Health Monitoring of Privilege and Deprivation with the Index of Concentration at the Extremes. *American Journal of Public Health*. 2016;106(2):256–263.

18. Massey DS. The Age of Extremes: Concentrated Affluence and Poverty in the Twenty-First Century. *Demography*. 1996;33(4):395–412.

19. Abraham L. *Mama Might Be Better Off Dead*. Chicago: University of Chicago Press; 1993.

20. Wilkinson RG, Pickett KE. Income Inequality and Socioeconomic Gradients in Mortality. *American Journal of Public Health*. 2008;98(4):699–704.

21. De Maio F. *Health and Social Theory*. Basingstoke: Palgrave Macmillan; 2010.

22. Jones C. The Impact of Racism on Health. *Ethnicity and Disease*. 2002;12(1):S2-10-13.

23. Jones CP. Toward the Science and Practice of Anti-racism: Launching a National Campaign against Racism. *Ethnicity and Disease*. 2018;28(Suppl 1):231–234.

24. Krieger N. *Epidemiology and the People's Health: Theory and Context.* Oxford: Oxford University Press; 2011.

25. Krieger N, Chen JT, Coull B, Waterman PD, Beckfield J. The Unique Impact of Abolition of Jim Crow Laws on Reducing Inequities in Infant Death Rates and Implications for Choice of Comparison Groups in Analyzing Societal Determinants of Health. *American Journal of Public Health.* 2013;103(12):2234–2244.

26. Pallok K, De Maio F, Ansell DA. Structural Racism—a 60-Year-Old Black Woman with Breast Cancer. *New England Journal of Medicine.* 2019;380(16):1489–1493.

27. Geronimus AT. To Mitigate, Resist, or Undo: Addressing Structural Influences on the Health of Urban Populations. *American Journal of Public Health.* 2000;90(6):867–872.

28. Hunt BR, Whitman S, Hurlbert MS. Increasing Black:White Disparities in Breast Cancer Mortality in the 50 Largest Cities in the United States. *Cancer Epidemiology.* 2014;38(2):118–123.

29. Hunt BR, Silva A, Lock D, Hurlbert M. Predictors of Breast Cancer Mortality among White and Black Women in Large United States Cities: An Ecologic Study. *Cancer Causes and Control.* 2019;30(2):149–164.

30. Rosenstock S, Whitman S, West JF, Balkin M. Racial Disparities in Diabetes Mortality in the 50 Most Populous US Cities. *Journal of Urban Health.* 2014;91(5):873–885.

31. Massey DS, Denton NA. *American Apartheid: Segregation and the Making of the Underclass.* Cambridge, MA: Harvard University Press; 1998.

32. Farley JE. Residential Interracial Exposure and Isolation Indices. *Sociological Quarterly.* 2005;46(1):19–45.

33. Chambers BD, Baer RJ, McLemore MR, Jelliffe-Pawlowski LL. Using Index of Concentration at the Extremes as Indicators of Structural Racism to Evaluate the Association with Preterm Birth and Infant Mortality—California, 2011–2012. *Journal of Urban Health.* 2019;96(2):159–170.

34. Hunt B, Balachandran B. Black:White Disparities in Lung Cancer Mortality in the 50 Largest Cities in the United States. *Cancer Epidemiology.* 2015;39(6):908–916.

35. De Maio FG. Income Inequality Measures. *Journal of Epidemiology and Community Health.* 2007;61(10):849–852.

36. Gillis M, Perkins DH, Roemer M, Snodgrass DR. *Economics of Development.* New York: Norton; 1996.

37. Atkinson AB. *The Economics of Inequality.* Oxford: Claredon; 1975.

38. Champernowne DG, Cowell FA. *Economic Inequality and Income Distribution.* Cambridge: Cambridge University Press; 1998.

39. Campano F, Salvatore D. *Income Distribution.* Oxford: Oxford University Press; 2006.

40. Robinson WS. Ecological Correlations and the Behavior of Individuals. *American Sociological Review.* 1950;15(3):351–357.

41. Subramanian SV, Jones K, Kaddour A, Krieger N. Revisiting Robinson: The Perils of Individualistic and Ecologic Fallacy. *International Journal of Epidemiology.* 2009;38(2):342–360; author reply 370–343.

42. Pearce N. The Ecological Fallacy Strikes Back. *Journal of Epidemiology and Community Health.* 2000;54(5):326–327.

43. Ansell D. *The Death Gap: How Inequality Kills.* Chicago: University of Chicago Press; 2017.

44. Krieger N, Waterman PD, Batra N, Murphy JS, Dooley DP, Shah SN. Measures of Local Segregation for Monitoring Health Inequities by Local Health Departments. *American Journal of Public Health.* 2017;107(6):903–906.

45. Landrine H, Corral I. Separate and Unequal: Residential Segregation and Black Health Disparities. *Ethnicity and Disease.* 2009;19(2):179–184.

46. Lobmayer P, Wilkinson RG. Inequality, Residential Segregation by Income, and Mortality in US Cities. *Journal of Epidemiology and Community Health.* 2002;56(3):183–187.

47. Mehra R, Boyd LM, Ickovics JR. Racial Residential Segregation and Adverse Birth Outcomes: A Systematic Review and Meta-analysis. *Social Science and Medicine.* 2017;191:237–250.

48. Williams DR, Collins C. Racial Residential Segregation: A Fundamental Cause of Racial Disparities in Health. *Public Health Reports.* 2001;116(5): 404–416.

49. Feldman JM, Waterman PD, Coull BA, Krieger N. Spatial Social Polarisation: Using the Index of Concentration at the Extremes Jointly for Income and Race/Ethnicity to Analyse Risk of Hypertension. *Journal of Epidemiology and Community Health.* 2015;69(12):1199–1207.

50. Whitman S, Shah AM, Benjamins MR, eds. *Urban Health: Combating Disparities with Local Data.* New York: Oxford University Press; 2011.

51. DeSalvo KB, Wang YC, Harris A, Auerbach J, Koo D, O'Carroll P. Public Health 3.0: A Call to Action for Public Health to Meet the Challenges of the 21st Century. *Preventing Chronic Disease.* 2017;14:E78.

PART IV TRANSLATING DATA INTO ACTION: PRACTICAL APPROACHES TO HEALTH EQUITY

We have to regard this problem as if it was a problem in our family, and we have to fight like hell to change it.

—Steve Whitman, PhD
Quoted in "An Ethical Indictment
on Disparities," *Science Life*, 2010

In earlier parts of this book, we documented inequities and attempted to understand the patterns of extensive variation in health outcomes across the largest US cities. We recognize that these are necessary, but not sufficient, steps for achieving health equity. To continue moving forward, cities need to engage community members and other stakeholders to help interpret the findings, make the complicated data accessible, and disseminate it widely. To increase the effectiveness of potential new initiatives or policy changes, the information must be combined with relevant evidence-informed best practices and community input on priorities and existing resources. In this final part of the book, we offer a framework for addressing health inequities and provide two case studies that offer concrete examples of how local-level data on health inequities were disseminated and used to drive community action.

In chapter 7, "Using a Social Justice Framework to Help Achieve Health Equity," we describe a social-justice-oriented approach to mobilizing community health improvement. In order to create sustainable pathways to health equity, Silva, Rozier, and Homan contend that initiatives should be based on shared values and cultures of community members, conducted in partnership with communities, and include a focus on structural changes. More specifically, the authors suggest an iterative approach involving six distinct but interrelated steps in which we (1) learn about a community's lived experiences, (2) engage with the community, (3) understand the context and circumstances that allow inequities to occur, (4) reflect on what we have learned, (5) collectively choose a set of actions aimed at transforming the community, and (6) evaluate whether those actions improved health and ameliorated inequities. The process must also include an evaluation of the efforts and be done using a health equity lens.

In chapter 8, "Data Are Not Enough: Moving toward Solutions-Focused Communication," Monnard and colleagues discuss considerations related to the framing and dissemination of health (and health equity) information to all relevant stakeholders. They highlight the need for authentic engagement with community members to guide dissemination, as well as to accurately identify priorities, potential partners, and existing resources before developing new policies or programs. Monnard et al. review multiple strategies for collaborating with community members, creating accessible data products, and disseminating information to multiple audiences. A real-world example demonstrates how findings from a local health survey were translated into actionable information, shared broadly, and used to motivate and support a variety of initiatives designed to improve health equity in Chicago.

In chapter 9, "Mobilizing to Action: Overcoming Chicago's 14-Year Life Expectancy Gap," Roesch et al. explore how data can be balanced with evidence-based best practices, community priorities, and existing assets to improve health equity in large urban areas. The authors introduce West Side United, a large, multisector initiative that was developed to address the racial gap in life expectancy seen across Chicago communities. They provide specific information on how this group visualized health inequities, structured the collaboration, and gained support from institutional, community, and philanthropic partners, mobilizing collective action with the objective of making Chicago a more equal city.

Together, these three chapters support cities in the quest for improving urban health and health equity through community-engaged approaches.

SEVEN

Using a Social Justice Framework to Help Achieve Health Equity

ABIGAIL SILVA, MICHAEL ROZIER, AND SHARON HOMAN

I**N THIS PART OF THE BOOK**, we use case studies to highlight how data are being used to mobilize collective efforts for health equity in Chicago. As the following chapters will show, these initiatives acknowledge, as has long been recognized, that community engagement is a critical and effective strategy for harnessing community potential, including health improvement.[1,2] Although there are practical frameworks that outline the steps needed for effectively engaging with community partners,[3] an overarching framework is also necessary to convey the purpose and direction of the proposed efforts.

Social justice is achieved when resources and opportunities are equitably distributed to *all* persons. Therefore, we cannot achieve health equity without social justice.[4] In this chapter, we describe a social justice framework that can be used to undergird health equity initiatives. We argue that any path to health equity should (1) involve *structural change* through the creation of a dynamic, transformative *partnership with the community*; (2) reflect *shared values* and cultures of community members; and (3) have a goal of *reducing, if not eliminating, inequities* in health and the adverse determinants. To achieve this, we propose using a praxis approach, that is, a process involving critical thinking, reflection, and committed action.[5] Each step is done by the community, for the community, and with the community. In doing so, the plan that is collectively created to improve community health and attain health equity is embraced by the community with conviction.

Toward Structural Change: Using Social Analysis to Drive a Social-Justice-Oriented Praxis

As pointed out in chapter 2, public health researchers have often examined the role of individual-level, downstream factors that may be contributing to poor health and health inequities. However, after decades of research, there is a widespread consensus among public health practitioners and researchers that social determinants, upstream structural factors, play a considerable role in the health of individuals and communities.[6,7] These structural factors, including racism, help produce, maintain, and in some cases exacerbate health inequities.[8-10] We cannot improve community health and eliminate inequities without addressing the social determinants of health. Therefore, in addition to a traditional epidemiologic study, it is critical to also conduct a social analysis in the context of a praxis framework. A social analysis is a systematic assessment of the cultural, political, economic, and social factors that promote or sustain a social problem.[11] Social analysis leads to critical consciousness, which is essential for prompting transformative social change.

The social-justice-oriented praxis approach begins by obtaining insight into the *experiences* of living with poor health, community disinvestment, and health inequities as a result of injustices. Although the "praxis" originally emerged from both Christian liberation theology and Marxist political commitments, we do not consider it a method that implies or requires any set of religious or political values, such as sin, oppression, or repression.[11,12] Instead, we are using praxis as a tool for locating the work of community-driven health initiatives in the geography of the lived experiences of individuals and communities and for valuing participative processes, sustainable partnerships organized around a shared definition of the common good.[11] This praxis framework incorporates the best-practice *Principles of Community Engage-*

ment, which are grounded in the social justice principles of fairness, justice, empowerment, participation, and self-determination.[3] We emphasize the value of putting into the hands of community members and collaborators (1) place-based data and community-tailored analyses of health inequities and the structural and social determinant roots, particularly through accessible formats such as infographics and dashboards; (2) information about evidence-informed programs and policies to consider; and (3) tools of program planning and evaluation to strengthen learning, outcomes, and sustainability. Further shaped by the hands in which they are placed, these resources help mobilize communities toward more effective collective action. Additionally, as stated earlier, the community action must involve *structural change* if we want every community member to have a fair and just opportunity to be as healthy as possible.[10]

A focus on structural change is critical to advancing health equity. In chapter 2, De Maio and Benjamins thoughtfully describe the theoretical approaches that help us understand the causes of health inequities. They point out that the emerging consensus from decades of research points toward social and structural determinants as the root causes of health inequities. More specifically, they highlight the detrimental effect of structural racism. Structural racism refers to "the totality of ways in which societies foster [racial] discrimination, via mutually reinforcing [inequitable] systems . . . (e.g., in housing, education, employment, earnings, benefits, credit, media, health care, criminal justice, etc.) that in turn reinforce discriminatory beliefs, values, and distribution of resources, [reflected in history, culture, and interconnected institutions]" (p. 650).[13] For instance, residential and educational segregation of Black Americans reduces their economic and social opportunities, which in turn adversely impacts health.[14,15]

The structural change needed requires that we admit that any structures in need of change likely came into being through the exertion of power, often of one group over others.[13,15] These structures likely persist through the active maintenance of a power differential and/or the passive acceptance that nothing can dislodge what has been. Because the structures themselves are wed to the economic, political, or social powers that initiated them, it is impossible to imagine them changing without also changing the power differentials that uphold them. This means, as we explain later in the praxis framework, that transformation requires that we go beyond public health interventions to addressing the underlying dynamics of power, voice, and representation. We must consider not just what we do but who we are. It speaks to our moral character. This relationship between doing and being relies on insight from virtue ethics, which asks us not just to evaluate rightness or wrongness of actions or outcomes but also to think of how we cultivate the right dispositions and intentions.[16,17] This encourages a *stance of commitment*, which deepens over time as doing and being reinforce one another. It is this dispositional change that makes sustained transformation possible.

From Entrenched Health Inequities to Health Equity: A Pursuit of Hope and Shared Praxis

Braveman describes the pursuit of health equity as "striving for the highest possible standard of health for all people and giving special attention to the needs of those at greatest risk of poor health, based on social conditions" (p. 6).[18,19] In part I, Benjamins and De Maio impress on us the level of entrenched racial inequities in US cities by exploring the historical and structural relationships of health inequities to our economic, political, social, and cultural institutions. Part II features data on the significant Black:white gaps in mortality, life expectancy, and premature mortality present across our largest US cities. Overcoming those inequities requires a concerted effort, in partnership with Black communities, to fix policies and systems that have created and maintained racial inequalities over time.

Cognitively, civic leaders, public health researchers, and practitioners can process these statistics that illustrate the magnitude of the entrenched, persistent racial inequities of mortality. Our individual and collective understandings of health inequities can mobilize action and inform our pathways to reducing them. For instance, the significant racial inequities observed in breast cancer and infant mortality motivated specific efforts, like the breast cancer navigation programs and Back-to-Sleep campaigns, respectively.[20,21] Furthermore, data show that racial inequities in health vary by place and time,[22-24] thus illustrating that the patterns are not universal or static and as such are amendable to change. Indeed, it is not difficult to find examples of how community-wide mobilization efforts have successfully tackled health inequities.[25-27] However, in order to obtain and sustain community-engaged action, an expression of hope is necessary. Hope is a catalyst to action, and thus keeping hope alive is part and parcel of the action step of praxis.[28] Hope emphasizes the element of *transformation* that can only arise out of social solidarity and a shared struggle for social justice, a shared commitment to the necessary social and political reform.[28]

Reshaping the future in our urban neighborhoods and cities must be about the reconstruction of hope in solidarity and partnership. Chapter 5 illustrated the staggering racial inequities in homicide mortality. In Chicago, the Black rate is more than 25 times higher than the white rate. Gun violence helps drive this inequity. In response, the Chicago Gun Violence Research Collaborative was launched to bring local hospitals, universities, and researchers together to have an impact on gun violence using a community-driven approach. The collaborative participated in listening sessions with community members on the West and South Sides of Chicago. The purpose was to gain insight into the community's lived experiences and listen to their ideas for reducing gun violence and the associated homicides and suicides among young people. The community members prioritized getting school youth engaged and teaching them about community activism. They felt that such experiences would give them a sense of hope, purpose, and even confidence that they can succeed in college.[29]

Socially just action requires attention to the needs of individuals while working for the common good, that is, "that which contributes to the unity of society and to the needs of that unified whole" (p. 105).[30] The common good is a good to which all members of society (e.g., all youth in our neighborhood) have access (e.g., safe, well-equipped park space without exposure to guns or drugs), and no one is excluded from enjoyment of that good. Working toward the common good of health equity can be accomplished through a shared commitment to practical action that responds to the lived experience of disadvantage, an understanding of the social determinants (and deeper structural roots) of health inequities, and a shared commitment to social change of structures that further disadvantage socially disadvantaged groups. This is what we mean by social-justice-oriented praxis.

Using a Social-Justice-Oriented Praxis Framework: Working Together for Health Equity

In the introduction to this chapter, we state that any path to health equity requires effort toward structural change in a transformative partnership with communities that reflects shared values. The "Circle of Praxis" can guide us on how to achieve our shared goal; it is an iterative process of decision and action that can be used to mobilize a place (e.g., West Side of Chicago) toward structural change for social justice. This structural change is essential for tackling health inequities, transforming policy making and social systems that perpetuate inequity, and significantly improving quality of life and life expectancy.

Praxis, as developed by Brazilian educator and philosopher Paulo Freire in his classic text *Pedagogy of the Oppressed*, is a hermeneutic, or interpretive, method that sees new questions of justice continually raised by new situations.[31] Each iteration of the praxis circle breaks new ground and moves people forward toward a vision of the common good. It helps identify our *shared values*.

Oppression can render persons passive in the world. It can leave us accepting and taking for granted gross inequities in mortality. Praxis calls us to take a more active and substantive role in matters of social justice, by developing critical consciousness in the world in which we live. One way that we can ignite this consciousness is by documenting the extent to which mortality experiences of Americans vary by race and place as we did in part II of this book. These data can empower cities (and other public health stakeholders) and activate communities to more strategically pursue specific policy and programmatic changes to improve health equity. Praxis informs and mobilizes work for the common good.

Praxis begins with the lived experience of community members. Praxis emphasizes taking a systemic view of any situation, probing root causes of injustices, thinking critically, and using dialogue and reflection as tools to move toward evidence-informed action. Praxis is an iterative process that involves experience, stance of commitment, social analysis, reflection, action, and evaluation (figure 7.1).

Experience

First, we must seek to "see more widely," that is, start with a deep desire to see and understand the *lived experience and knowledge of community members*. For example, in seeking to establish program and research priorities to address homicide inequities in the predominantly Black communities on the West and South Sides, the Chicago Gun

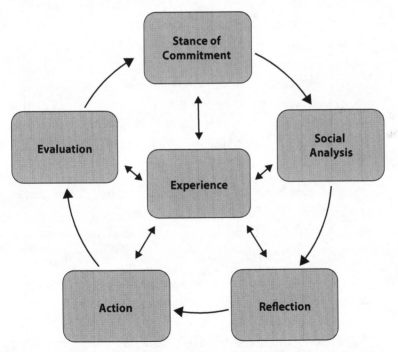

Figure 7.1. "Circle of Praxis": A Six-Step Social-Justice-Oriented Approach to Collectively Improving Community Health. *Note:* Informed by the work of Holland and Henriot, *Social Analysis: Linking Faith and Justice* (1983).

Violence Research Collaborative first conducted listening sessions and interviews with approximately 140 community members.[29] When we asked them to identify the root causes of gun violence, they shared some of the following:

- Concentration of severe economic hardship and unemployment in communities of color: "The majority of young males are unemployed. They don't have anywhere to go, and education isn't an option, so they develop hopelessness. This is concentrated in brown and black communities."
- Housing inequities, including high rates of homelessness, redlining, segregation, gentrification, public housing relocation, taxation policies, and high costs of living: "Redlining and segregation are root causes. There were a lot of racist and discriminatory practices by the housing market that had a huge impact on the community."
- Long-term disinvestment in schools located in Latino and African American communities: "You don't get what you need in school. You get an education, but you know it wasn't as good as other people's. You get less, and you know it."
- Pervasiveness of intergenerational trauma and violence: "In this community, there are just two main gangs. There has been a huge rivalry between those two gangs for decades. This hatred gets passed down generation to generation and you don't really know the other people."

Community members were also encouraged to provide the team with recommendations for future research studies and to refine our community-driven research model.[29] They provided suggestions, including the following:

- Commit to addressing the structural causes of violence: "You need to create whole communities with good schools and opportunities for community residents."
- Work collaboratively and collectively with those on the ground in communities: "My role is boots on the ground. I'm already in the community. I can find out what you want to know."

- Use community-driven and community-owned cross-sectoral approaches: "Need to look at a village approach. Bring law enforcement, churches, different programs, businesses together. Need to bring together all the smaller efforts to have a greater impact—a collective/collaborative effect."

It is critical that, with each of the subsequent steps, we stay grounded in the experience of the community.

Stance of Commitment

Engaging with community members and entities and learning about their experiences requires that we immerse ourselves in the community from a *stance of commitment to a common purpose*. This stance includes what we do, who we are, and our disposition toward each other and our communities. This leads to personal connectedness to people as neighbors and kindles a desire to see "more widely" and probe root causes to social problems. This achieves a level of connectedness through active back-and-forth communication that demonstrates open appreciation, a sense of inquisitiveness, and an acknowledgment of the struggle. Over time, engagement inspires yet other virtues, such as hope and collective self-determination.[32,33] The *Principles of Community Engagement* provide guidance for how we can insert ourselves into the lived community experience, grow trust, and increase the potential to collectively work toward health equity and achieve measurable results (box 7.1). Through stance of commitment, we help direct the process of change toward dynamic transformation in partnership with the community.

Social Analysis

The "Circle of Praxis" entails examining the determinants and root causes of the situation, including the structural barriers. Because we immerse ourselves into the community and their experiences, we can then use social analysis to systematically examine the present situation. This type of exploration gives us a wider lens and a deeper understanding.

Box 7.1. PRINCIPLES OF COMMUNITY ENGAGEMENT

Before Starting a Community Engagement Effort

1. Be *clear about the purposes* or goals of the engagement effort and the populations and/or communities you want to engage.
2. Become *knowledgeable about the community's* culture, economic conditions, social networks, political and power structures, norms and values, demographic trends, history, and experience with efforts by outside groups to engage it in various programs. Learn about the community's perceptions of those initiating the engagement activities.

For Engagement to Occur, It Is Necessary to:

3. Go to the community, *establish relationships, build trust,* work with the formal and informal leadership, and seek commitment from community organizations and leaders to create processes for mobilizing the community.
4. Remember and accept that *collective self-determination* is the responsibility and right of all people in a community. No external entity should assume that it can bestow on a community the power to act in its own self-interest.

For Engagement to Succeed:

5. *Partnering with the community* is necessary to create change and improve health.
6. All aspects of community engagement must *recognize and respect the diversity of the community.* Awareness of the various cultures of a community and other factors affecting diversity must be paramount in planning, designing, and implementing approaches to engaging a community.
7. Community engagement can only be sustained by identifying and *mobilizing community assets and strengths and by developing the community's capacity and resources* to make decisions and take action.
8. Organizations that wish to engage a community, as well as individuals seeking to effect change, must be prepared to *release control of actions or interventions to the community* and be flexible enough to meet its changing needs.

Source: Butterfoss, F., and Kegler, M. 2002. Toward a comprehensive understanding of community coalitions: Moving from practice to theory. In *Emerging Theories in Health Promotion Practice and Research,* ed. R. DiClemente, R. Crosby, and M. Kegler 157–93. San Francisco: Jossey-Bass.

We are able to ask questions such as the following: What is the *history* of this situation (e.g., gang activity, youth violence)? What are the major *structures* that influence this situation (e.g., lack of economic investment)? What key *values* are operative in these structures? What is the future direction of this situation? Can we overcome structural impediments of bureaucracy, lack of empowerment, and other barriers to constructive action?

Social analysis is not something done on a community, but an iterative exercise done by, for, and with a community. In a praxis approach, social analysis is about creating a knowledge ecology, to move beyond simply using a knowledge management strategy. Knowledge management is about converting data to usable information and then to actionable knowledge in order to mobilize strategic action. Taking the next step, cocreating a knowledge ecology engages and mobilizes community partners, puts the data and knowledge tools in the hands of community members and partners, and integrates the qualitative analyses of the social, political, and historical roots with the epidemiologic analyses of health, social, and economic inequities (as exemplified in the case study in chapter 9).

A social analysis is needed to generate an understanding of the diverse contexts in which health inequities take place and obtain insight into the ways in which needs and priorities are identified and addressed. As an example, in chapter 9 Roesch et al. present the sociocultural, economic, and political factors that have contributed to the unacceptably low life expectancy of community members on the West Side of Chicago. However, they also point out the assets found in the community, including its strong past and present history of activism and resilience. Other valuable resources that could be leveraged to help effect change include health care and public health institutions, community organizations, and agencies that support housing, commercial, and economic development. A social analysis can help us to begin creating a dynamic transformation in partnership with communities, one that reflects shared values and cultures of community members. This is an imperative if we are to create structural changes that reduce, if not eliminate, inequities in health and their adverse determinants.

Reflection

This part of the cycle requires us to engage in reflective practice, to develop, as Schön describes, the ability to reflect on one's actions, thus enabling us to engage in continuous learning.[34] Thus, via reflective practice, we cultivate the sharing of knowledge and deeper learning of each iteration of praxis, and we intentionally aim to build a knowledge ecology by, for, and with the community partnership and community at large. As such, critical reflection entails thoughtfully seeking to understand the situation and choose a course of action by using professional and personal skills and by evaluating evidence using theories of justice, moral reasoning, ethical principles, and empirical data.

For example, in part II of this book the authors highlight the racial differences in life expectancy at birth, with Black Americans expected to live shorter lives and be more likely to die from heart disease, cancer, stroke, diabetes, and kidney disease. Even starker are the unequal burdens of HIV and homicide on Black Americans. And while opioid mortality rates are taking a huge toll on all Americans, in our nation's capital the Black rate of opioid mortality is 438% higher than the white rate. The burdens of HIV, opioids, homicides, and early deaths from chronic health problems concentrate within our Black neighborhoods and community areas that are economically and socially challenged.[35-38] In the United States, racism has become embedded as a structural phenomenon incorporating the whole social system, that is, the economic, political and cultural life of communities, cities, states, and our nation.[13] Surely we cannot tackle the health burdens of these race inequities without a social justice lens and analyses.[9,10]

Over 20 years ago, Professors Daniels, Kennedy, and Kawachi argued for the need for an account of justice that would help us answer these questions: "When is an inequality in health status between different socioeconomic groups unjust? . . . Is every health inequality that results from unequally distributed social goods unjust?" (p. 216).[39] The questions they raise are the ingredients for engaging professionals and community partners in thoughtful reflection:[39] If there is an irreducible health gradient across socioeconomic groups, does that make the very existence of those inequalities unjust? Alternatively, are some health inequalities the result of acceptable trade-offs? Perhaps they are simply an unfortunate by-product of inequalities that work in other ways to help worse-off groups. For example, it is often claimed that permitting economic inequality provides incentives to work harder, thereby stimulating growth that will ultimately benefit the poorest groups. To whom must these trade-offs be acceptable if we are to consider them just? Are they acceptable only if they are part of a strategy aimed at moving the situation toward a more just arrangement? Does it matter in our judgments about justice exactly how social determinants produce inequities in health status?

Action

Taking action is the step of the praxis cycle with which people are most comfortable, although it often occurs absent the other steps previously outlined. It is important to recognize that taking action without the preceding steps of experience, stance of commitment, analysis, and reflection reduces the likelihood that the changes we seek can be sustained. Without the preceding steps, those who suffer, such as Black Americans across our 30 largest cities, are the objects of rather than the agents of change. In this model, action must be broad-based and leadership must be shared.

The praxis model provides another way of conceptualizing evidence-based work. It takes the core concepts of evidence-based public health and requires the most robust interpretation possible.[40] The "best peer-reviewed evidence," for example, is not limited to intervention data but includes evidence on history, sociology, communications, and more. "Engaging the community in decision-making" means going beyond standard community forums or stakeholder roundtables and actually ensuring that the community has meaningful power over the process. For example, in the first round of the Sinai Community Health Survey (discussed in chapter 8), the Sinai Urban Health Institute created a community advisory committee and gave them broad authority, including the power to include or exclude any survey questions. In the 2002 survey, the committee vetoed questions on social capital and drug use owing to concerns about the potential value and use of the data.[41] And "disseminating what is learned" requires not only sharing the results of the evaluation process, as well as what worked and what did not on a technical level, but also sharing the fruits of the experiential steps, including stance of commitment and critical reflection. We can fail to bring about sustained progress by either ignoring evidence altogether or having too narrow a conception of evidence, the latter of which is discussed too infrequently in public health.

One model of action that incorporates many of the principles mentioned in this section is known as collective impact.[42] Its five conditions—a common agenda, shared measurement, mutually reinforcing activities, continuous communication, and backbone support organization—require organizations to look beyond themselves in all the right ways. Note that collective impact can include organizations that represent the elite or powerful in a community. However, for collective impact to be transformative, the coalition must be committed to including a wide range of stakeholders, especially those directly from the communities in most need. Such a coalition, West Side United, is described in the final chapter of the book.

The kind of action advocated in this model admittedly has downsides that can make it challenging for some to fully embrace. For example, other approaches to action can be implemented more quickly because they require less relationship building, less need for consensus, less iterative learning, and less time. Yet such interventions fail to transform communities and rarely lead to long-term, broad-based reductions in inequities. Speed is sometimes a great virtue, such as in emergencies or acute crises. But we must fight the temptation that faster is always better when acting to achieve heath equity.

Evaluation

Many different evaluation strategies, methodologies, metrics, and tools can be employed to guide, inform, evaluate, and support efforts to use evidence and best practices in program and policy planning. For instance, logic models can be used to illustrate how a program's resources and activities are intended to produce particular results.[43,44] Web-based interactive data dashboards can be very effective in providing metrics on population health outcomes and risk factors that help inform the direction of population health improvement initiatives.[45] In addition, *The Community Guide* is a free resource that provides evidence-based findings and recommendations on programs and interventions that have shown to be effective at improving population health.[46] However, in a social-justice-oriented community collaboration, the evaluation efforts must focus on the effects of policy and programmatic interventions on the community's health and on addressing health inequities.

A Practitioner's Guide for Advancing Health Equity, from the Centers for Disease Control and Prevention, illustrates how evaluations can be designed to understand what works, for whom, and under what conditions and to reveal whether health inequities have decreased, increased, or remained the same.[47] It provides guidance on incorporating health equity into each phase of evaluation from logic model to dissemination, and it builds in the reflective practice (box 7.2).

Another valuable resource includes HealthEquityGuide.org, which provides examples of community partnerships that incorporate health

---

Box 7.2. QUESTIONS FOR REFLECTION WHEN EVALUATING EFFORT TO ADDRESS HEALTH INEQUITY

1. Where are we now? How are we currently assessing the effect(s) of our efforts to address health equity?
2. How do we start the evaluation process with health equity in mind?
3. How can we consider health equity in evaluation questions and design?
4. How can we integrate health equity principles in the data-gathering process?
5. How can we understand our effect on health equity through our analysis plan?
6. How can we share our evaluation efforts with diverse stakeholders?
7. What are our next steps?

Source: Centers for Disease Control and Prevention. *A Practitioner's Guide for Advancing Health Equity: Community Strategies for Preventing Chronic Disease.* Atlanta, GA: US Department of Health and Human Services. 2013.

---

equity into their collective impact health initiatives. The Human Impact Partners, in consultation with national health equity experts and with support from the California Endowment, developed this e-resource to orient and support local health departments with their efforts to advance health equity. Specifically, this e-resource provides concrete steps on strategic practices (e.g., mobilizing data, building organization capacity, engaging in movements) that aim to *transform* how local health departments work internally, with communities and other government agencies, to systematically address structural factors. In chapter 9, the authors describe how the West Side United metrics workgroup used health equity principles when designing their evaluation.

Implementing programs and policies aimed at achieving health equity requires that we evaluate our efforts with a health equity lens.[48,49] In other words, evaluation plans need to effectively measure not just the impact of intervention on the overall improvement of the community but also its success in alleviating or eliminating health inequities. Fortunately, city stakeholders looking to improve their health equity can greatly benefit from existing examples and tools.

Conclusion

We named hope as an essential ingredient to tackling entrenched health inequities and promoting community health. We argued that socially just action requires active engagement across sectors (e.g., health care, academic, nonprofit, business, government, faith based) to create sustainable partnerships by, for, and with communities. We proposed the use of a social-justice-oriented praxis framework, for which social analysis is the engine, fueled by social justice values. The framework is inherently *place based* because, as laid out in chapter 2, improving community conditions (e.g., social supports, safety, economic opportunities) is integral to improving population health and attaining health equity.[50,51] As such, the approach requires local commitment and analysis of the lived experience of people residing in a specific area, and it cannot be activated without entering the process from a stance of long-term commitment and desire to build trust. Trust is built via the mutual processes of reflective practice and shared action and reinforced by the cocreated knowledge ecology.

The final chapter of this book illustrates how the social-justice-oriented praxis approach (involving experience, stance of commitment, social analysis, reflection, action, and evaluation) presented here is being used to create tangible, sustainable pathways to health equity on the West Side of Chicago. The creation, growth, and likely sustainability of West Side United, a multisector collaborative, have been made possible by using the *Principles of Community Engagement*.[3] The collaborative aims to achieve health equity by working toward structural change and practical work for social justice. Through the processes of experience, stance of commitment, and social analysis, the collaborative is creating pathways to health equity that are directed toward dynamic transformation in partnership with communities, in ways that reflect shared values and cultures of community members. Their processes of deliberate reflection, action, and evaluation will help ensure sustainability and create structural change that ultimately leads to reduction, if not elimination, of inequities in health and their adverse determinants.

References

1. Butterfoss FD, Kegler MC. Toward a Comprehensive Understanding of Community Coalitions. *Emerging Theories in Health Promotion Practice and Research.* 2002:157–193.

2. Cyril S, Smith BJ, Possamai-Inesedy A, Renzaho AM. Exploring the Role of Community Engagement in Improving the Health of Disadvantaged Populations: A Systematic Review. *Global Health Action.* 2015;8:29842.

3. National Institutes of Health. Clinical and Translational Science Awards Consortium Community Engagement Key Function Committee Task Force on the Principles of Community Engagement. *Principles of Community Engagement.* 2nd ed. Bethesda, MD: National Institutes of Health; 2011.

4. Benjamin GC. Health Equity and Social Justice: A Health Improvement Tool. *Grant Makers in Health Views from the Field.* 2015.

5. Street JL. A Shared Praxis Approach. *Religious Education.* 1988;83(2):234–242.

6. Daniel H, Bornstein SS, Kane GC. Addressing Social Determinants to Improve Patient Care and Promote Health Equity: An American College of Physicians Position Paper. *Annals of Internal Medicine.* 2018;168(8):577–578.

7. Magnan S. Social Determinants of Health 101 for Health Care: Five Plus Five. *NAM Perspectives*. 2017.

8. Palmer RC, Ismond D, Rodriquez EJ, Kaufman JS. Social Determinants of Health: Future Directions for Health Disparities Research. *American Journal of Public Health*. 2019;109(S1):S70–S71.

9. Ford CL, Airhihenbuwa CO. Critical Race Theory, Race Equity, and Public Health: Toward Antiracism Praxis. *American Journal of Public Health*. 2010;100(Suppl 1):S30–S35.

10. Thomas SB, Quinn SC, Butler J, Fryer CS, Garza MA. Toward a Fourth Generation of Disparities Research to Achieve Health Equity. *Annual Review of Public Health*. 2011;32:399–416.

11. Holland J, Henriot P. *Social Analysis: Linking Faith and Justice*. Maryknoll, NY: Orbis Books; 1983.

12. Lebacqz K. *Six Theories of Justice: Perspectives from Philosophical and Theological Ethics*. Minneapolis: Augsburg; 1986.

13. Krieger N. Discrimination and Health Inequities. *International Journal of Health Services: Planning, Administration, Evaluation*. 2014;44(4):643–710.

14. Pallok K, De Maio F, Ansell DA. Structural Racism—a 60-Year-Old Black Woman with Breast Cancer. *New England Journal of Medicine*. 2019;380(16):1489–1493.

15. Bailey ZD, Krieger N, Agenor M, Graves J, Linos N, Bassett MT. Structural Racism and Health Inequities in the USA: Evidence and Interventions. *Lancet*. 2017;389(10077):1453–1463.

16. Oakley J. Virtue Ethics and Bioethics. In: Russell DC, ed. *Cambridge Companion to Virtue Ethics*. Cambridge: Cambridge University Press; 2013:197–220.

17. Rozier MD. Structures of Virtue as a Framework for Public Health Ethics. *Public Health Ethics*. 2015;9(1):37–45.

18. Braveman P, Gruskin S. Defining Equity in Health. *J Epidemiol Community Health*. 2003;57(4):254–258.

19. Braveman P. What Are Health Disparities and Health Equity? We Need to Be Clear. *Public Health Rep*. 2014;129(Suppl 2):5–8.

20. American Academy of Pediatrics. Reducing Sudden Infant Death with "Back to Sleep." https://www.aap.org/en-us/advocacy-and-policy/aap-health-initiatives/7-great-achievements/Pages/Reducing-Sudden-Infant-Death-with-Back-to-.aspx.

21. Parks SE, Erck Lambert AB, Shapiro-Mendoza CK. Racial and Ethnic Trends in Sudden Unexpected Infant Deaths: United States, 1995–2013. *Pediatrics*. 2017;139(6).

22. Orsi JM, Margellos-Anast H, Whitman S. Black-White Health Disparities in the United States and Chicago: A 15-Year Progress Analysis. *American Journal of Public Health*. 2010;100(2):349–356.

23. Rust G, Zhang S, Malhotra K, et al. Paths to Health Equity: Local Area Variation in Progress toward Eliminating Breast Cancer Mortality Disparities, 1990–2009. *Cancer*. 2015;121(16):2765–2774.

24. Rust G, Zhang S, Yu Z, et al. Counties Eliminating Racial Disparities in Colorectal Cancer Mortality. *Cancer.* 2016;122(11):1735–1748.

25. Sighoko D, Murphy AM, Irizarry B, Rauscher G, Ferrans C, Ansell D. Changes in the Racial Disparity in Breast Cancer Mortality in the Ten US Cities with the Largest African American Populations from 1999 to 2013: The Reduction in Breast Cancer Mortality Disparity in Chicago. *Cancer Causes and Control.* 2017;28(6):563–568.

26. Grubbs SS, Polite BN, Carney J Jr, et al. Eliminating Racial Disparities in Colorectal Cancer in the Real World: It Took a Village. *Journal of Clinical Oncology.* 2013;31(16):1928–1930.

27. Itzkowitz SH, Winawer SJ, Krauskopf M, et al. New York Citywide Colon Cancer Control Coalition: A Public Health Effort to Increase Colon Cancer Screening and Address Health Disparities. *Cancer.* 2016;122(2):269–277.

28. Lane DA. *Keeping Hope Alive: Stirrings in Christian Theology.* Eugene, OR: Wipf & Stock; 2005.

29. Williamson C, Barth L, Lynch J. *Community Listening Session Report— April 2018.* Chicago Gun Violence Research Collaborative; 2018.

30. Schindler TF. *Ethics: The Social Dimension: Individualism and the Catholic Tradition.* Theology and Life Series, no. 27. Wilmington, DE: Glazier; 1989.

31. Freire P. *Pedagogy of the Oppressed.* Trans. Myra Bergman Ramos. New York: Herder; 1972.

32. Cargo M, Mercer SL. The Value and Challenges of Participatory Research: Strengthening Its Practice. *Annual Review of Public Health.* 2008;29:325–350.

33. Salsberg J, Macridis S, Garcia Bengoechea E, Macaulay AC, Moore S, Committee ObotKSTP. Engagement Strategies That Foster Community Self-Determination in Participatory Research: Insider Ownership through Outsider Championship. *Family Practice.* 2017;34(3):336–340.

34. Schön DA. *The Reflective Practitioner: How Professionals Think in Action.* New York: Routledge; 2017.

35. Centers for Disease Control and Prevention (CDC). Estimated HIV Incidence and Prevalence in the United States (2010–2016). July 5, 2019. https://www.cdc.gov/hiv/pdf/library/slidesets/cdc-hiv-incidence-prevalence-2010-2016.pdf.

36. Gomes T, Tadrous M, Mamdani MM, Paterson JM, Juurlink DN. The Burden of Opioid-Related Mortality in the United States. *JAMA Network Open.* 2018;1(2):e180217–e180217.

37. Ingram D, Chen LH. Age-Adjusted Homicide Rates, by Urbanization of County of Residence—United States, 2004 and 2013. *Morbidity and Mortality Weekly Report.* 2015;64(5):133.

38. Kawachi I, Daniels N, Robinson DE. Health Disparities by Race and Class: Why Both Matter. *Health Affairs (Millwood).* 2005;24(2):343–352.

39. Daniels N, Kennedy BP, Kawachi I. Why Justice Is Good for Our Health: The Social Determinants of Health Inequalities. *Daedalus.* 1999;128(4):215–251.

40. Brownson RC, Fielding JE, Maylahn CM. Evidence-Based Public Health: A Fundamental Concept for Public Health Practice. *Annual Review of Public Health*. 2009;30:175–201.

41. Whitman S, Shah A, Benjamins M. *Urban Health: Combating Disparities with Local Data*. New York: Oxford University Press; 2011.

42. Kania J, Kramer M. Embracing Emergence: How Collective Impact Addresses Complexity. *Stanford Social Innovation Review*. (1–14).

43. West JF. Public Health Program Planning Logic Model for Community Engaged Type 2 Diabetes Management and Prevention. *Evaluation and Program Planning*. 2014;42:43–49.

44. Tucker P, Liao Y, Giles WH, Liburd L. The Reach 2010 Logic Model: An Illustration of Expected Performance. *Preventing Chronic Disease*. 2006;3(1):A21.

45. Gourevitch MN, Athens JK, Levine SE, Kleiman N, Thorpe LE. City-Level Measures of Health, Health Determinants, and Equity to Foster Population Health Improvement: The City Health Dashboard. *American Journal of Public Health*. 2019;109(4):585–592.

46. Sabatino SA, Lawrence B, Elder R, et al. Effectiveness of Interventions to Increase Screening for Breast, Cervical, and Colorectal Cancers: Nine Updated Systematic Reviews for the Guide to Community Preventive Services. *American Journal of Preventive Medicine*. 2012;43(1):97–118.

47. Centers for Disease Control and Prevention. *A Practitioner's Guide for Advancing Health Equity: Community Strategies for Preventing Chronic Disease*. Atlanta, GA: US Department of Health and Human Services. 2013.

48. Heller J, Givens ML, Yuen TK, et al. Advancing Efforts to Achieve Health Equity: Equity Metrics for Health Impact Assessment Practice. *International Journal of Environmental Research and Public Health*. 2014;11(11):11054–11064.

49. Douglas MD, Josiah Willock R, Respress E, et al. Applying a Health Equity Lens to Evaluate and Inform Policy. *Ethnicity and Disease*. 2019;29(Suppl 2):329–342.

50. Dankwa-Mullan I, Perez-Stable EJ. Addressing Health Disparities Is a Place-Based Issue. *American Journal of Public Health*. 2016;106(4):637–639.

51. Amobi A, Plescia M, Alexander-Scott N. The Business Case for Investing in Place-Based Public Health Initiatives. *Journal of Public Health Manag and Practice*. 2019;25(6):612–615.

[EIGHT]

Data Are Not Enough

Moving toward Solutions-Focused Communication

KRISTIN MONNARD, JANA HIRSCHTICK, MAUREEN R. BENJAMINS,
AND PAMELA T. ROESCH

PREVIOUS CHAPTERS provided clear evidence of racial health inequities and introduced theories to explain the drivers of these inequities. Specifically, the data show that (1) geographic and racial inequities in mortality exist across the largest US cities; (2) although Black individuals generally have shorter life expectancies, more premature mortality, and higher mortality rates for most leading causes of death compared to whites, the size of the inequities varies substantially by city; and (3) city-level factors, such as median household income and income inequality, are associated with overall mortality and mortality inequities. These findings, particularly the ecological results, support our understanding that health inequities are rooted in structural biases and policies that drive socioeconomic inequities—leading to excess deaths of Black people.

These compelling findings raise the fundamental dilemma: how to translate these data into action. City leaders and other stakeholders now have access to an unprecedented amount of data relevant to their jurisdictions. But without context, framing, and collaboration, change may remain elusive. To help those eager to move forward, this chapter outlines practical ways to engage communities in data interpretation and catalyze a wider net of stakeholders by translating data into knowledge using solutions-focused communication.

Communicating findings in a way that inspires dialogue about health inequities and facilitates solutions-focused action is an imperative component of the research endeavor, yet that is the step most often overlooked. As Whitman notes, if we think it morally shameful that persistent racism and structural inequities cut Black lives short, "we have an obligation to say so, and to respond with anger to a situation that demands anger" (p. 398).[1] Some contend that studies that merely document health inequities without offering solutions are unethical.[2] At the very least, we maintain that findings must be communicated in a way that balances a description of the problem with an envisioning of the solutions.[2]

This chapter will help cities understand how to more effectively communicate and disseminate sensitive health data to the public and relevant decision-makers. The solutions-focused approach we outline will suggest how to engage and motivate community members and other key stakeholders in collectively envisioning the changes needed to improve health. Take, for example, the 3,341 excess Black deaths that occurred annually (2013–2017) in Chicago owing to the racial inequity in all-cause mortality rates (as seen in chapter 3). How can a local health department or nonprofit effectively communicate this incredibly important information in a way that convinces the public that the root causes of inequities are at play? And how can they share data in a way that will inspire action by multiple stakeholders to address these enduring structural determinants, in a way that avoids unintentionally harming the Black community further by reinforcing stereotypes? How can they tailor their communication to different audiences to inspire them to mobilize and join with all the other stakeholders necessary to effect change? We will discuss in this chapter why data on their own are insufficient to solve the problem of inequities. We will argue for a solutions-focused approach to communication that engages a wide range of audiences, highlighting insights gained from a past dissemination approach. For researchers, health departments, city officials, nonprofits, or others interested in undertaking this much-needed work, we hope this chapter will offer a pathway for pursuing community-based solutions to inequities in your city.

Data Alone Are Not Enough

Data collection and analysis of population health trends are critical for documenting and understanding health inequities. However, data alone cannot drive change. As a society, we have more access to data than ever before and increasingly sophisticated tools to identify trends.[3-5] At the same time, we live in an age of staggering inequities. Despite documented racial inequities for as long as records have been kept, people of color in the United States continue to face worse outcomes across practically all health outcomes.[6] We can logically expect inequities to persist unless we change how we use data to pursue structural change.

Public health officials and other advocates now have an important opportunity to be bold in their messaging and intentional in their communication to redirect discussion about the true drivers of unequal health outcomes for communities of color. As discussed in previous chapters, clear and long-standing evidence supports the role of racism in perpetuating inequities and poor health.[7] Thoughtful messaging based on data like those found in this book can help elevate public discourse and educate key stakeholders about the origins and legacy of inequities still driving current health outcomes and how to disrupt them.

A Movement toward Solutions-Focused Communication

Traditionally, much public health communication about health inequities has been "problem-focused," identifying and explaining the structures that perpetuate inequities. "Solutions-focused" communication, in contrast, is grounded in an exploration of strategies and interventions to remediate these structures.[2] While it is important for audiences to understand the structural drivers of inequities, we must also make sure the conversation does not stop with the diagnosis. Previous chapters in this book have described these structural drivers by showing the links between varying mortality rates and socioeconomic inequities. To move forward, solutions-focused communication shifts the emphasis from the problem to envisioning potential solutions that lead to just and equitable health outcomes for all communities.

A solutions-focused communication approach differs from traditional research dissemination in other important ways. Typically, public health researchers disseminate their findings primarily through peer-reviewed journals or academic conferences within specific disciplines and give little thought to communicating the results to public health practitioners, health care providers, advocacy groups, or civic leaders.[8-10] The approach we advocate calls for translating findings into practice by driving political, institutional, and organizational change locally. While federal-level policy and systems changes are critical for correcting entrenched societal inequities, change at the local level can happen more quickly where proposed changes can be directed toward the precise drivers producing inequities in that local jurisdiction. The growing literature on place-based health demonstrates that much of health is created locally.[11-13] Those who wish to act on health inequities will need locally focused communication as well.

Expanding Our Audiences

To utilize findings in a way that drives change, we must also engage the broader civic community. We need to create useful evidence for and collaborate with cross-sector leaders, as well as community members themselves, in city planning, policy, and community organizing.[14-17] Not surprisingly, these different audiences will require different communication approaches.

Cross-sector leaders are important partners in catalyzing action at the city level. Consider Braveman's definition of health equity: "Health equity means that everyone has a fair and just opportunity to be as healthy as possible. This requires removing obstacles to health, such as poverty, discrimination, powerless, and their consequences, including lack of access to good jobs with fair pay, safe environments, and quality education, housing, and health care" (p. 5).[18] The breadth of obstacles identified in this definition underscores the range of participants and partnerships needed to tackle the problem—from sectors including housing, social services, civil rights, education, urban planning, and health care. Each of these sectors shares equity priorities with public health. That includes urban planners who must consider commercial growth, infrastructure development, and health and quality of life for residents when designing community environments. Housing advocates are invested in ensuring safe, accessible, and affordable housing. Educators are committed to bringing high-quality educational opportunities within reach of all children regardless of socioeconomic background. The principles of collective impact demonstrate the advantages of reaching broader networks of stakeholders and establishing shared priorities and language to achieve common goals.[19]

Engaging Communities in Knowledge Cocreation

Community members are another vital stakeholder to reach through solutions-focused health communication. First, cities and researchers have a responsibility to share data findings with the communities they concern and were collected from. Further, while we all have an obligation to address injustice in health outcomes, the communities most affected by it have the right to lead the way in envisioning solutions. Work done on behalf of communities without their involvement perpetuates the same racist power structures that created the health inequities initially. Worse, it can generate misguided or even racist interpretations and top-down solutions. Rather, the remediation of racial inequities must be undertaken in concert with communities and must prioritize the right of communities of color to tell their story and author their future.

Too often, those in positions of power, such as researchers or city governments, leave marginalized communities completely out of such dialogues or provide only token opportunities that "check the box" on informing the public and seeking their feedback. Figure 8.1 demonstrates the continuum of community engagement as defined by the International Association for Public Participation. As shown here, simply informing or seeking input is the very least of our obligation to the public. To truly engage communities, we should strive to move as far along the continuum as possible.

Engaging disproportionately impacted communities to participate in dialogue around data can also ground any interpretations in local

	INFORM	CONSULT	INVOLVE	COLLABORATE	EMPOWER
PUBLIC PARTICIPATION GOAL	To provide the public with balanced and objective information to assist them in understanding the problem, alternatives, opportunities and/or solutions.	To obtain public feedback on analysis, alternatives, and/or decisions.	To work directly with the public throughout the process to ensure that public concerns and aspirations are consistently understood and considered.	To partner with the public in each aspect of the decision including the development of alternatives and the identification of the preferred solution.	To place final decision-making in the hands of the public.
PROMISE TO THE PUBLIC	We will keep you informed.	We will keep you informed, listen to and acknowledge concerns and aspirations, and provide feedback on how public input influenced the decision.	We will work with you to ensure that your concerns and aspirations are directly reflected in the alternatives developed and provide feedback on how public input influenced the decision.	We will look to you for advice and innovation in formulating solutions and incorporate your advice and recommendations into the decisions to the maximum extent possible.	We will implement what you decide.

Figure 8.1. International Association for Public Participation's Spectrum of Public Participation. *Source:* International Association for Public Participation. www.iap2.org. Reprinted with permission.

knowledge and lived experience.[20] Solutions reached through such interpretations are likely to prove more feasible and lasting because they will have the buy-in of the community. The field of knowledge management suggests that knowledge occurs through an exchange of information that results in action.[21,22] Turning data into knowledge thus requires a bidirectional exchange, in which knowledge is cocreated through dialogue and collective meaning making between researchers and communities. Those in positions of power, such as researchers, public health professionals, and city governments, can work together with community members to turn data into knowledge by collaborating to interpret data and craft broader messaging.

Working in solidarity with marginalized communities demands that we respect their right to self-determination and highlight their voices and experiences in this exchange.[23] As Vogel explains, much of the persistent racial injustice in our country flows from "the denial of [Black people's] basic right to full and meaningful participation in the social, economic and political life of the republic on terms that represent their wishes coupled with the support needed to carry out those wishes, rather than to impose a solution from the top-down" (p. 202).[24] Self-determination, then, recognizes the right of communities of color to exert authority and control over their lives and respectfully supports them in realizing the solutions to injustice that they put forth. By featuring the voices of communities most impacted by inequitable and racist structures, we put their perspectives and their solutions at the center of all our dialogue. Centering marginalized communities means that our messengers, messages, and proposals for rectifying injustices are generated within those communities.

Just as data alone are not enough to solve health inequities, our actions will not improve health unless they are grounded in deep, local understanding and unless they are accepted by the communities they aim to help. As we have seen from past public health interventions, actions to improve health can actually increase inequities by improving health for more privileged populations while failing to reach more socially disadvantaged groups. For example, highly active antiretroviral therapy (HAART) treatment for HIV is very effective in reducing viral load for HIV positive patients, but the requirement for daily treatment administration has led to underutilization in populations with higher barriers to care access and disproportionate benefits for those with fewer access barriers.[25] Even policies designed to benefit the population equally can have a disproportionate advantage for more privileged people. Legislation prohibiting smoking in bars and restaurants is less likely to be enforced in areas with lower socioeconomic status, for example, leading to greater smoking cessation and subsequent health outcomes for those living in areas with more socioeconomic advantage where smoking bans are more strictly enforced.[26] Approaching data interpretation and solution generation as a process in which knowledge is cocreated and the experience of those most affected by health inequities is incorporated will produce more effective solutions that do not perpetuate structural barriers to health. The following sections provide an example of how one organization applied these principles in practice. They offer lessons learned and practical steps to guide users toward more achievable and feasible outcomes.

Case Study: Sinai Community Health Survey 2.0

While this book has thus far taken a macrolevel focus to examine health inequities *across* cities, we will now shift our perspective to see how a local public health research institute sought to understand and communicate inequities *within* one city. "Big picture" city-level data are valuable for highlighting comparisons between cities, but more local data provide users with additional support to motivate and guide action for a specific city.

Sinai Urban Health Institute (SUHI) is a unique community-driven public health research center located in a safety net health care system in Chicago. For 20 years, SUHI has worked to identify and address health inequities across Chicago's underserved neighborhoods through epidemiologic data collection and analysis, community-based interventions, and the translation of data into actionable knowledge for community members, policy makers, and other stakeholders. In all its work, SUHI strives to engage the community in partnership.

One notable example of SUHI's efforts to spur change through data is the Sinai Community Health Survey (Sinai Survey; box 8.1). First conducted in 2002, the Sinai Survey was a community-driven effort designed to document neighborhood-level health inequities within select Chicago communities.[27] Participating communities were chosen because they represented some of Chicago's most vulnerable communities and allowed researchers to examine findings for four separate racial and ethnic groups (Black, white, Mexican, and Puerto Rican). All but one were low-income communities of color. Survey findings underlined the importance of "hyperlocal" health data, as they uncovered substantial inequities in health outcomes by neighborhood.

Driven by demand from community-based organizations and other stakeholders, SUHI conducted the Sinai Survey 2.0 in 2015 to provide an updated snapshot of health outcomes across communities and to better understand the social determinants of health.[28] All coauthors of this chapter participated in the design, implementation, or dissemination of the survey. This second iteration provides an example of how health findings can be communicated through a solutions-focused framework.

Box 8.1. SINAI COMMUNITY HEALTH SURVEY 2.0
(SINAI SURVEY)

Overview
Sinai Survey 2.0, a project of the Sinai Urban Health Institute, was a community-driven, cross-sectional survey of adults (18+ years) and children (0–12 years) living in nine officially designated community areas in Chicago, Illinois.[28]

Methods
Trained interviewers (who reflected the demographics of the participants) conducted the survey face-to-face within people's homes in English and Spanish from 2015 to 2016. The survey included over 500 questions related to health outcomes, such as obesity and diabetes, and the social determinants of health, such as insurance status, income, and neighborhood safety. In total, 1,543 adult and 394 child surveys were administered in collaboration with the University of Illinois at Chicago Survey Research Laboratory and the Sinai Survey Community Advisory Committee (CAC).

Sinai Survey Community Advisory Committee
The CAC was composed of representatives from each surveyed community and included both community organizers and leaders, as well as lay community members with an interest (but no formal training) in health. For 4 years, the CAC guided many aspects of the survey, from design, to data collection, to dissemination. They reviewed over 700 proposed questions and approved, denied, added, and/or amended questions depending on cultural appropriateness and perceived importance. CAC members from each community also prioritized findings from their respective communities to highlight in the dissemination process and oversaw the development of appropriate messaging for different audiences.

Sinai Survey Findings and Communication Materials
For more detailed information on the survey methods and results, visit the Sinai Survey website, www.sinaisurvey.org.

As part of our dissemination efforts, we developed a plan to reach various priority audiences, using tailored messaging and methods to meet the unique needs of each audience.[29] Our strategy was motivated by principles of community engagement and knowledge transfer and focused on improving data accessibility in five areas: message, audience, messenger, communications process and infrastructure, and impact of the knowledge transfer.[30-32] A summary of the audiences engaged, our dissemination activities, and key audience-specific messages appears in table 8.1.

Steps for Success

The Sinai Survey dissemination process yielded several overarching lessons for designing and implementing a community-engaged, solutions-focused communication approach. Here we outline steps that city leaders, researchers, and other community health stakeholders can take to implement a similar strategy. We discuss the importance of centering marginalized voices and using trusted messengers to solicit community input in order to devise local solutions to health inequities. We discuss how prioritizing dissemination, engaging our audiences, and tailoring messages to meet the unique needs of the stakeholders helped us reach a broader array of people. Finally, we zero in on action-oriented communication, which is key to mobilizing stakeholders to initiate change. While we offer our experience and lessons learned here, many toolkits are available to help cities and communities develop a multifaceted communication strategy. Box 8.2 highlights some excellent resources for those interested in beginning this work.

Centering Marginalized Voices

First and foremost, public health researchers documenting and addressing health inequities should center the voices of marginalized communities throughout the entire course of the process. This applies not only to research on racial inequities but also to inequities related to gender identity, disability status, age, income, documentation status, religion, and all other marginalized groups. Authentically engaging marginalized communities most affected by inequities is critical to dismantling the systems that perpetuate them.

For the Sinai Survey, we purposely made sharing our findings with community residents a priority by holding community forums in each community we surveyed. Forums took place in easily accessible

Table 8.1. Dissemination Activities for Sinai Community Health Survey 2.0

Audience	Message/Goal	Messenger (Dissemination Mechanism)	Communication Process and Infrastructure
All audiences	Provide central hub for all audiences to access survey findings and dissemination products.	Sinai Survey website	A website (www.sinaisurvey.org) provided information on Sinai Survey methodology, findings, and dissemination activities.
Community residents	Share Sinai Survey findings in an accessible format. Gather community members' insights to better contextualize data.	Community forums	SUHI hosted seven forums to share findings with residents through roundtable co-learning sessions.
	Share information on community prevalence, signs, symptoms, and risk factors for an important health issue. Provide action steps and local resources.	Health infographics	Nine infographics that highlighted one priority health topic per community.
	Present brief introduction to Sinai Survey and initial findings.	Community health video series	Nine animated videos highlighted findings from each community, including quotes from residents.
Community-based organizations and service providers	Demonstrate the link between social determinants of health and health outcomes. Help community organizations tell the story of their community to funders/policy makers.	Community health profiles	Nine community health profiles integrated and contextualized findings. Each briefly summarized the physical environment, social and economic factors, clinical care, health behaviors, and health outcomes impacting community well-being.
Decision-makers	Identify leading community health issues. Explain social factors contributing to health. Compare health inequities by race/ethnicity, gender, and community area.	*Community Health Counts* booklet	Booklet of 16 data snapshots of health and social determinants presented prevalence data by community, race/ethnicity, and gender. Covered topics such as diabetes, health insurance, and food insecurity.
Public health researchers and professionals	Provide access to Sinai Survey prevalence data.	City Health Department data portal	Made findings publicly available through city health department's data portal.
	Provide access to raw data to generate new research.	Data housing through ICPSR	Made raw data available to all researchers (with IRB clearance).
	Describe emerging health inequities and survey methods. Provide lessons learned from survey approach.	Academic presentations	Shared survey methodology, findings, and lessons learned via traditional oral presentations.
Members of the press and other organizations	Share key findings from Sinai Survey more broadly.	Media event	Held media event at a community-based organization to formally release and briefly summarize findings.

Notes: ICPSR = Inter-university Consortium for Political and Social Research; IRB = institutional review board. Table ordered according to the framework defined in Lavis JN, Robertson D, Woodside JM, McLeod CB, Abelson J, How Can Research Organizations More Effectively Transfer Research Knowledge to Decision Makers?, *Milbank Quarterly* 2003;81:221–248.

Box 8.2. SELECTED COMMUNICATION RESOURCES
TO SUPPORT LOCAL HEALTH EQUITY EFFORTS

Communications to Promote Interest and Participation
Community Tool Box, University of Kansas Center for Community
Health and Development
www.ctb.ku.edu/en/promoting-interest-and-participation-initiatives

Communications Guide
Government Alliance on Race & Equity
www.racialequityalliance.org/tools-resources/communication-tools/

Community Engagement Toolkit
Collective Impact Forum
www.collectiveimpactforum.org/sites/default/files/Community%20
Engagement%20Toolkit.pdf

Unnatural Causes Action Toolkit
California Newsreel
www.unnaturalcauses.org/assets/uploads/file/UC_Toolkit_All.pdf

Health Equity Guide
Human Impact Partners
www.healthequityguide.org

A Conversation Guide for Health Equity
Reos Partners and Robert Wood Johnson Foundation
www.reospartners.com/wp-content/uploads/2017/07/AConversationGuide
forHealthEquity_Feb2017.pdf

American Opportunity: A Communications Toolkit
The Opportunity Agenda and the SPIN Project
https://community-wealth.org/content/american-opportunity
-communications-toolkit

---

community settings, such as churches, libraries, and community centers. Within the forums, we used a rotating roundtable format and distributed posters and handouts with relevant community health findings. Each forum lasted approximately two hours and included four
roundtable discussions (about 20 minutes each) covering the four com-

munity priority topics. Each roundtable began with a short overview of the findings, followed by facilitated discussion among attendees, who were asked to contribute their insights, personal interpretations, and proposed solutions to the health issues in their community.[33]

We made dissemination to community residents the priority based on the understanding that data on communities should ultimately belong to those communities. Additionally, we knew we would need the input of community members to accurately contextualize the data, shape their community's narrative on health problems and solutions, and build partnerships in order to move forward. For example, one of the surveyed communities receives disproportionate media attention related to gun violence. An outsider might assume that the community forum we held with residents from this community would be focused on understanding and addressing violence. That was not the case. Instead, community members reported feeling stigmatized and overpoliced as a result of the disproportionate amount of negative media attention given to their community. They further reported that the media portrayals brought fear and eroded trust among neighbors, which negatively affected local community-building efforts, business development, and overall quality of life. Many forum participants interpreted public attention on "community safety" as coded language perpetuating a racist stereotype. In response to this feedback, we crafted our subsequent messaging to avoid any images of the community that residents would find unfair, objectionable, or counterproductive.

Elevating marginalized voices in the processes of interpreting and disseminating data can also produce more appropriate interventions. Two communities in the Sinai Survey, North Lawndale and South Lawndale, border one another and have similar rates of poverty and food insecurity. However, conversations with residents revealed that the barriers to food access, and consequently the solutions to addressing food insecurity, were quite different. In North Lawndale, a predominantly non-Hispanic Black and relatively sparsely populated community, the barriers to finding affordable and healthy food were physical. It lacked adequate grocery stores, emergency food providers, and accessible transportation to utilize resources in other communities. In South Lawndale, a densely populated, predominantly Mexican community with a substantial immigrant population, undocumented residents cannot access government programs like the Supplemental Nutrition Assistance Program. Many are also deterred from seeking emergency food sources like food pantries because funding sources require food providers to ask for identification, spurring fears of deportation among immigrants frightened by anti-immigrant political rhetoric regardless of their status. Both communities identified demanding job schedules as an additional barrier to accessing emergency food sources, which were often available only during daytime hours. Given these varied pathways to food insecurity, effective solutions would also be expected to vary between these two communities, geographically adjacent but differently affected.

For cities with high levels of Black:white mortality inequities (documented within this book), an important first step in shaping messaging designed to elicit workable solutions is to engage those communities and residents most affected by these inequities. Community-generated solutions may differ from those conceived by stakeholders located farther from the problem; communities are often better poised to connect the dots between structural inequities and health outcomes.

Use Trusted Messengers

Choosing the right messenger to convey the message is another critical component for effectively reaching the intended audience. For our community forums, we used SUHI's staff of community health workers to present our data and facilitate dialogue about the Sinai Survey findings. Community health workers are trusted frontline public health employees who know their communities intimately and have experience communicating with community members about health in an understandable, approachable way.[34] Using trusted community messengers who reflected the demographics of the communities was also crucial in our efforts to cocreate knowledge. For cities newer to this work, trusted messengers may be less readily available. Building relationships with community-based organizations can help identify these messengers, while also developing connections within the community. Of course, over the long term, cities should also strive to hire a staff that reflects the demographics of the communities they serve.

Trusted messengers will vary across stakeholders and therefore must be selected with care and an eye toward the targeted audience. Among many professional groups, physicians may be the most trusted messenger when talking about health and mortality. Hospital executives may also be fitting messengers to articulate the need to improve health at the population level. To mobilize stakeholders at the city level, a local elected official such as a city council representative, mayor, or state legislator may be the most valuable messenger. For messaging about economic investment, a representative from the local business sector may be most persuasive. Whenever possible, leverage voices from a variety of sectors and perspectives to articulate the need for action.

Invest in Dissemination
Even if researchers or individuals in positions of power recognize the significance of dissemination in using data to motivate action, it has to be acknowledged that following a multilevel, community-engaged communication approach generally requires a substantial commitment of staff time and resources. Dissemination activities often demand skill sets unavailable within public health departments and research institutes. Our SUHI staff came from diverse backgrounds, allowing us to leverage individuals' skills in project management, health education, and community organizing. However, we still needed to contract with outside experts in graphic design, data visualization, and media relations.

For Sinai Survey 2.0, a three-member team coordinated dissemination activities and monitored consistency across messaging and audiences. Each activity entailed extensive preparation and planning to ensure that the messages were packaged in usable, easy-to-interpret formats. We also had to allocate additional time for our Community Advisory Committee (CAC) (box 8.1) to review our materials and messages for their appropriateness, understandability, grounding in community member experiences, and focus on solutions.

Engage Your Audiences

Chapter 2 highlighted the diverse determinants of health that are often social and political. Thus, mortality inequities should concern those working in housing, transportation, urban planning, education, and other sectors beyond health departments. The audiences shown in table 8.1 may also be helpful in generating a list of target populations. To the extent possible, those disseminating results should consult representatives from target audiences to fashion the most useful and compelling messages and the most effective and acceptable modes of communication.[35,36]

Despite the greater availability of automatically generated data reports, such standardized products may be perceived by the targeted audiences as lacking authenticity and relevance, and thus less authentic, relevant, and acceptable. Codesigning communication materials will avoid this pitfall and yield approachable language customized for that particular audience and products that will be useful for moving their work forward.

Working with stakeholder groups to codesign our products for various audiences of the Sinai Survey, we asked CAC members from each community to prioritize health topics for their community. They helped us develop relevant and approachable wording and images for the information being shared and emphasized the need to highlight local community resources offering residents help for a particular health issue. As one CAC member explained, "Don't just give people bad news without telling them what they can do about it." Stakeholders told us that the most valuable aspect of the survey for community organizations was the availability of local-level data that they could use to demonstrate need to funders in grant applications. With this in mind, materials for this audience were designed to articulate the connection between social and environmental factors and health outcomes, offering organizations a more holistic picture of their communities to present to potential funders.

Use Language That Resonates

Customizing our messaging and using an array of dissemination mechanisms allowed us to successfully reach multiple stakeholder groups and provide them with the resources they needed to understand and turn findings into plans for action. We worked hard to develop language that felt relevant and relatable for each audience. That meant avoiding jargon or terminology more familiarly heard within the public health community, like *equity*, *social determinants*, or *adverse childhood experiences*; this language may put off or elude more general audiences.[37] Using straightforward, explicit language that clearly describes the problems and solutions will help your audiences grasp and relate to the issues more readily. Messages are also more powerful if they do not overwhelm the audience with data, but instead focus on a few compelling facts that audiences will remember.

Carefully consider the audience you are trying to reach before crafting your message, and be mindful of your own biases. In recent years, some communities have begun naming racism as a cause for health inequities. Madison, Wisconsin, Milwaukee County, Wisconsin, and Cook County, Illinois, have all formally proclaimed that racism is a public health crisis, for instance.[38,39] For conservative-leaning audiences who may not readily accept that racism is a structural driver of health outcomes, the messaging issues are more complex. There may be debates over interpretation of data points, and heated arguments over causal pathways and policy implications. There will be groups that look for genetic explanations for racial health inequities, and groups that will place the onus on cultural (rather than structural) differences. One strategy for overcoming these divides would be to appeal to our shared patriotic ideal of working together to create a strong country where every child has a chance to succeed.[40,41] Messages pitched in terms of "us" convey the sentiment that we are all affected by and benefit from the creation of a more just society.[41] Yet, at the same time, the truth is that racism disadvantages some while advantaging others; "us" statements may well ring hollow to groups and communities that have experienced disinvestment, exploitation, and discrimination. Health equity work requires a more just distribution of resources, opportunities, and power. We should not waver in calling out racism as a structural driver of health outcomes, even if that message is unwelcome by some.

Communicate with Action in Mind

Communication materials should frame data in a way that empowers the target audiences and guides them toward a path for action. Calls to action will vary by stakeholder. Communication directed toward community residents might highlight local resources for health or social assistance. For community-based organizations, communications might feature information on how to join an existing task force or collaborative working on the issue. Whatever the audience, all communication should include information on where to learn more. For Sinai Survey 2.0, all our communication materials directed audiences to our website, www.sinaisurvey.org, for additional information about the survey, findings for their community, and an invitation on how to contact SUHI staff with questions and get involved in next steps.

Conclusion

In this chapter, we have offered specifics on how public health advocates and city leaders can communicate health findings in a way that engages the community, generates deeper understanding of the data, and mobilizes stakeholders in solutions-focused dialogue, all while keeping community perspectives and community-generated solutions at the fore. When we have communicated our findings successfully and enlisted the support of community and stakeholders in dialogue to understand the implications and jointly agree on potential solutions, the groundwork has been laid to motivate stakeholders to act. The next chapter will outline one local coalition's place-based, multisector, community-driven approach to mobilizing around the issue of geographic inequities in life expectancy along racial lines on the West Side of Chicago. The authors explore how data can be balanced with evidence-based best practices, community priorities, and existing community assets to address health equity in large urban areas, even in the face of enduring, historically based inequities.

References

1. Whitman S. Racial Disparities in Health: Taking It Personally. *Public Health Reports*. 2001;116(5):387–389.

2. Muntaner C, Sridharan S, Solar O, Benach J. Commentary: Against Unjust Global Distribution of Power and Money: The Report of the WHO Commission on the Social Determinants of Health: Global Inequality and the Future of Public Health Policy. *Journal of Public Health Policy.* 2009;30(2):163–175.

3. Glaeser EL, Kominers SD, Luca M, Naik N. Big Data and Big Cities: The Promises and Limitations of Improved Measures of Urban Life. *Economic Inquiry.* 2018;56(1):114–137.

4. Zhenshan Y, Ying L, Douay N. Opportunities and Limitations of Big Data Applications to Human and Economic Geography: The State of the Art. *Progress in Geography.* 2015;34(4):410–417.

5. Philip TM, Schuler-Brown S, Way W. A Framework for Learning about Big Data with Mobile Technologies for Democratic Participation: Possibilities, Limitations, and Unanticipated Obstacles. *Technology, Knowledge and Learning.* 2013;18(3):103–120.

6. Haines MR. Ethnic Differences in Demographic Behavior in the United States: Has There Been Convergence? *Historical Methods.* 2003;36(4):157–195.

7. Williams DR, Lawrence JA, Davis BA. Racism and Health: Evidence and Needed Research. *Annual Review of Public Health.* 2019;40:105–125.

8. Brownson RC, Jacobs JA, Tabak RG, Hoehner CM, Stamatakis KA. Designing for Dissemination among Public Health Researchers: Findings from a National Survey in the United States. *American Journal of Public Health.* 2013;103(9):1693–1700.

9. Carpenter D, Nieva V, Albaghal T, Sorra J. Development of a Planning Tool to Guide Research Dissemination. *Advances in Patient Safety: From Research to Implementation.* 2005;4:83–91.

10. Kerner J, Rimer B, Emmons K. Introduction to the Special Section on Dissemination: Dissemination Research and Research Dissemination: How Can We Close the Gap? *Health Psychology.* 2005;24(5):443–446.

11. Branas CC, MacDonald JM. A Simple Strategy to Transform Health, All over the Place. *Journal of Public Health Management and Practice.* 2014;20(2):157.

12. Dannenberg AL, Frumkin H, Jackson RJ, eds. *Making Healthy Places. Designing and Building for Health, Well-Being, and Sustainability.* Washington, DC: Island; 2011.

13. Poland B, Lehoux P, Holmes D, Andrews G. How Place Matters: Unpacking Technology and Power in Health and Social Care. *Health and Social Care in the Community.* 2005;13(2):170–180.

14. Glasgow RE, Vinson C, Chambers D, Khoury MJ, Kaplan RM, Hunter C. National Institutes of Health Approaches to Dissemination and Implementation Science: Current and Future Directions. *American Journal of Public Health.* 2012;102(7):1274–1281.

15. Nandi A, Harper S. How Consequential Is Social Epidemiology? A Review of Recent Evidence. *Current Epidemiology Reports.* 2015;2(1):61–70.

16. O'Campo P, Dunn J. *Rethinking Social Epidemiology: Towards a Science of Change.* Dordrecht: Springer; 2012.

17. Wallerstein NB, Yen IH, Syme SL. Integration of Social Epidemiology and Community-Engaged Interventions to Improve Health Equity. *American Journal of Public Health*. 2011;101(5):822–830.

18. Braveman P, Arkin E, Orleans T, Proctor D, Plough A. *What Is Health Equity? And What Difference Does a Definition Make?* Princeton, NJ: Robert Wood Johnson Foundation; 2017.

19. Kania J, Kramer M. Collective Impact. *Stanford Social Innovation Review*. Winter 2011.

20. Baum F, MacDougall C, Smith D. Participatory Action Research. *Journal of Epidemiology and Community Health*. 2006;60(10):854–857.

21. Por G, Molloy J. Nurturing Systemic Wisdom through Knowledge Ecology. *Systems Thinker*. 2018:1–18.

22. Garfield S. Knowledge & Knowledge Management Defined. April 13, 2015. https://www.linkedin.com/pulse/knowledge-management-defined-stan-garfield/.

23. Wallerstein N, Duran B. Theoretical, Historical and Practice Roots of CBPR. In: Wallerstein N, Duran B, Oetzel J, Minkler M, eds., *Community-Based Participatory Research for Health: Advancing Social and Health Equity*. San Francisco: Jossey-Bass; 2017.

24. Vogel HJ. African Americans and the Right to Self-Determination in a Christian Context. *Journal of the Society of Christian Ethics*. 2002;22:201–228.

25. Gebo KA, Fleishman JA, Conviser R, et al. Racial and Gender Disparities in Receipt of Highly Active Antiretroviral Therapy Persist in a Multistate Sample of HIV Patients in 2001. *JAIDS Journal of Acquired Immune Deficiency Syndromes*. 2005;38(1):96–103.

26. Tabuchi T, Iso H, Brunner E. Tobacco Control Measures to Reduce Socioeconomic Inequality in Smoking: The Necessity, Time-Course Perspective, and Future Implications. *Journal of Epidemiology*. 2017:JE20160206.

27. Whitman S, Shah A, Benjamins M. *Urban Health: Combating Disparities with Local Data*. New York: Oxford University Press; 2011.

28. Hirschtick JL, Benjamins M, Homan S. *Community Health Counts: Sinai Community Health Survey 2.0*. Sinai Urban Health Institute, Sinai Health System; March 2017.

29. Monnard K, Benjamins MR, Hirschtick JL, Castro M, Roesch PT. Co-creation of Knowledge: A Community-Based Approach to Multilevel Dissemination of Health Information. *Health Promotion Practice*. 2019:1524839919865228.

30. Lavis JN, Lomas J, Hamid M, Sewankambo NK. Assessing Country-Level Efforts to Link Research to Action. *Bulletin of the World Health Organization*. 2006;84(8):620–628.

31. Lavis JN, Robertson D, Woodside JM, McLeod CB, Abelson J. How Can Research Organizations More Effectively Transfer Research Knowledge to Decision Makers? *Milbank Quarterly*. 2003;81(2):221–248.

32. Reardon R, Lavis JN, Gibson J. *From Research to Practice: A Knowledge Transfer Planning Guide*. Institute for Work & Health; 2006.

33. Woolf SH, Purnell JQ, Simon SM, et al. Translating Evidence into Population Health Improvement: Strategies and Barriers. *Annual Review of Public Health*. 2015;36:463–482.

34. American Public Health Association. Community Health Workers. https://www.apha.org/apha-communities/member-sections/community-health-workers.

35. Broughton HO, Buckel CM, Omvig KJ, Mullersman JL, Peipert JF, Secura GM. From Research to Practice: Dissemination of the Contraceptive Choice Project. *Translational Behavioral Medicine*. 2017;7(1):128–136.

36. Scullion PA. Effective Dissemination Strategies. *Nurse Researcher*. 2002;10(1):65–77.

37. Srivastav A, Spencer M, Thrasher JF, Strompolis M, Crouch E, Davis RE. Addressing Health and Well-Being through State Policy: Understanding Barriers and Opportunities for Policy-Making to Prevent Adverse Childhood Experiences (ACEs) in South Carolina. *American Journal of Health Promotion*. 2019:0890117119878068.

38. Committee to End Discrimination in Chicago Medical Institutions. What Color Are *Your* Germs? In: De Maio F, Shah RC, Mazzeo J, Ansell DA, eds. *Community Health Equity: A Chicago Reader*. Chicago: University of Chicago Press; 2019 [1954].

39. University of Wisconsion Population Health Institute. Sign-On: Racism Is a Public Health Crisis 2019. https://uwphi.pophealth.wisc.edu/match/match-wisconsin-healthiest-state-initiative/racism-is-a-public-health-crisis-in-wisconsin/#current-list-of-organizational-signers.

40. *GARE Communications Guide*. Government Alliance on Race & Equity; May 2018.

41. American Opportunity: A Communications Toolkit. https://www.racialequitytools.org/resourcefiles/opportunity.pdf.

NINE

Mobilizing to Action

Overcoming Chicago's 14-Year Life Expectancy Gap

PAMELA T. ROESCH, BRITTNEY S. LANGE-MAIA, EVE SHAPIRO, DARLENE OLIVER HIGHTOWER, VEENU VERMA, NIKHIL G. PRACHAND, EMILY LAFLAMME, AYESHA JACO, DAVID ANSELL, SHARON HOMAN, AND THE WEST SIDE UNITED METRICS WORKING GROUP

THE PREVIOUS THREE CHAPTERS of this book have demonstrated that most US cities experience substantial inequities in overall and cause-specific mortality, as well as inequalities in life expectancy by race. Across US cities, Black residents face disproportionately burdensome outcomes that cannot be explained solely by disparities in health care access or quality. Despite this trend, the epidemiologic patterns also illustrate the unique nature of inequities by city. Each city examined faces unique challenges related to overall mortality and life expectancy. This chapter presents a detailed case study of the efforts of one collaborative, West Side United (WSU), to mobilize toward health equity on Chicago's West Side. WSU began in 2017 when Rush University Medical Center, a longtime institution located on the West Side of Chicago, presented data on the overwhelmingly poor life expectancy and health outcomes in their service area with the aim of mobilizing a diverse stakeholder group to take action. The WSU case study creates an argument that sustainable pathways to health equity in US cities must be place-based and multisector, be rooted in social justice, and engage the most disadvantaged communities and their residents.

The History of Chicago's West Side

The West Side's history, population, challenges, and assets are reflected in the nearly 640,000 people (out of a total city population of 2.7 million) who live in the 10 West Side community areas served by WSU (Austin, Belmont Cragin, East and West Garfield Park, Humboldt Park, Lower West Side, Near West Side, North and South Lawndale, and West Town).[1] Most of these community areas (herein referred to as "communities") are low-income neighborhoods of color, with four consisting of predominantly Black populations and four of predominantly Hispanic/Latinx populations. Notwithstanding the unique histories of individual West Side neighborhoods, certain common events are identified as the drivers of extreme racial and economic segregation across the West Side[2] and the resulting poor health outcomes.

Originally a landing spot for European immigrant groups, the West Side began assuming its contemporary demographic makeup during and after World War II with the arrival of Mexican and African American immigrants attracted to the area's available manufacturing jobs and thriving residential and retail districts. As the Great Migration swelled Chicago's Black population,[3] unscrupulous and racist real estate practices, such as "blockbusting,"[4] contract buying, restrictive covenants,[5] and redlining,[6] heavily restricted where Black Chicagoans could live.[7] Systematic actions deliberately pursued by powerful, white, and racist institutions escalated in the 1950s, catalyzing white violence and intimidation against Black residents and, eventually, white flight. Purposeful economic disinvestment soon followed.[3] A case in point is the city's construction of an expressway in 1949 going from downtown through the West Side to the suburbs, bisecting and displacing communities along its path.[8] Local actions and policies of this sort, occurring amid an environment of federal policies that systematically made suburban homeownership unavailable to Blacks, dramatically changed the demographics of Chicago's neighborhoods, particularly the West Side. In West Garfield Park, the population changed from 0.05% Black in 1950 to 97.9% Black in 1970,[8] and in North Lawndale, the number of white residents dropped from 87,000 in 1950 to less than 11,000 in the 1960s, while the number of Black residents increased from 13,000 to nearly 125,000 over the same period.[9]

By the 1960s, Chicago had become a national epicenter of racially discriminatory practices in housing, employment, education, and policing, and its residents of color who clustered on the West and South Sides faced systemic barriers to wellness and economic vitality at every turn. In 1966, Martin Luther King Jr. and his family moved to the West Side to participate in the Chicago Freedom Movement, a northern extension of the civil rights movement, and to call attention to the plight facing his neighbors there.[10] Following King's assassination in April 1968, many cities experienced internal rebellions by residents. In Chicago, West Side commercial corridors in North Lawndale and East Garfield Park were especially impacted.[11] The departure of businesses, which had already begun due to a loss of white workers, increased over time.[10] The number of manufacturing jobs available in companies such as International Harvester and Sears in the Lawndale and Austin neighborhoods fell from nearly 25,000 in 1970 to less than 4,000 by 2015.[10,12] East and West Garfield Park went from over 18,000 retail jobs in 1970 to fewer than 400 by 2015.[12] The exodus of white residents, combined with business and economic flight, resulted in a population loss of 70% in communities like East Garfield Park.[13] The subsequent extreme concentrations of poverty and disadvantage continued, and in some areas increased, throughout the rest of the century.[14]

The long-standing segregation between Black and Latinx communities on the West Side has its origins in this period. As North Lawndale faced extreme business disinvestment, Eastern European residents from South Lawndale, directly south, worked to retain their local businesses and to separate their neighborhood's image from that of their neighbor to the north, renaming their community "Little Village."[15] This intentional segregation of a white neighborhood from a Black neighborhood eventually led to a strong Black/Latinx divide as Mexicans were pushed into South Lawndale when the University of Illinois at Chicago expanded its campus and the original Eastern European residents moved farther west.[15,16]

The impact these events had on the well-being of residents of color cannot be overstated. As of 2017, four West Side neighborhoods—

Austin, East and West Garfield Park, and North Lawndale—had life expectancies at or below 70 years of age (figure 9.1), compared to 81 years in Chicago's downtown Loop community. At the extreme, life expectancy in 2017 varied by up to 14 years when East Garfield Park and North Lawndale were compared with Chicago's affluent, predominantly white downtown Loop neighborhood. Additionally, predominantly Latinx communities with higher life expectancies (e.g., South Lawndale, Lower West Side) have seen downward trends in life expectancy over time, likely because of economic challenges facing Latinx in Chicago and demographic changes due to gentrification pressures.

Amid the challenges, West Side neighborhoods have demonstrated continued activism and resilience.[17] The West Side hosts a bevy of social

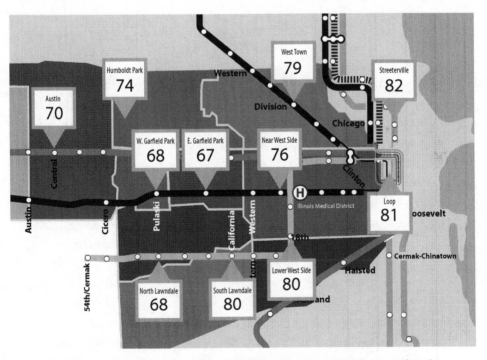

Figure 9.1. Life Expectancy in West Side United Communities Compared to the Downtown Loop Community (Chicago, IL). *Note:* Data are displayed for 2017 and are accessible at www.chicagohealthatlas.org/indicators/life-expectancy. *Source:* Rush University Medical Center.

service organizations, advocacy groups, religious organizations, and churches designed to support community needs. Throughout its neighborhoods, both vibrant and struggling commercial corridors are found, including the second-highest-grossing retail district in Chicago,[18] as well as varying access to community resources such as health and financial services. In addition, the West Side is home to numerous health care institutions and includes the Illinois Medical District, an area of over 560 acres encompassing four major hospitals, two major universities, and other health care- and biotechnology-related facilities.[19]

WSU: Moving toward Solutions-Focused Work on Chicago's West Side

I love the fact that the West Side already has everything it needs to be amazing. We just need to put it to work.

Participant, Coalition of Hope 2017
West Side United Listening Session

West Side United is a social justice response to the glaring life expectancy inequities evident on Chicago's West Side (figure 9.1). WSU and its partners operate from the assumption that the gaps witnessed in life expectancy stem from historic and ongoing structural racism rooted in societal and institutional laws, policies, and practices that have advantaged white populations over people of color. Chicago's West Side is filled with examples of structural racism, from real estate practices limiting home ownership in Black neighborhoods, to overaggressive and discriminatory policing tactics targeting communities of color, to long-standing disinvestment from local business communities. WSU recognizes the impact of these long-standing injustices on health and well-being and uses a social justice and health equity framework to collaboratively address structural racism in the health care sector and beyond. Particularly notable is how WSU involves West Side community residents as true partners and leaders in its efforts to coordinate across sectors and magnify its impact.

Building on the West Side's existing capacity of community and institutional resources, WSU is a collaborative of six major health and hospital systems, community residents, education providers, the faith community, businesses, government, and other organizations, such as the Illinois Medical District, aimed at improving health and economic vitality in 10 West Side communities (see table 9.1 for key partners). These partners serve a population nearly as large as the city of Las Vegas (the smallest city included in this book) and larger than Miami, St. Louis, and Oakland. Although WSU was initially spearheaded by health care institutions, stakeholders recognized early on that addressing clinical factors alone would be inadequate to impact health and life expectancy. Instead, WSU uses a place-based approach to achieve its vision of improving neighborhood health by addressing inequities in four domains: Education, Economic Vitality, Neighborhood and Physical Environment, and Health and Healthcare. Its mission is to build community health and economic wellness on Chicago's West Side and to build healthy, vibrant neighborhoods.

Many believe health equity means equal access to care, but it truly means every man, woman, and child has the chance to lead a long and healthy life. What drives the large gaps in life expectancy you see in Chicago are actually differences in social conditions under which people live, play, and work. Structural racism, a lack of community investment, and concentrated poverty are examples of social and structural conditions that contribute to health inequities. There are solutions, but it's not just health care alone. The most effective way is to improve neighborhoods. We are taking a holistic approach with West Side United. The goal is to reduce the overall life expectancy gap [with the downtown Loop neighborhood] by 50 percent by 2030.

David Ansell, MD, MPH, Senior Vice President for Community Health Equity and Associate Provost for Community Affairs, Rush University Medical Center; WSU Cofounder; and Executive Committee Member of the WSU Leadership Council

Table 9.1. West Side United (WSU) Key Stakeholders and Partners by Sector

Sector	Key Partners
Health/health care	Access Community Health Network Alivio Medical Center American Heart Association American Medical Association AMITA Health (*anchor hospital*) Ann and Robert H. Lurie Children's Hospital of Chicago (*anchor hospital*) CommunityHealth Consortium to Lower Obesity in Chicago Children Cook County Health and Hospital System (*anchor hospital*) Enlace Erie Family Health Center Esperanza Health Centers Illinois Medical District Lawndale Christian Health Center Local Federally Qualified Health Centers (FQHCs) Loretto Hospital Metropolitan Family Services National Alliance on Mental Illness Northshore Hospital Rush University Medical Center (*anchor hospital*) Sinai Health System (*anchor hospital*) TLSG University of Chicago Hospital University of Illinois Hospital and Health Sciences System (*anchor hospital*)
Public health	Alliance for Health Equity Center for Community Health Equity Chicago Department of Public Health HEAL Initiative Illinois Public Health Institute Sinai Urban Health Institute UIC School of Public Health
Corporate	A. T. Kearney Bain & Company Boston Consulting Group Canon CIBC U.S. Civic Consulting Alliance Kivvit KPMG McKinsey & Company Now Pow PwC Root, Inc. SG2 Verizon Wireless
Small business/local economy/employment	Accion Chicago Austin African American Business Networking Association Chicago Anchors for a Strong Economy Chicago Community Loan Fund

Sector	Key Partners
	Chicago Cook Workforce Partnership
	Chicagoland Healthcare Workforce Collaborative
	Economic Strategies Development Corporation
	IFF
	Little Village Chamber of Commerce
	Local Initiatives Support Corporation
	North Lawndale Employment Network
	Pilsen Alliance
	Pilsen Community Market Thresholds
	West Town Bikes
	Women's Business Development Center
	World Business Chicago
Education	Academy of Scholastic Achievement
	Austin College and Career Academy
	Benito Juarez High School
	Chicago Department of Family & Support Services
	Chicago Hope Academy
	Chicago Partnership for Health Promotion
	Chicago Public Schools
	ChiCat
	Christ the King College Prep
	City Colleges of Chicago
	Collins Academy High School
	Community Christian Alternative Academy
	Crane Medical Preparatory High School
	David G. Farragut Career Academy
	Douglass Library
	Frederick A. Douglass Academy High School
	George Westinghouse College Prep
	Hammond Elementary School
	Illinois Student Assistance Commission
	Infinity Math Science and Technology High School
	Instituto Health Science Career Academy High School
	ITW David Speer Academy
	John Marshall Metropolitan High School
	Kids First Chicago
	Kelvyn Park High School
	Legal Prep Charter Academy
	Little Village Lawndale High School
	Lozano Public Library
	Malcolm X College
	Manley Career Academy High School
	Maria Saucedo Scholastic Academy
	Michele Clark Academic Prep Magnet High School
	Noble DRW College Prep
	North Grand High School
	North Lawndale College Prep—Christiana
	North Lawndale College Prep—Collins
	Ombudsman Chicago West
	One Million Degrees
	Orr Academy
	Partnership for Resilience
	Phoenix Military Academy High School
	Project Exploration

(continued)

Table 9.1. (Continued)

Sector	Key Partners
	Prosser Career Academy
	Roberto Clemente Community Academy High School
	Skills for Chicagoland's Future
	Thrive Chicago
	UIC College Prep
	Urban Autism Solutions
	Whitney M. Young Magnet High School
	World Language High School
Housing	Chicago Coalition for the Homeless
	La Casa Norte
	Northwest Side Housing Center
Funders/philanthropy/government	The Ballmer Group
	Chicago Community Trust
	Chicago Workforce Funders Alliance
	Cook County Land Bank Authority
	Department of Business Affairs and Consumer Protection
	JPMorgan Chase & Co.
	Michael Reese Health Trust
	Northern Trust
	Polk Bros. Foundation
Community organizations	Austin Coming Together
	Austin Rising
	Chicago Access Network Television (CAN TV)
	The Community Builders
	Democracy Collaborative
	European American Association Pantry
	Farm on Ogden
	Forty Acres Fresh Farm
	Foxglove Alliance
	Garfield Park Community Council
	Greater Chicago Food Depository
	Harmony Community Church Pantry
	The Hatchery
	Hektoen Institute
	Homan Square Foundation
	Iglesia Evangelica Emmanuel Pantry
	Lawndale Christian Development Corporation
	MAAFA Redemption Project
	Marillac House Pantry
	Marshall Square Resource Network
	New Morning Star Food Pantry
	North Lawndale Community Coordinating Council
	Oak Park River Forest Food Pantry
	Pilsen Food Pantry
	Puerto Rican Cultural Center
	The Resurrection Project
	West Side Forward
	Windy City Dolphins
	Windy City Harvest
	YogaCare
	Youth Outreach Services

Sector	Key Partners
Faith community	Catholic Charities The Leaders Network New Mount Pilgrim Missionary Baptist Church St. Stephen AME Church
Residents	WSU Community Advisory Council Members
Small business grantees	6978 Soul Food Ad Hoc Property Services, LLC All the Details Cleaning Amazing Edibles Catering Back of the Yards Coffee, LLC (Pilsen Coffee House) BLK Building Solutions, LLC Chef's on the Go'Go, LLC La Chilangueda Colemans BBQ 2 The Corner Store Deli DermaPhilia DLV Printing Service, Inc. The Exodus Drum and Bugle Corp. Fitt City The Goodie Shop It Takes a Village The Lighthouse Café, LLC LiveEquipd, LLC Madison Ethos, Inc. McCanna Videography Metaphrasis Language and Cultural Solutions, LLC Rose and Jaad Construction, Inc. Salsedo Press, Inc. Smooth and Social Roots Social Impact Films Strickland Brothers BBQ & Jerk Sweet Beginnings, LLC A Taste of Nostalgia Terra Bites TheJumperStore.com, Inc. Thomas Mechanical Corporation Twenty Eleven Construction, Inc. US Veterans Security, LLC Worthy One Designs
Nonprofit grantees	Bethel New Life Foundation, dba West Side Forward Chicago Botanic Garden/Farm on Ogden Children's Home & Aid Erie Neighborhood House Garfield Park Community Council New Moms, Inc. North Lawndale Employment Network Project Exploration Telpochcalli Community Education Project United for Better Living, Inc.

Note: Current as of April 2020.

A Place-Based Approach Rooted in Social Justice

As noted, West Side United uses a cross-sector, place-based approach to pursue social justice and health equity. Place-based initiatives based on multisector collaboration and the engagement of community residents are gaining popularity as an increasingly strong body of emerging evidence highlights the role of social and economic factors in health outcomes.[20,21] Overall, place-based solutions seek to improve social and economic conditions within a particular geographic area, taking into account the area's unique history, needs, and assets.[20] Success depends on the involvement of key community stakeholders (e.g., residents, institutions, businesses) in identifying solutions that address the structural determinants of health, such as housing, education, economic vitality, health care, and policy.[20,22,23]

> *Each community should have [a] Planning Committee. Part of my concern is that person over in Humboldt Park . . . they might not know what the concerns over here [in Austin] are.*
>
> *Participant, Austin Coming Together*
> *2017 West Side United Listening Session*

Place-based solutions are still in their early stages; however, they have strong potential on account of their alliance with community residents and focus on the unique determinants of health in a particular place. Specifically critical for WSU's success is its coordination of institutions and community assets by a single entity and its concurrent focus on both the entire West Side and the West Side's 10 unique communities. WSU's focus on the whole service region without neglecting individual neighborhoods allows WSU to consider equity on the West Side overall and within each West Side neighborhood. From the outset, WSU leadership affirmed its desire to bring in community residents from each West Side community as experts and leaders to help develop its work. This commitment is built into all WSU does—from its organizational structure to the identification of initiatives to the selection of grantees.

[West Side communities] have programs and programs and programs, another program to add to the programs and we are still not getting anywhere.

Participant, Greater Galilee Baptist Church, 2017 West Side United Listening Session

Another element that distinguishes place-based change from traditional project-based work is its consideration of the interaction of these programs in people's lives. At its core, WSU is a collaborative of six anchor hospital and health care systems that encompass academic medical centers, safety net systems, and religiously affiliated entities. Combining these systems, along with residents and organizations, as true partners to address health, social, and economic issues offers an exciting avenue for creating communities where individuals can thrive. WSU lessens fragmentation by building synergies across projects and programs already operating in target communities, expanding successful approaches, and pursuing innovative and new solutions to long-standing challenges. The goal of this cross-sector, multipartner approach is to maximize impact at a larger scale.

We don't want to come together to "fix" the West Side. To be successful, we must build upon the collective power of residents, community-based organizations, the faith community, institutions, and government. Harnessing the work and ideas of this multisector group will move us beyond individual issues to address the assortment of challenges affecting health on the West Side. We can make our neighborhoods healthy and vibrant places to live. However, the work is bigger than any one person, organization, or institution.

Ayesha Jaco, Master of Art in Management (MAM), Executive Director of West Side United

Implementing a Place-Based Approach

Forming a Multisector Collaborative

In 2016, Rush University Medical Center (hereafter Rush), an academic medical center located on Chicago's West Side, was particularly concerned about the life expectancy inequities occurring in its own backyard. Rush's 2016 Community Health Needs Assessment (CHNA) focused on life expectancy gaps, the most illustrative statistic of the systemic inequities in neighboring communities. In response, Rush leadership, including its board of directors, changed the health facility's mission to focus on health equity and strengthen its commitment to community partnership. This system-wide strategy triggered Rush to rethink its approach to business operations (hiring, procurement, investing, etc.) and community programming. The revamped team quickly realized that reversing the effects of long-standing disinvestment and structural racism would require a more holistic, collective approach; one hospital alone could not address the life expectancy gaps identified in Rush's needs assessment.

Acknowledging the West Side's existing assets, particularly the health care and economic resources of local anchor hospital and health care systems, Rush forged a relationship with the Civic Consulting Alliance (CCA) to convene stakeholders around the innovative idea of taking a community-driven, collaborative, place-based approach to addressing systemic inequities. As an affiliate of the Civic Committee of the Commercial Club of Chicago, CCA is a nonprofit organization that draws on their experienced staff, best-in-class corporate pro bono partners, and deep public and private sector relationships to focus solutions at a systems level and create real impact that benefits the entire region.

> *What began as support to Rush University Medical Center to develop an internal anchor strategy has grown into West Side United, the nation's most ambitious multi-anchor community development initiative. The private sector has played a critical role in establishing and growing West Side United; Civic Consulting Alliance and our partners have contributed nearly $10 million in pro bono services to the effort since its inception in late 2016. But when the history of West Side United is written, I believe it will be the way that these (and other) institutional resources were brought together to work with and support community organizations and priorities, creating a new model of community AND institutions working together, that will be most important. In*

today's polarized world, models like West Side United are too few
and far between. Civic Consulting Alliance has been honored to
be part of the work from the beginning.

> Brian Fabes, Chief Executive Officer,
> Civic Consulting Alliance

Strong individual support among top leadership at Rush enabled the group to approach other hospitals, and in December 2016 Rush contacted two nearby hospital systems to ask them to join its growing partnership. Over the next year, three other West Side hospital systems joined. Several factors made this unique alliance possible. First, like Rush, many hospitals identified similar intractable health challenges on the West Side in their own CHNAs. Despite decades of individual efforts by these hospitals to alleviate local health inequities, they had seen little change. Additional support came from the Chicago Department of Public Health (CDPH), which provides rich neighborhood-level data as part of its Healthy Chicago 2.0 community health improvement plan.[24] Its data and neighborhood-level reports helped West Side hospitals understand the depth of these challenges.

Many leaders at the time were ready to take a different approach to pursue health improvement. In addition, Chicago hospitals had already started working together through an entity called the Alliance for Health Equity, which facilitated the undertaking of joint CHNAs. This collaboration provided a foundation that showed hospitals how they could pool resources to address shared aims. The opportune timing, the urgency revealed by the data, and the Alliance's demonstrated success helped persuade often-competing health care institutions of the value of joint partnerships.

> *Lurie Children's Hospital's mission is to improve the health and*
> *wellbeing of children. And we know that health is more than*
> *healthcare. We were honored to join West Side United, because to*
> *truly address the social influencers of health in Chicago, we need a*
> *data-driven, community-engaged, multi-sector collaborative.*
>
> Mary Kate Daly, MBA, Vice President,
> Lurie Children's Healthy Communities;

Cochair, WSU Anchor Committee; and, Member,
WSU Impact Investing and Small Business
Grant Pool Working Groups

Pursuing True Community Engagement

Place-based approaches put community residents in the lead as the drivers of these multisector initiatives. From the outset, West Side United institutions worked with community residents to develop strategies to tackle the effects of historically racist policies and systems that were still adversely affecting well-being throughout the West Side. Figure 9.2 provides a detailed timeline of WSU's formation and highlights key community-focused activities in its foundational years.

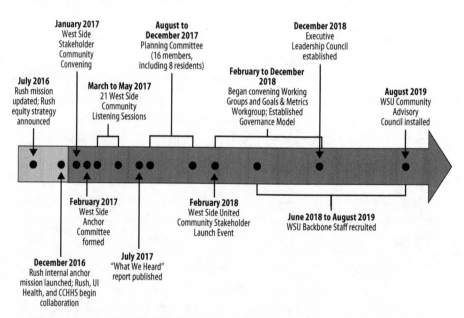

Figure 9.2. West Side United (WSU) High-level Timeline of Key Activities (July 2016 to August 2019). *Note:* Rush: Rush University Medical Center; UI Health: University of Illinois Hospital & Health Sciences System; CCHHS: Cook County Health and Hospital System.

The community has to be the ones to do it. It has to come from within.

> Participant, Oakley Square Apartments
> 2017 WSU Listening Session

The first step in the process was a series of discussions with community residents about the links between structural racism and well-being. WSU kicked off activities by convening several local organizations and stakeholders in early 2017. It then held 21 smaller community listening sessions with residents, community-based organizations, social service agencies, educational institutions, public sector agencies, foundations, and others. The sessions encouraged attendees to share their feedback about creating an inclusive, equitable, and representative collaborative.

[We need to] cultivate relationships first, have one-on-ones, and learn what are the concerns from those at the table. Don't make top-down decisions and then invite everyone to something that has been already decided.

> Katya Nuques, Executive Director,
> Enlace Chicago, at January 2017 WSU Convening

The sessions reaffirmed several key tenets of WSU's approach: its commitment to assets-based approaches and community engagement that recognizes residents as key decision-makers, its focus on collaboration, and its aim to harness the diversity and unique neighborhood identities of the West Side in solutions.[25]

Presence, trust, and consistency are the three things that are going to be the most important in sustaining this program.

> Participant, Salvation Army, 2017
> WSU Listening Session

WSU felt that it was imperative to publicly share the feedback coming from these sessions to let participants see their contributions and voices reflected in the work to follow. WSU published a "What We Heard" report that was shared with participants by mailing and hand-delivering hard copies to listening session hosts and by posting it online.[25] It also used the suggestions as a foundation for resulting initiatives and to develop a WSU Planning Committee of 16 members, who were in part nominated by those who attended the listening sessions (8 West Side residents and 8 representatives from local organizations that had a strong presence on the West Side, such as CDPH, NAMI Chicago, and Metropolitan Family Services, among others). The Planning Committee and WSU leadership worked together from August to December 2017 to develop 10 initiatives that were announced at a Community Stakeholder Launch the following February. The remainder of 2018 was spent forming Working Groups to incubate the 10 initiatives, develop a governance structure, and determine a metrics and evaluation approach. WSU also hosted 25 more community listening sessions that year. This work culminated in the organizational structure and strategic approach in place today.

Organizing to Ensure Ongoing Partnership

Early on, WSU leadership carefully considered how to structure itself to ensure transparency among partners, institutionalize continued executive and community leadership, and facilitate ongoing momentum and participation of stakeholders, residents, and institutions. The planners were guided by three principles in developing WSU's operational and governance structure:

1. *Equity*: Community representation would be part of every level of governance and operations, guaranteeing community residents a central role in the decision-making process from the start.
2. *Distributed Leadership*: Accountability and leadership would be distributed across the hospitals, with each offering its unique strengths and assets.
3. *Flexibility*: Governance would remain flexible, agile, and adaptable to respond to evolving needs; this meant an openness toward new institutions, partners, initiatives, and practices that could further progress toward their goal of improving life expectancies.

WSU anchor hospitals, leadership, and Working Group members were committed to these driving principles in determining the organizational structure. It took about a year to create the structure, throughout which the organizers responded to continuing feedback and changed course when it meant closer alignment with the founding principles. Table 9.2 outlines the resulting organizational structure. A key element is the

Table 9.2. West Side United (WSU) Organizational Structure

Role	WSU Entity	Description	Responsibilities
Strategy	Leadership Council	Includes six executive-level reps. from anchor hospitals, six community reps. from CAC and ex officio members Includes three-person Executive Committee	Defines WSU's long-term vision, success, and priorities; secures resources to support WSU; decides funding allocation (operations vs. programmatic areas)
Management	Operations Committee	Staff reps. (community engagement or government relations staff) from all six anchor hospitals Group met until Q1 2018, when Backbone WSU Staff assumed much of its role; group still provides ad hoc support as needed	Supports, augments, and coordinates WSU's work within their own organizations; links Leadership Council to WSU's original Planning Committee; in early years, planned WSU strategy, events, funding approaches, and other infrastructure activities
	CAC	Council of 18 West Side community residents	Provides critical feedback to and participates on Leadership Council and Working Groups; provides a link between WSU and community residents and organizations
Execution	Backbone WSU Staff	Nine WSU staff members	Provides day-to-day infrastructure and support to execute WSU strategies; manages and coordinates Working Groups; coordinates community engagement events
	Working Groups	Individual groups aligned to specific WSU initiatives and domains (e.g., Anchor Strategy Steering Committee, Metrics Working Group); led by hospital cochairs and supported by other hospital practitioners, WSU staff, initiative partners (e.g., CBOs, service providers), and CAC members	Designs and implements initiatives across WSU's domains (Education, Economic Vitality, Neighborhood and Physical Environment, and Health and Healthcare); includes WSU Metrics Working Group

Notes: reps.: representatives; CBO: community-based organization; CAC: Community Advisory Council.

development of the Community Advisory Council (CAC) to facilitate community resident inclusion as decision-makers in all of WSU's work.

I love seeing the beauty of working together, and institutions becoming a part of the community. I am sitting at the table with heroes, owning their part in the disparity of a community and taking action to correct it.

Angela Taylor, Wellness Coordinator, Garfield Park Community Council; and Member, WSU Community Advisory Council

Building Synergy among Stakeholders

Taking its lead from the 2016 CHNA findings and feedback from hospital and community partners in 2017, West Side United targets improvement in the structural determinants of health across four domains: Education, Economic Vitality, Neighborhood and Physical Environment, and Health and Healthcare. WSU's primary assumption is that collective action taken to achieve equity within these four domains will improve the overall well-being and life expectancy of residents. Initiatives within each domain complement each other, creating the potential for broader, complementary community change. For example, as part of the Economic Vitality domain, WSU administers the Small Business Grant (SBG) program, which awards grants and provides capacity-building support to small West Side businesses and entrepreneurs. Within this domain, WSU also leads a hospital procurement initiative that works with hospitals to connect local businesses to hospital supply chains. In an effort to create synergy between these two Economic Vitality initiatives, WSU works with hospitals to specifically connect small businesses that have been funded through the SBG program to hospital supply chains—increasing the success of both programs in strengthening the local business community. Complementary to Economic Vitality activities, WSU initiatives in its Neighborhood and Physical Environment domain aim to improve the built environment through strategic investment. By creating an environment where small businesses can flourish and that consumers feel enticed to frequent, initiatives within the Economic Vitality and Neighborhood and Physical Environment domains create synergistic movement toward the goal of building a thriving West Side business community.

> *Vibrant small businesses are key to boosting commercial activity in a neighborhood, creating jobs for local residents and building a prosperous community. At JPMorgan Chase, we are committed to supporting small business activity, with a focus on entrepreneurs of color, as part of our $40 million investment to connect South and West Side residents with economic opportunity.*
>
> Charlie Corrigan, Head of Midwest
> Philanthropy, JPMorgan Chase

To accelerate progress across domains, WSU focuses on four strategies that capitalize on the unique assets provided by anchor hospitals:

1. accelerate hospital anchor strategies;
2. coordinate hospital community efforts;
3. unite the West Side; and
4. pilot new ideas across domains.

Activities within the strategies are driven by feedback gathered from residents and organizations in the initial years of planning (2017 and 2018), as well as data from hospital CHNAs about key areas of need on the West Side. Each strategy includes several key initiatives that also align with the domains.

The first strategy, *accelerating hospital anchor strategies*, fast-tracks existing WSU and hospital efforts to use hospitals' own economic resources to increase economic vitality on the West Side. This focus acknowledges that hospitals are part of the systems that may perpetuate inequitable outcomes. A key feature of the first strategy is an acknowledgment that hospitals employ community residents and invest substantial capital within their neighborhoods. The health care industry hires a large number of entry-level workers, many of whom have no opportunity to advance further within the industry. A key initiative within this strategy is the development of streamlined career pathways that offer full-time, low-wage hospital staff access to higher-paid positions as trained and certified clinical professionals while continuing to work. Other key initiatives focus on hospital- and partner-funded grant investments to small, for-profit local businesses (the SBG program previously described) and the overhaul of hospital procurement strategies to source equipment and services from West Side businesses and/or vendors (also previously described).

The second strategy, *coordinating hospital community efforts*, aims to increase coordination between existing hospital health improvement initiatives, often through coordination with community stakeholders, to minimize duplication and increase effectiveness. As partner hospitals serving the same communities, many target the same health and social challenges. Coordinating efforts can maximize capacity and potential effectiveness by pooling resources, expertise, and best practices. Current activities coordinated by WSU include a cross-hospital effort to strengthen the emergency food safety net by connecting food-insecure patients with local pantries, the joint development of community health worker capacity building, and the aggregation of hospital hypertension control quality metrics to identify best practices and facilitate shared learning.

The third strategy, *uniting the West Side*, positions WSU as the entity to unite existing improvement efforts by reducing silos and competition between programs. Here the focus is on convening stakeholders involved in all relevant West Side initiatives and augmenting the resources and partnerships of successful existing efforts. Activities include a regular convening of community listening sessions and supporting local nonprofits by awarding small hospital- and partner-funded grants (another element of the SBG program).

The fourth and final strategy, *piloting new ideas across domains*, targets life expectancy through innovation. Currently, the strategy's key activity is a community hub partnership with Chicago Public Schools. Following a series of workshops and the participation of a diverse team focused on educational outcomes, WSU identified a need for community hubs in West Side schools. These hubs provide a broad range of wraparound support services to students, including access to primary care and mental health services, trauma-informed training for teachers, exposure to health care career opportunities, and other programs.

Using Data to Measure Progress

Accountability is the largest barrier with collaboratives. Who's going to get credit and who's accountable when things go wrong?
Darnell Shields, Executive Director of Austin
Coming Together, January 2017
WSU Convening

As West Side United established its organizational structure, governance, and key initiatives, the group recognized the need to assess their collective impact over time and to measure their progress in meeting their goal of reducing the life expectancy gap between West Side communities and Chicago's downtown Loop neighborhood by 50% by 2030. All parties understand that life expectancy cannot be improved over night, and WSU is committed to a long-term approach. However, WSU realized that a mechanism to show short- and long-term progress would help keep activities on track and foster ongoing participation. WSU created a Metrics Working Group to identify an assessment approach that would

1. tie specific outcomes of individual WSU initiatives to WSU's overarching life expectancy goal through a series of iterative metrics showing short-, medium-, and long-term progress;
2. guide WSU's ongoing strategic decisions and initiatives; and
3. coalesce anchor hospitals and stakeholders around shared goals.

Beyond these aims, it was vital to develop a measurement approach rooted in health equity that took into account equity on the West Side as a whole without losing sight of equity across and within WSU's 10 unique neighborhoods. The approach also needed to be readily understandable to a broad group of stakeholders without losing sight of the complex network of factors that influence life expectancy. Finally, the approach needed to inform and embrace midcourse strategic changes that could accommodate the expansion of successful initiatives and the refinement of those not meeting desired aims.

The WSU Metrics Working Group

The WSU Metrics Working Group comprised public health experts from partner hospitals and stakeholder institutions such as CDPH, CCA, WSU program managers, and CAC. Members had technical expertise in epidemiology, community-based and behavioral interventions, program evaluation, community-based participatory research, community engagement, survey design/administration, and health inequities research, as well as content expertise in a variety of health-related areas (e.g., social determinants of health, aging, psychology, maternal and child health, infectious disease, chronic conditions, and substance use). The participation of CDPH was particularly helpful because of the department's strong commitment to health equity and its wealth of community-specific data and epidemiologic expertise. Furthermore, CDPH was in the process of conducting its own Healthy Chicago 2025 Community Health Assessment, which allowed both entities to better align their longer-term aims for improved health. While WSU focuses on the West Side, the issues it targets are the same as those that the city is grappling with—having alignment with the city is vital because WSU and CDPH are now working to address similar underlying issues. The Working Group's leadership was made up of WSU's director of data and evaluation, Eve Shapiro, MPH; CCA representative Veenu Verma, who was familiar with WSU's history and aims; and two public health epidemiologists from participating anchor hospitals, Pamela Roesch, MPH (from Sinai Health System), and Brittney Lange-Maia, PhD, MPH (from Rush University Medical Center), who were well versed in racial health inequities and community-level health research.

If we are to make any progress towards reversing the widening racial gaps in life expectancy we see in Chicago today, the public health system needs to squarely acknowledge the effects of social and institutional racism as the root cause of the city's most glaring health inequities. The successful implementation of Chicago Department of Public's Health call to action—Healthy

Chicago 2025, which brings a racial equity focus to the improvement of conditions in which people live—has benefited greatly from strongly aligned efforts like the West Side United to affect measurable change across the communities that have most greatly endured historical disinvestment and social exclusion.
Nikhil Prachand, MPH, Director of Epidemiology,
Chicago Department of Public Health

Tiers of Impact: Measuring Progress toward Equity

The following sections outline how the Metrics Working Group developed West Side United's final assessment approach using evidence-based best practices.[26] The resulting Assessment Framework is first described to provide an end point for readers before summarizing the steps taken to define it. At a broad level, the WSU Assessment Framework tracks the progress of individual initiatives in meeting WSU's overarching goal to reduce the life expectancy gap through three levels, or tiers, of impact (figure 9.3). The three-tiered approach is essential for tracking incremental progress toward WSU's overarching goal as it works upward from the measurement of initiative-level metrics (e.g., SBG program outputs and outcomes), to domain-related community-wide metrics (e.g., unemployment rates by community), to health-related community-wide metrics that influence life expectancy (e.g., cause-specific mortality rates by community).

The framework is based on the assumption that to reduce the life expectancy gap, meaningful improvement must be demonstrated in health and disease-specific mortality (Tier I). Progress in these areas requires evidence of improvement across metrics in the four domains: Education, Economic Vitality, Neighborhood and Physical Environment, and Health and Healthcare (Tier II). Ideally, evidence of improvement within the four domains should predict improvement in the mortality and life expectancy metrics in Tier I. It is notable that within Tiers I and II, measurements are at the community level, such as rates of unemployment within each WSU community (rather than among just the participants in

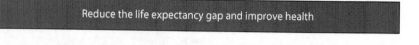

Tier I. WSU Overarching Goal (Community-Level Health, Mortality, and Life Expectancy Metrics)

Reduce the life expectancy gap and improve health

Tier II. WSU Domains of Impact (Domain-Related, Community-Level Metrics)

| Education | Economic Vitality | Neighborhood & Physical Environment | Health and Healthcare |

Tier III. WSU Initiatives (Initiative-Level Metrics)

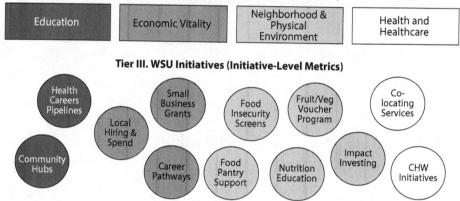

Figure 9.3. West Side United (WSU) Three-Tiered Assessment Framework. *Notes:* Circles in Tier III represent examples of existing initiatives. CHW: community health workers.

WSU programs). Tier III incorporates initiative-level assessment metrics. At this level, the same community-level metrics identified in Tiers I and II (e.g., unemployment) are tracked, but just among participants. Additionally, the team tracks initiative process, output, and outcome metrics to facilitate ongoing evaluation and encourage continuous improvement. The three-tiered WSU Assessment Framework connects the dots between individual initiatives and WSU's overarching goal and facilitates ongoing monitoring and refining as WSU moves toward this goal.

> We created the WSU Metrics Working Group to mobilize neighborhood-level data, research and evaluation expertise, and community knowledge to make the case for, assess, and inform our health equity strategies and initiatives. We believe the resulting Framework, data, and tools will enable us to work with community residents, as well as the WSU partners,

and use metrics of interest to measure progress toward our shared goals.

Sharon Homan, PhD, Former President, Sinai Urban Health Institute, Sinai Health System; and, Former Member, WSU Executive Leadership Council

Developing a Framework: Identifying Tier I Community-Level Life Expectancy and Mortality Metrics

West Side United's first step in understanding life expectancy inequities on the West Side was to examine the causes of premature death. To start, the Metrics Working Group coordinated with its CDPH members to use the results of an existing CDPH analysis that used Arriaga's decomposition method to compare the causes and ages of death in each of the 10 West Side communities with those of the Near North community (a downtown, high-income, predominantly non-Latinx white neighborhood).[27] While WSU's overarching goal is relative to the downtown Loop community, that community's smaller population was not amenable to the Arriaga assessment. However, the demographics and overall life expectancies of the two communities (Loop and Near North) are very similar. The decomposition analysis revealed, for example, that between 2012 and 2016 a disproportionate number of heart-disease-related deaths in Austin were responsible for 2.4 years of the overall 11.4-year life expectancy gap between Austin and Near North. In other words, if Austin's heart-disease-related death rate were brought down to that seen in the Near North, one would expect to see a 2.4-year decrease in the life expectancy gap between these two neighborhoods. In the CDPH analysis, cardiometabolic diseases were the largest contributors to the life expectancy gaps in all West Side communities. When considering years of life lost, a small number of individuals who die very young from causes like infant mortality and homicide will affect life expectancy rates disproportionately, comparable to the effect of a large number of people who die just below the age of average life expectancy as a result of chronic disease (e.g., diabetes or heart disease). To identify mortality drivers to target in Tier I, the Metrics Working Group compared the key contributors to premature mortality, such as heart-disease-related deaths, cancer-related deaths, and homicides, within the 10 West Side communities. The group examined deaths by age group to determine those having a disproportionately negative impact on life expectancy rates and the life expectancy gap; for example, deaths caused by infant mortality, homicide, and opioid overdose have a greater effect on rates in the aggregate because of their relatively young ages individually. Finally, the Metrics Working Group incorporated other publicly available focus group data from the West Side and community feedback from WSU planning activities (2017 and 2018) to confirm that there was a level of community momentum and support around the final set of key mortality drivers. This step was taken to incorporate both empirical data and community feedback into the final Assessment Framework, balancing WSU's data-driven and community-driven approaches.

Five mortality drivers were ultimately identified for Tier I: *cardiometabolic disease* (heart-disease-, diabetes-, and stroke-related deaths), *cancer, infant mortality* (including maternal mortality), *homicide*, and *opioid overdose*. Depending on the community, these mortality drivers explained anywhere from 48% to 73% of the life expectancy gap between each WSU neighborhood and the city's downtown area (table 9.3).

Table 9.3. Gap in Life Expectancy between West Side United (WSU) Communities and Downtown Near North Community Explained by Five Mortality Drivers

WSU Community	Life Expectancy	Total Gap with Near North (years)	Gap Explained by Five Mortality Drivers (years)	Gap Explained by Five Mortality Drivers (%)
West Garfield Park	70.45	13.15	9.56	73
East Garfield Park	70.77	12.83	9.14	71
North Lawndale	71.07	12.53	8.36	67
Austin	72.18	11.43	7.79	68
Humboldt Park	75.45	8.15	5.22	64
Near West Side	78.06	5.55	3.74	67
West Town	79.91	3.70	1.92	52
Belmont Cragin	80.67	2.94	1.95	66
South Lawndale	81.08	2.53	1.21	48
Lower West Side	81.19	2.42	1.41	58

Notes: Data from 2012–2016. Near North life expectancy: 83.61. Mortality drivers: cardiometabolic disease (heart-disease-, diabetes-, and stroke-related deaths), cancer, infant mortality (including maternal mortality), homicide, and opioid overdose.

While the decomposition analysis revealed these results to WSU prior to the publication of this book, the data seen for Chicago in earlier chapters would lead to a similar output (Chicago had the fifth-largest racial inequity for cancer mortality of the 29 included cities and the third-highest inequity for opioid-related deaths). Therefore, WSU's experience suggests that other cities may not need to go about a local decomposition analysis to identify key drivers of the Black:white life expectancy gaps identified in this book. The results within previous chapters should provide a quick idea of key mortality areas of focus to decrease Black:white gaps in life expectancy and premature death.

After confirming the five mortality drivers, the Metrics Working Group identified Tier I metrics available by community to assess improvement in disease-specific mortality rates over time. The criteria used to select the metrics (e.g., coronary heart disease death rate and gun-related homicide rate) are outlined in table 9.4; however, disease-specific mortality rates derived from public health surveillance data provided regularly by CDPH were mostly used.[28]

Developing a Framework: Identifying Tier II Community-Level Domain Metrics

With the five mortality drivers and associated metrics identified, the Metrics Working Group moved into the four domains in Tier II: Education, Economic Vitality, Neighborhood and Physical Environment, and Health and Healthcare. They began by gathering a list of metrics available from national, state, and citywide sources that could be calculated at the community level. Sources included vital statistics from the Illinois Department of Public Health, Healthy Chicago Survey[29] data from CDPH, crime statistics from the Chicago Police Department, data on community socioeconomic factors from the American Community Survey (US Census), and hospital data from the Illinois Hospital Association. The list of over 150 metrics was initially developed by CDPH for its Healthy Chicago 2025 Community Health Assessment. It allowed the Metrics Working Group to have a universal view of the metrics that could be measured.

Table 9.4. West Side United (WSU) Selection Criteria for Tier II (Domains of Impact) and Tier I (Overarching Goal) Assessment Framework Metrics

Criteria	Question	Description	Example
Cross-cutting	"Do the metrics reflect community sentiment, and is the metric applicable across communities?"	To facilitate collaboration and alignment, chose metrics (a) supportive of overarching goals, (b) reflective of community sentiment and areas of concern, (c) prevalent across the diverse communities, (d) aligned to City initiatives, such as CDPH's Healthy Chicago 2.0	Economic Vitality: Unemployment and Individual Poverty Neighborhood and Physical Environment: Perceptions of Safety and Violent Crime
Changeability	"How feasible is it for WSU and its partners to solve the problem/improve the metric by 2030?"	Focused on activities WSU could directly change given its current resources, four domains of impact, and four strategies	Despite clean air's link to health, this is not a direct focus of WSU's strategies; therefore, eliminated this from final list of metrics
Impact	"If we see improvement in this metric over time, will it impact downstream health outcomes and our drivers of the life expectancy gap? If we see improvement in this metric over time, how great of an impact would it have on our other downstream health outcomes and the five drivers?"	Focused on metrics with greatest potential impact rather than several metrics promising smaller effect; based decisions partly on research identifying driver-specific logic models	Educational attainment is closely related to subsequent employment and income, as well as to various improvements in health outcomes
Repeatability	"Is this measure continually tracked over time?"	Included previously published metrics that would be collected continually at the community level moving forward	Local jobs availability was not included in final list because the data source was not updated regularly
Sensitivity	"Will changes in this metric truly reflect that there are underlying community changes taking place?"	Gave priority to metrics that are sensitive to change from interventions and will move over time (up and/or down)	Third-grade reading levels and child poverty are closely linked to high school graduation rates
Understandability	"Is this metric easily understood and broadly acceptable to stakeholders and community residents?"	Indices encompassing multiple metrics can be difficult to interpret and to assess change over time, so examined individual variables rather than entire indices to aid interpretation	Economic hardship index compiles metrics (e.g., unemployment, level of education, crowded housing) into a composite score useful to describe community economic conditions, but changes in this relative index are hard to interpret, and the index is not widely recognized by a lay audience

Note: CDPH: Chicago Department of Public Health.

Working Group members assessed existing research regarding the metrics most closely linked to poorer health across the five mortality drivers, particularly those related to mortality inequities between racial/ethnic groups. For each mortality driver (e.g., cardiometabolic disease), the Metrics Working Group identified the most influential factors of the mortality inequity. For example, they found that living in areas of high poverty and living in areas of high unemployment were key factors explaining the Black:white preterm birth inequity in Illinois,[30] that food insecurity was associated with increased risk of type 2 diabetes[31] and cardiovascular disease,[32] and that homelessness was associated with higher all-cause mortality.[33] The Working Group members then identified key metrics within each domain (e.g., Economic Vitality) that predicted the mortality drivers, creating five mortality-driver-specific logic models. After identifying a large list of potential metrics within the mortality-driver-specific logic models, the group used the criteria in table 9.4 to select a curated set of metrics seen in figure 9.4. In addition to setting the metrics, the group included superscripts in figure 9.4 (i.e., CM, CN, IM, H, OO) to indicate which of the five mortality drivers were tied to each Tier II metric, a reflection of the mortality-driver-specific logic models created by the team.

Tier I and Tier II Goal Setting

Once the Tier I and Tier II community-level metrics were established, the team baselined its values for 2017, the year preceding WSU's first initiatives within each West Side community. Because the Working Group focused on place-based change and equity, it did not aggregate metrics *across* the West Side. From there, it set goals for each metric, keeping in mind WSU's overarching goal to reduce the life expectancy gap by 50%, as well as existing WSU initiatives that already targeted some metrics. In setting short- and long-term goals (for 2025 and 2030), the Working Group used Healthy People 2030's goal-setting approach,[34] had discussions with CDPH about the Healthy Chicago 2.0 goal-setting approach,[24] and considered both national and Healthy Chicago 2.0 targets for the same metrics.[24,35] In addition, although it collected data by community, for simplicity's sake the Metrics Working Group limited itself to one goal

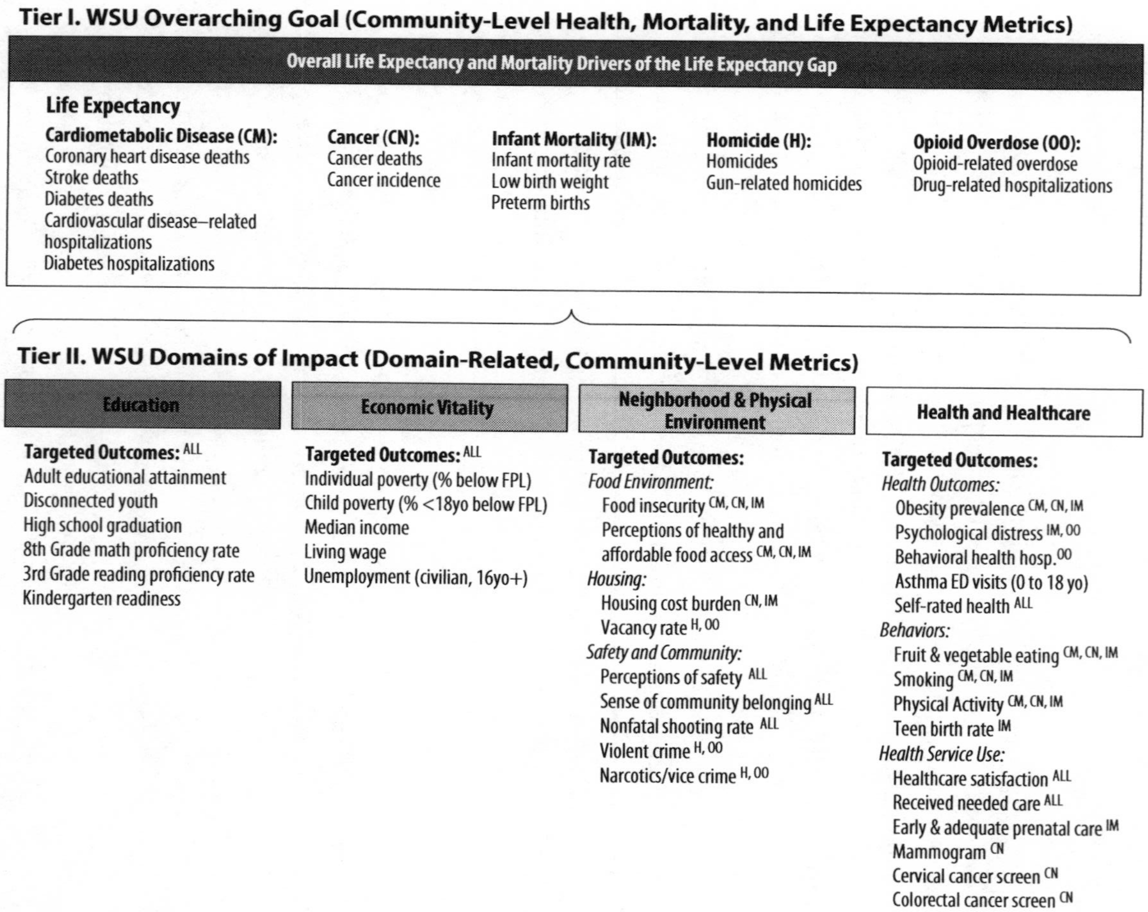

Tier I. WSU Overarching Goal (Community-Level Health, Mortality, and Life Expectancy Metrics)

Overall Life Expectancy and Mortality Drivers of the Life Expectancy Gap

Life Expectancy

Cardiometabolic Disease (CM):
Coronary heart disease deaths
Stroke deaths
Diabetes deaths
Cardiovascular disease–related hospitalizations
Diabetes hospitalizations

Cancer (CN):
Cancer deaths
Cancer incidence

Infant Mortality (IM):
Infant mortality rate
Low birth weight
Preterm births

Homicide (H):
Homicides
Gun-related homicides

Opioid Overdose (OO):
Opioid-related overdose
Drug-related hospitalizations

Tier II. WSU Domains of Impact (Domain-Related, Community-Level Metrics)

Education	Economic Vitality	Neighborhood & Physical Environment	Health and Healthcare

Education

Targeted Outcomes: ALL
Adult educational attainment
Disconnected youth
High school graduation
8th Grade math proficiency rate
3rd Grade reading proficiency rate
Kindergarten readiness

Economic Vitality

Targeted Outcomes: ALL
Individual poverty (% below FPL)
Child poverty (% <18yo below FPL)
Median income
Living wage
Unemployment (civilian, 16yo+)

Neighborhood & Physical Environment

Targeted Outcomes:
Food Environment:
Food insecurity CM, CN, IM
Perceptions of healthy and affordable food access CM, CN, IM
Housing:
Housing cost burden CN, IM
Vacancy rate H, OO
Safety and Community:
Perceptions of safety ALL
Sense of community belonging ALL
Nonfatal shooting rate ALL
Violent crime H, OO
Narcotics/vice crime H, OO

Health and Healthcare

Targeted Outcomes:
Health Outcomes:
Obesity prevalence CM, CN, IM
Psychological distress IM, OO
Behavioral health hosp. OO
Asthma ED visits (0 to 18 yo)
Self-rated health ALL
Behaviors:
Fruit & vegetable eating CM, CN, IM
Smoking CM, CN, IM
Physical Activity CM, CN, IM
Teen birth rate IM
Health Service Use:
Healthcare satisfaction ALL
Received needed care ALL
Early & adequate prenatal care IM
Mammogram CN
Cervical cancer screen CN
Colorectal cancer screen CN

Figure 9.4. Selected West Side United (WSU) Tier I and II Metrics for the WSU Three-Tiered Assessment Framework. *Note:* FPL: federal poverty level; yo: years old; ED: emergency department.

per metric, rather than 10 individual goals for each target community. For nine of these metrics, including infant mortality, housing cost burden, and obesity, WSU's 2025 goals were aligned with the citywide 2025 goals set forth in the Chicago Community Health Improvement Plan, Healthy Chicago 2.0.[24] An exception to setting a single goal across communities was WSU's overarching life expectancy goal, which was set at a 50% reduction in the life expectancy inequity between each West Side community and the downtown Loop community using 2017 baseline values. For example, 2017 life expectancy in Austin was 70.1, compared to 81.6 in the Loop; therefore, to reduce this gap by 50% by 2030, the difference between the two communities (81.6 − 70.1 = 11.5 years) was divided in half (11.5/2 = 5.75) and then added to Austin's 2017 life expectancy to reach the 2030 goal of 75.9 (70.1 + 5.75 = 75.9). Table 9.5 shows the

Table 9.5. West Side United (WSU) 2025 and 2030 Goals for Adult Obesity (Tier II: Domains of Impact) and Life Expectancy (Tier I: WSU Overarching Goal) by Community

WSU Communities	Adult Obesity Prevalence[a]			Life Expectancy	
	Baseline[b]	2025 Goal	2030 Goal	Baseline[c]	2030 Goal
Belmont Cragin	32.4	27.6	10.4	79.7	80.7
Humboldt Park	35.4	27.6	10.4	74.7	78.1
West Town	18.7	27.6	10.4	80.0[d]	80.8
Austin	38.9	27.6	10.4	70.1	75.9
West Garfield Park	44.6	27.6	10.4	68.5	75.1
East Garfield Park	33.4	27.6	10.4	67.7	74.7
Near West Side	19.8	27.6	10.4	76.3	79.0
North Lawndale	46.8	27.6	10.4	68.1	74.9
South Lawndale	42.5	27.6	10.4	80.5	81.0
Lower West Side	24.2	27.6	10.4	80.2	80.9
Downtown Loop	10.4	N/A	N/A	81.6	N/A
City of Chicago	30.8	N/A	N/A	77.2	N/A
Goal-setting method	Healthy Chicago 2.0 Goal in 2025; Loop 2017 value in 2030			Reduce 2017 gap between each WSU community and the Loop by 50% by 2030	

[a] Percentages weighted to represent the population from which the sample was drawn (household population of adults 18 years of age and older residing in Chicago); obesity is defined as a body mass index of 30 or greater, based on self-reported height and weight.
[b] Community estimates are pooled 3-year estimates for 2015–17; Chicago estimate is 1-year estimate for 2017.
[c] Estimated for the year 2017.
[d] Life expectancy is <80 years (79.9984), so it is reported as 79 elsewhere in this chapter (figure 9.1); however, when rounded in this table, it rounds to 80.

difference between the overarching life expectancy goal and the individual metrics goals (e.g., adult obesity).

The goal setting demonstrated that each community on the West Side had different baseline levels of risk factors and therefore would require different strategies to achieve the goals. This was particularly important to the assessment of WSU's success, whose overarching life expectancy goal was not a combined average across the West Side, but rather a community-specific goal. In other words, to be successful, each community would have to see progress in reducing the gap in life expectancy between itself and the downtown Loop community by 50% by 2030.

Developing a Framework: Assessing Tier III Initiatives and Programs

One aim of the WSU Assessment Framework was to create a culture of learning that accommodated both the growth of successful initiatives and ongoing adjustments to initiatives not meeting desired aims. The assessment of initiatives and programs within Assessment Framework Tier III is critical for this approach. Tier III, which measures the progress of individual initiatives, ties together all three tiers of impact by linking WSU's initiatives on the ground to changes within its domains of impact (Tier II) and health (Tier I). Resource constraints prevented the Metrics Working Group from undertaking quality improvement and evaluation activities for every WSU initiative. Therefore, Metrics Working Group members work closely with WSU's initiative-focused Working Groups and Backbone Staff to build capacity to measure progress. The Metrics Working Group members advise these groups to develop logic models and data collection plans for all WSU initiatives that connect WSU's on-the-ground work to the metrics in the Assessment Framework. Table 9.6 offers examples of this linkage for four initiatives. For example, investment in local small businesses is expected to produce an increase of living wage jobs for West Side residents. A measurement component built into the SBG program enables WSU to assess whether the funded business increased local hiring and provided living wage jobs. If not, an assessment will be made to determine why and suggest ideas for

Table 9.6. Linking West Side United (WSU) Initiative Metrics (Tier III) to Domain-Level (Tier II) and Health-Related (Tier I) Metrics

| Domain/ Strategy | Initiative/ Programs | Tier III. Initiatives/Programs (Initiative-/Participant-Level Metrics) | | Tier II. Domains (Community-Level Domain Metrics) | Tier I. Overarching Goals (Community-Level Health Metrics) |
| | | Activities | Outputs | Outcomes | | |

Domain/ Strategy	Initiative/ Programs	Activities	Outputs	Outcomes	Tier II. Domains (Community-Level Domain Metrics)	Tier I. Overarching Goals (Community-Level Health Metrics)
Domain: Economic Vitality Strategy: accelerate hospital anchor strategies	Small Business Grant Pool	Fund West Side small businesses (SB) with small business grants; provide technical assistance (TA) and coaching to small businesses on West Side; connect funded businesses to hospital supply chains	Number of SB applicants; number of grants provided; amount ($) of SB grants provided; number of SBs participating in TA/ coaching; number of SB contracts with hospitals	Increase SB revenue and net income; increase number of living-wage jobs given to West Side residents; increase SB employee wages	Decrease individual and child poverty on the West Side; increase median income; increase percent of adults making a living wage; decrease unemployment	Expect improvement in various health metrics across the five drivers of the life expectancy gap; increase life expectancy
Domain: Neighborhood and Physical Environment Strategy: coordinate hospital community efforts	WSU Food Voucher Program	Identify food insecure patients at hospitals; provide vouchers and make referrals for fresh fruits/ vegetables; provide nutrition education	Number of patients identified as food insecure; number of referrals; number of vouchers accepted; number of vouchers redeemed	Increase knowledge about food preparation; lower levels of food insecurity; increase consumption of fruits/vegetables	Decrease food insecurity; increase perceptions of healthy and affordable food access; increase self-rated health; increase fruit and vegetable consumption; lower levels of obesity	Decrease in diabetes- and cardiovascular-disease-related hospitalizations; decrease deaths due to coronary heart disease, diabetes, and stroke; decrease cancer incidence and death; decrease complications related to infant mortality; increase life expectancy

(continued)

Table 9.6. (Continued)

Domain/ Strategy	Initiative/ Programs	Tier III. Initiatives/Programs (Initiative/Participant-Level Metrics)			Tier II. Domains (Community-Level Domain Metrics)	Tier I. Overarching Goals (Community-Level Health Metrics)
		Activities	Outputs	Outcomes		
Domain: Education Strategy: pilot new ideas across domains	Community Hub Partnership (Chicago Public Schools)	Wraparound support services; access to primary care and mental health services; trauma-informed teacher training; health career exposure	Number of students accessing services; number of teachers trained; number of events	Improve student attendance; improve student behavior; improve student academic performance	Improve third-grade reading proficiency rate; improve eighth-grade math proficiency rate; increase high school graduation	Expect improvement in various health metrics across the five drivers of the life expectancy gap; increase life expectancy
Domain: Health and Healthcare Strategy: coordinate hospital community efforts	Target: Blood Pressure Program	Physician education, community partnerships, establishment of new practices for hypertension control	Number of newly identified individuals with high blood pressure (HTN); number of individuals with HTN that receive evidence-based care; number of providers trained	Increase adherence to HTN control protocols; decrease cardiovascular complications; improve self-rated health	Decrease levels of obesity; improve self-rated health; improve health care satisfaction; increase number of adults receiving needed health care	Decrease in diabetes- and cardiovascular-disease-related hospitalizations; decrease deaths due to coronary heart disease, diabetes, and stroke; decrease complications related to infant mortality; increase life expectancy

Note: Lists of activities, outputs, and outcomes are not exhaustive and serve as examples only.

program improvements. Data collection approaches will vary by initiative on account of the wide range of programs that span content areas, populations, and approaches; however, all will be fed into a centralized WSU infrastructure to facilitate transparency, shared learning, and quality improvement.

Disseminating the Framework

To ensure that the three-tiered WSU Assessment Framework was integrated across WSU and responsive to the needs and considerations of other stakeholders, the Metrics Working Group shared it throughout the entire WSU organization and with CAC. When early feedback made clear that the initial list of metrics was too long, the Working Group trimmed the list and prioritized certain, short-term metrics. Notably, one CAC member emphasized that systemic racism should be acknowledged as the root of inequities and encouraged the group to find ways to measure WSU's impact in that regard. The feedback highlighted that a full understanding of WSU's impacts might require the collection of new community-level data to supplement the data already gathered.

WSU is also committed to bringing the Assessment Framework and data to everyone, not just those who work with data all the time. To increase and promote transparency, it developed an interactive, multi-layered dashboard via the WSU website to share the Assessment Framework, key metrics, and program progress. The dashboard was designed with a broad range of stakeholder groups in mind (residents, organizations, medical professionals, etc.) and thus includes layers of accessible data depending on users' needs. The Metrics Working Group also worked with WSU leadership to develop a data infrastructure plan for the regular reporting of these metrics.

Using Data Moving Forward

The final Assessment Framework allows WSU to meet its three aims of using data to demonstrate short- and long-term progress, guide ongoing strategic decision-making, and coalesce a broad, diverse group of stakeholders around shared goals. In particular, it measures progress overall, while also accounting for each community's unique priorities. Looking ahead, the reframing of community-level data in this three-tiered fashion presents an exciting opportunity to use data in a new way. Over time, Working Group members expect the Assessment Framework to become a crucial mechanism for more fully pinpointing the most influential factors in moving the needle on community vibrancy and well-being. WSU recognizes that the Assessment Framework is a living product that will evolve as new information becomes available and factors emerge for measuring progress toward community vitality in more meaningful ways. The Metrics Working Group has already identified several gaps in the existing data's ability to inform place-based approaches, and its members will continue to explore ways to address these gaps on Chicago's West Side and beyond.

Having laid out a set of roles and responsibilities for overseeing the WSU assessment across the three tiers, the Metrics Working Group will focus next on building capacity within WSU Working Groups, Backbone Staff, Leadership Council, and community partners by sharing the Assessment Framework, data, and evaluation and quality improvement techniques so they can take an active role in the evaluation of their own initiatives. WSU is determined to change the narrative on "evaluation" and to make WSU a learning community where data are used to highlight successful initiatives and also indicate areas needing course correction without the fear of being perceived as failing. By institutionalizing an assessment culture of learning, transparency, and continuous improvement, WSU hopes it can move more rapidly toward its ultimate goals of addressing structural racism and increasing well-being and life expectancy for all West Siders.

Lessons Learned

West Side United's efforts provide lessons for pursuing place-based, social-justice-minded approaches to address health equity and structural racism. The substantial financial and in-kind support required to pursue an endeavor of WSU's size must be emphasized. Place-based initiatives are not short-term, 3- or 5-year programs but decades-long endeavors. Thus, funding is also not a one-time need but a long-term requirement that warrants the development of a strategic plan for ongoing financial stability. Philanthropic organizations and other stakeholders who fund collective impact approaches targeting the social and structural determinants of health must be made aware of and acknowledge the substantial resources needed to pursue these forms of meaningful change. In late 2017, WSU received a $1 million grant from a local anonymous foundation to launch its early work, including the recruitment and hiring of its Backbone Staff and support for initial initiatives. These seed funds and subsequent operational funding have been critical to ongoing success and stability. However, the speed of WSU's achievements was only possible because of the extensive in-kind support provided by anchor hospital systems, community partners, and corporations. In particular, WSU's relationship with CCA and the attention given by hospital leadership allowed the initial idea to grow into the significant entity it is today. Not only hospital leadership but also Working Group members—including hospital staff, residents, and partners—provided hours, weeks, and months of in-kind support to ensure that WSU and its initiatives were operationally set to thrive (see table 9.1). The in-kind support would not have been possible without the intentional fostering of existing relationships and the pursuit of new, innovative partnerships.

To secure this level of financial and in-kind support from a broad array of stakeholders, WSU leadership set out to intentionally recruit and organize stakeholders of all types (table 9.1). From the outset, Rush and WSU leadership understood that gaining the necessary level of collaboration required trust among and between stakeholders, particularly institutional partners and residents. Once initial trust was established, maintaining that trust became an ongoing process that required attention and thoughtfulness. WSU's transparent communication about aims and constraints has been critical for maintaining that trust, enabling all stakeholders to understand WSU's future plans and provide feedback. WSU uses various forms of communication to regularly share its accomplishments, progress, setbacks, and future plans: a centralized website, emailed newsletters and announcements, ongoing community listening sessions, an annual stakeholder convening, and social media.

Another successful effort that fostered community and stakeholder trust from the start was WSU's focus on immediate action—even before it began planning the organizational structure. Taking action demonstrated that WSU was serious about collaborating with residents, organizations, and hospitals. For example, WSU committed to creating a Planning Committee to steer WSU's early directions. In addition, WSU began pursuing the initiatives developed through stakeholder feedback. Immediate action also established buy-in from anchor hospitals as they started to see how combining efforts advanced their own goals. Very early on, WSU established a Career Pathways program between hospitals that would not have been as feasible for any one hospital to pursue. The program has proven crucial for retaining hospital employees and filling needed medical positions. In taking accountability seriously, WSU leadership achieved the aims it set out to accomplish, inspiring long-term commitment from community residents and organizations, hospital partners, and other stakeholders.

To build momentum and mobilize wider participation within diverse stakeholder groups, WSU leaders focused on life expectancy. This is an easily understood, comprehensive measure of health that embodied the structural racism and social factors underlying a wide array of inequitable health outcomes. WSU leadership found it effective to facilitate ongoing participation by demonstrating early wins and progress, using both data and community feedback. The WSU Assessment Framework shares WSU's road map to success, coalesces stakeholders around shared aims, and shows how short-term wins relate to the overarching life expectancy goal. By broadly sharing its Assessment Framework, WSU has demonstrated to residents and stakeholders that it is invested for the long haul. The Assessment Framework shares short-term accomplishments in order to demonstrate progress toward longer-term goals, helping to continuously engage stakeholders. By intentionally aligning many of the Assessment Framework's goals with the metrics and strategies of the city health department's community improvement plan, WSU has also increased the buy-in and ongoing participation of stakeholders already involved in Healthy Chicago 2.0.[24]

Including residents as leaders in all of WSU's work has been a major component of the social justice and place-based framework. It is foundational to WSU's success and sets it apart from other collaboratives. From the outset, residents helped choose WSU initiatives, nominate the initial Planning Committee, determine recipients of community grants, and identify the social impact investing approach. CAC members serve all WSU Working Groups, where they provide local insights. In reaching out to audiences beyond its organizational structure, WSU regularly conducts community listening sessions to gather ongoing feedback from a broader set of residents to learn about their challenges, to discover their community assets, and, most importantly, to share WSU's plans and progress with them. This engagement solicits the continuing support of both WSU and residents in pursuit of mutually agreed-upon activities, leading to potentially more lasting impact.

Also early on, Rush and WSU leadership appealed to anchor institutions to examine their internal business units to determine how they could positively impact community well-being from a financial standpoint. The commitment of anchor hospitals to change the way they did business was fundamental in demonstrating WSU's seriousness about addressing health equity and social justice. Without the courage and willingness of anchor hospitals to recognize the impact their own internal policies had on inequitable community outcomes, WSU could not have focused on improving health equity in the surrounding communities. Once anchor hospitals began the ongoing process of working with each other, community residents, organizations, and other partners, their understanding of why certain policies and practices may not be community friendly also changed. For example, Rush shortened its 45-day vendor payment policy to seven days to accommodate local, small businesses that could not afford to wait so long to be paid.

WSU Assessment Framework Development

The development of an Assessment Framework offers several lessons for others interested in using a place-based approach to address life expectancy and mortality inequities in their communities. One of WSU's first revelations was the merit of striking a balance between the large number of metrics needed to get a well-rounded view of the community and the small number of metrics needed to provide focus. The Metric Working Group took a data-driven approach (the decomposition data analysis) to help identify five mortality drivers, but it synthesized the results of the decomposition analysis with other critical factors, such as other publicly available data on trends and community resident feedback, to balance its use of both data- and community-driven approaches.

> *More important than quantitative data is the qualitative data*
> *that comes from knocking on doors and speaking to individuals.*
> Norman Kerr, Vice President for
> Violence Prevention, UCAN, January 2017
> WSU Convening

The Metrics Working Group needed to consider both quantitative data (decomposition analysis results or results similar to those found in this book) and qualitative data (community feedback from WSU planning activities and other sources) to select drivers. The use of two approaches also secured community and stakeholder buy-in. For example, in final mortality driver decisions, the Metrics Working Group considered the impact of extremely premature deaths, such as those occurring in the first year of life or before age 25, on community-wide wellness, mental health (and its associated physical repercussions), stability, and disinvestment. Feedback from residents underlining safety and poor birth outcomes in Black communities also factored into choosing the five drivers. The Working Group incorporated infant mortality (including maternal mortality) and homicide into its final set of Tier I drivers because of existing momentum around these issues in West Side communities. The group chose opioid overdose rather than HIV/other infectious disease based on a consideration of trends CDPH had identified. Annual data from CDPH indicated that the increasing opioid-related death rate had tripled over the past 10 years in Chicago, with the West Side experiencing the highest numbers.[36] Concurrently, the incidence of HIV-related deaths had declined in Chicago overall and in West Side communities.

WSU singles out the diversity of its Metrics Working Group, which included representatives from the local health department (CDPH), public health professionals, epidemiologists, subject matter experts, and community residents with local expertise. Including epidemiologists and public health professionals knowledgeable about the strengths and limitations of available data sources was invaluable in identifying useful and fitting metrics. WSU acknowledges the ongoing, special role CDPH has played by providing both epidemiologic expertise and highly accessible neighborhood data needed to steer large initiatives focused on health. The Metrics Working Group also has the skill sets to critically consider current data limitations and how they could be addressed in the future. Certain concepts, such as the neighborhood-built environment and social cohesion, are not fully captured by a single number; therefore, the Metrics Working Group had to decide whether to accept the best surrogate data or to acknowledge the gap and note a need to further address it in the future. WSU feels confident that it is well equipped and positioned to respond to changes over time in the data, research, and even its strategies and domains.

Although the WSU Metrics Working Group has just begun disseminating the Assessment Framework and baseline data, moving forward, as metrics change, it is imperative that the Working Group not link the changes specifically to WSU. For example, improvements seen in the community-level metrics may actually be capturing temporal trends caused by a variety of factors, such as policy-level changes. Further, shifts in community outcomes could result from gentrification's impact on underlying population demographics. Such seemingly positive changes are troubling because they are caused by the displacement of, rather than health improvements within, the original population. Therefore, it is imperative to collect not only underlying population data but also initiative-level metrics to determine whether WSU programs are contributing to community-wide outcomes. WSU's ongoing listening sessions are a key component of the assessment. Maintaining community engagement will enable WSU to keep its finger on the pulse of changes in community sentiment and lived experiences not captured by quantitative data.

Conclusion

This chapter went beyond analyses of life expectancy and mortality inequities to describe how a local collaborative in one of the largest US cities uses a place-based approach to pursue social justice and reduce geographic and racial inequities in life expectancy. It outlined how West Side United uses data to evaluate place-based, equity-focused initiatives targeting the structural determinants of health. While it is not expected that all cities adapt this approach, this multisector, place-based, and data-driven method to address inequities in life expectancy and mortality provides a promising foundation that can be modified for use by collective efforts in other US cities. Hopefully, detailing WSU's experience will suggest ideas that could be used to marshal action elsewhere in order to ameliorate unjust geographic inequities in life expectancy along racial lines. Specific initiatives will differ based on local issues and priorities, but this place-based approach offers universally applicable lessons.

Ultimately, WSU formed because the data about local inequities in life expectancy and mortality gaps—like those presented in this book—were too unjust to overlook. The data revealed an urgency that mobilized institutions, community organizations, and residents to think beyond business as usual and to pursue social justice and health equity in a collaborative, holistic, and community-driven fashion.

References
   1. City of Chicago. Chicago Health Atlas, Community Areas. 2020. https://www.chicagohealthatlas.org/community-areas.
   2. Metropolitan Planning Council. *The Cost of Segregation.* Chicago: Metropolitan Planning Council; March 2017.
   3. Seligman AI. *Block by Block: Neighborhoods and Public Policy on Chicago's West Side.* Chicago: University of Chicago Press; 2005.
   4. Hirsch AR. Blockbusting. *The Electronic Encyclopedia of Chicago.* 2005. http://www.encyclopedia.chicagohistory.org/pages/147.html.

5. Hirsch AR. Restrictive Covenants. *The Electronic Encyclopedia of Chicago*. 2005. http://www.encyclopedia.chicagohistory.org/pages/1067.html.

6. Hunt DB. Redlining. *The Electronic Encyclopedia of Chicago*. 2005. http://www.encyclopedia.chicagohistory.org/pages/1050.html.

7. Ralph JR. *Northern Protest: Martin Luther King, Jr., Chicago, and the Civil Rights Movement*. 1st ed. Cambridge, MA: Harvard University Press; 1993.

8. Loerzel R. Displaced: When the Eisenhower Moved in, Who Was Forced Out? https://interactive.wbez.org/curiouscity/eisenhower/.

9. Steans Family Foundation. North Lawndale History. 2009–20. http://www.steansfamilyfoundation.org/lawndale_history.shtml.

10. Seligman AI. North Lawndale. *The Electronic Encyclopedia of Chicago*. 2005. http://www.encyclopedia.chicagohistory.org/pages/901.html.

11. Chicago Historical Society (ICHI-19851). West Madison Street, 1968. *The Electronic Encyclopedia of Chicago*. 2005. http://www.encyclopedia .chicagohistory.org/pages/6354.html.

12. Cordova TL, Wilson MD. *Abandoned in Their Neighborhoods: Youth Joblessness amidst the Flight of Industry and Opportunity*. Chicago: Great Cities Institute, University of Illinois at Chicago; January 2017.

13. Seligman AI. East Garfield Park. *The Electronic Encyclopedia of Chicago*. 2005. http://www.encyclopedia.chicagohistory.org/pages/404.html.

14. Sampson RJ. *Great American City: Chicago and the Enduring Neighborhood Effect*. Chicago: University of Chicago Press; 2012.

15. Magallon FS. *Images of America: Chicago's Little Village, Lawndale-Crawford*. Charleston, SC: Arcadia; 2010.

16. Reed CR. South Lawndale. *The Electronic Encyclopedia of Chicago*. 2005. http://encyclopedia.chicagohistory.org/pages/1174.html.

17. Hermida A. Mapping the Black Panther Party in Key Cities, Mapping American Social Movements through the 20th Century. 2015–20. http://depts .washington.edu/moves/BPP_map-cities.shtml#Chicago.

18. Gerasole V. Little Village Retail Strip Is Second Highest Grossing in City. *CBS Chicago*. October 14, 2015.

19. Illinois Medical District Commission. Facts & Figures. 2013. https:// archive.ph/20130415003926/http://www.imdc.org/facts.htm.

20. Dankwa-Mullan I, Perez-Stable EJ. Addressing Health Disparities Is a Place-Based Issue. *American Journal of Public Health*. 2016;106(4):637–639.

21. Yen IH, Kaplan GA. Neighborhood Social Environment and Risk of Death: Multilevel Evidence from Alameda County Study. *American Journal of Epidemiology*. 1999;149(10):898–907.

22. Flood J, Minkler M, Hennessey Lavery S, Estrada J, Falbe J. The Collective Impact Model and Its Potential for Health Promotion: Overview and Case Study of a Healthy Retail Initiative in San Francisco. *Health Education and Behavior*. 2015;42(5):654–668.

23. Boyce B. Collective Impact: Aligning Organizational Efforts for Broader Social Change. *J Acad Nutr Diet*. 2013;113(4):495–497.

24. Dircksen JC, Prachand NG, Adams D, et al. *Healthy Chicago 2.0: Partnering to Improve Health Equity (2016–2020)*. Chicago: Chicago Department of Public Health; March 2016.

25. Rush University Medical Center, University of Illinois Hospital and Health Sciences System, Cook County Health and Hospitals System, Presence Health, Civic Consulting Alliance. *What We Heard: Coming Together to Improve Health and Wellness on the West Side*. Chicago; July 2017.

26. W. K. Kellogg Foundation. *The Step-by-Step Guide to Evaluation: How to Become Savvy Evaluation Consumers*. November 29, 2017.

27. Auger N, Feuillet P, Martel S, Lo E, Barry AD, Harper S. Mortality Inequality in Populations with Equal Life Expectancy: Arriaga's Decomposition Method in SAS, Stata, and Excel. *Ann Epidemiol*. 2014;24(8):575–580.e571.

28. City of Chicago. Chicago Health Atlas, Indicators. 2020. https://www.chicagohealthatlas.org/indicators.

29. City of Chicago. Healthy Chicago Survey. 2020. https://www.chicago.gov/city/en/depts/cdph/supp_info/healthy-communities/healthy-chicago-survey.html.

30. Le J, Bennett A. *Illinois Infant Mortality Data Report*. Illinois Department of Public Health, Office of Women's Health and Family Services; January 2018.

31. Abdurahman AA, Chaka EE, Nedjat S, Dorosty AR, Majdzadeh R. The Association of Household Food Insecurity with the Risk of Type 2 Diabetes Mellitus in Adults: A Systematic Review and Meta-analysis. *Eur J Nutr*. 2019;58(4):1341–1350.

32. Redmond M, Dong F, Goetz J, Jacobson L, Collins T. Food Insecurity and Peripheral Arterial Disease in Older Adult Populations. *J Nutr Health Aging*. 2016;20(10):989–995.

33. Baggett TP, Hwang SW, O'Connell JJ, et al. Mortality among Homeless Adults in Boston: Shifts in Causes of Death over a 15-Year Period. *JAMA Internal Medicine*. 2013;173(3):189–195.

34. US Department of Health and Human Services. *Secretary's Advisory Committee Report #4: Target-Setting Methodologies for Objectives in Healthy People 2030*. Washington, DC: US Department of Health and Human Services; July 23, 2018.

35. US Department of Health and Human Services. Healthy People 2020: Leading Health Indicators. 2020. https://www.healthypeople.gov/2020/Leading-Health-Indicators.

36. Turner B, Arwady A, Jasmin W, et al. *Annual Opioid Surveillance Report—Chicago, 2018*. Chicago; January 2020.

CONCLUSION

Next Steps on the Path to Health Equity

MAUREEN R. BENJAMINS AND FERNANDO G. DE MAIO

POPULAR DISCOURSE often depicts "urban" issues very negatively, and often in a way that generalizes across cities. Lost in that discourse are the considerable differences between our largest cities. Inequality exists both *within* and *between* large cities in the United States. This dual inequality maps on to gaps in mortality rates.

Our book is a testament to a basic but powerful idea: both race and place matter to health. Although race is a social, not a biological, construct, the color of your skin can predict how long you will live and the likely cause of your death. Despite decades of attention to racial differences in mortality, the national picture remains stark: Blacks in the United States continue to have a shorter life expectancy and die more frequently from most of the leading causes of death compared to whites in this country. This is clear from the analyses presented in this book and also evident in the emerging data on mortality inequities related to COVID-19. However, hidden within the national picture lies an important issue: place matters too. We discovered a difference in life expectancy of more than 10 years between residents of the healthiest and unhealthiest large cities. This statistic and other striking findings from this book are shown in box C.1. Looking further, we show that race and place interact to produce varying levels of racial inequities between

269

Box C.1. SELECTED STATISTICS HIGHLIGHTING GEOGRAPHIC AND RACIAL INEQUITIES IN THE LARGEST US CITIES

 The average life expectancy varied by more than a decade within the largest US cities, with San Francisco and San Jose having the longest life expectancy at 82.9 years.

 The life expectancy for a white baby born in Washington, DC, was 86 years, while a Black baby born in many big cities cannot even expect to live to age 72.

 Several cities had mortality rates near or over 1,000 per 100,000, while two cities had rates under 600.

 Chicago and New York each had over 3,000 excess Black deaths annually.

 Almost 30% of all excess Black deaths in the United States occurred in these big cities.

 Cause-specific mortality inequities varied significantly, with many cities having inequities 40%–50% higher than what is seen nationally.

 All of the big cities had significant racial disparities in diabetes mortality, with the most extreme inequities seen in Washington, DC, where the Black rate was 582% higher than the white rate.

 In Chicago, the Black homicide mortality rate was 26.4 times the white rate.

 Opioid-related mortality rates varied more than 24-fold among the largest cities (from 2 per 100,000 in Philadelphia to 49 in Baltimore).

Notes

Based on 2013–2017 data. indicates racial inequities, while represents geographic inequities.

the cities. In some of our largest cities, Blacks and whites have similar longevity; in others, the racial life expectancy gap is a full decade. There is nothing natural about this.

The data shown in this book emphasize how important it is for local health department leaders and other health advocates to consider—and have supporting data for—overall outcomes *and* levels of equity within them, since our largest cities often performed well in one but not both areas. Certainly, we could rank the cities included here and identify which performed best for the outcomes at hand. Cities such as Boston, New York, and El Paso tended to have better mortality and equity outcomes than the others, for instance. However, the path those cities followed to attain their distinguished results may not be applicable for other cities intent on improving their outcomes. Cities clearly vary by more than just location; they have different histories, cultures, government structures, demographic compositions, public and private leadership, assets, and competing priorities.

Complex problems often have complex causes. That is the case here, where few clear geographical patterns emerged across the wide range of mortality outcomes we examined. Although we would have loved to uncover a tidy set of "model" cities, the real story is messier and more nuanced. To begin understanding how city-level features are related to mortality outcomes and the inequities hiding within, we examined numerous structural factors suggested by the theoretical models outlined in chapter 2. Our analyses revealed that cities may want to consider attributes such as income inequality and racial segregation in any efforts to improve mortality outcomes (chapter 6). We showed that income inequality is associated with Black:white differences in all-cause mortality, life expectancy, and premature mortality, as well as racial differences in the two leading causes of death, heart disease and cancer. Surprisingly, a city's level of poverty showed very little explanatory power in our analyses—adding to the growing body of literature that points toward inequality (and not just poverty) as a fundamental cause of poor health. We found that racial segregation does not necessarily explain differences between cities, although evidence does link racial segregation and mortality within cities, as evidenced by our experiences in Chicago.

The Imperative to Act on These Data

The data presented in this book make it clear that the United States has an equity problem, which is reflected in most, but not all, of our largest cities. Yet how many people living in the United States know about these health inequities? A recent national survey found that only 45% of adults knew that Blacks had a lower life expectancy than whites.[1] Think about that: Black babies can expect to live 4 years less than white babies born at the same time (and, as we have shown, this number is up to three times as large in some cities). However, less than half of Americans realize there is an inequity, reflecting "colorblind" ideology that minimizes the existence and strength of racism in contemporary society. We believe that in order to make real progress, we must first document the levels of Black:white inequities in mortality across the United States and name the fundamental causes of those inequities in structural and social conditions. Knowing how difficult it will be to motivate and sustain the political will to act on these issues without greater public awareness of the problem, it behooves all of us who work in health equity to prioritize intentional communication efforts around findings like these. As Dr. Steve Whitman, the noted Chicago equity researcher and founding director of the Sinai Urban Health Institute, asserted in 2001, "I cannot see how we will make progress against racial disparities unless we reveal them and proclaim their destructiveness" (p. 388).[2]

In chapters 3–5, we took the first step, by "revealing" city-level racial inequities. As outlined by Monnard and colleagues in chapter 8, public health leaders and researchers need to make information like this accessible to the public, taking special care to disseminate results to people in a position to make changes. Fortunately, those in charge, such as mayors and health commissioners, appear to be better informed about inequities than the general public; unfortunately, 30% of mayors and 10% of health commissioners believed that city policies have little or no impact on inequities.[3]

These findings highlight the importance of having a deliberate communication plan for disseminating this type of information. Health equity findings must be framed correctly to motivate change effectively.

Framing determines how values and meaning are communicated and conceptualized, giving people a context to interpret a specific message.[4] As discussed in chapter 2, the traditional way of viewing health—as one's personal responsibility—is limited in both its accuracy and its ability to effect change. Thus, public health messages about health inequities cannot be framed using a "portrait" perspective that puts the focus on individual behaviors and knowledge.[4] This narrow view centered on a single person or activity ignores the broader structures that can facilitate (or constrain) individuals' health-related behaviors and outcomes. Discussions of health inequities can have more impact when described from a "landscape" perspective that includes the social and economic environments in which people live. This wide view calls attention to the underlying upstream factors, like racism, public policies, and living conditions, which ultimately are the most powerful determinants of health.

This stance was reiterated in chapter 7, where Silva and colleagues discussed how city-level efforts to address health inequities like those documented in the book could employ a social justice framework. They argued that equity work requires not only a "landscape" orientation, focused on structural changes and broad determinants, but also iterative efforts, undertaken in partnership with communities and based on shared values. Again, such a framework emphasizes the long-standing economic, political, social, and cultural structures underlying inequities. Using an approach that acknowledges the historical roots and current manifestations of racism is more likely to produce sustained changes through genuine engagement of the relevant communities and the creation of a shared commitment to social and political change.

In other words, actions to address city-level inequities should incorporate a wide, societal view and a "value-driven" perspective. Or, as the prominent physician, policy researcher, and advocate Dr. Vanessa Gamble put it, "to be effective, research must not only reveal problems but also frame them in a way that they are perceived as bad situations and moral wrongs that government can and should fix" (p. 95).[5] Dr. Whitman poignantly stated a similar viewpoint: "I would suggest that one of the most important things we can do is to take the matter of disparities in health personally. If the existence of these racial disparities, indeed their growth, is a national shame, then each of us should say so. . . . It is time to respond with anger to a situation that demands anger." (pp. 388–389).[2] It is with this perspective that we chose to write this book and why we have dedicated it to the memory of Dr. Whitman. We hope readers encountering these data will feel something themselves—perhaps anger, perhaps a moral conviction—compelling them to work together, to do something about the problem.

Acknowledging that the paramount burden of human suffering produced by inequities falls on communities of color, the substantial economic toll of inequities on society at large should also be recognized. Researchers have estimated that health inequities cost the United States approximately $230 billion in extra health care expenditures for the years 2003–2006.[6] With the addition of indirect costs, such as reduced productivity, the total climbs to more than $1 trillion in excess expenditures. Over half of this cost is related to health inequities for Blacks. At a more local level, a recent study from Minnesota confirmed this substantial economic impact, concluding that the state could save $1.2 to $2.9 billion per year if racial inequities in preventable deaths were eradicated.[7] Perhaps public officials should make this point more frequently, to provide a pragmatic complement to the social justice framework and values-fueled approach described above.

Where Can Cities Go from Here?

Just as our country has a long history of racial health inequities, it also has a history of efforts to address them (albeit much more recent), as summarized in chapter 1. Although several examples show promising signs of success, it must be underscored that actions cities (or other levels of government) might take to improve the health of the overall population differ from the actions required to improve health equity.[8–10]

One valuable first step toward improving both overall mortality outcomes and equity in mortality is to supplement the mortality data provided here with city-level data on other health outcomes and determinants of health. These types of data are increasingly available through initiatives such as 500 Cities, City Health Dashboard, and CityHealth.

Once local stakeholders can see the full picture of their city's health, they can then begin the work of disseminating the data, engaging communities, prioritizing goals, and building partnerships.

Cities that would like to specifically focus on improving overall health outcomes (rather than inequities) have a plethora of resources offering guidance and examples. For example, the Centers for Disease Control and Prevention's Health Impact in 5 Years (HI-5) initiative highlights potential city-level interventions shown to improve health outcomes within a 5-year period and save costs.[11] A wider array of options can be found in their Community Health Improvement Navigator database, which provides tools for any organization or agency looking to embark on multisector, collaborative health initiatives.[12] The database includes resources from *The Community Guide* from the Community Preventive Service Task Force and *What Works for Health* from the County Health Rankings and Roadmaps project, among others. Both of these resources present community-based interventions along with user-friendly ratings of the supporting evidence. Another resource, the Build initiative, offers extensive insight into systems change for communities.[13] Dr. Denise Koo and colleagues helpfully reviewed these and other efforts and toolkits, relieving communities from having to start from scratch.[14]

In addition, Health in All Policies is a framework to help city governments (and other levels of jurisdiction) improve health outcomes by focusing on social determinants of health and extending the responsibility for our nation's population health goals beyond public health into other sectors, such as housing, education, regional planning, transportation, and workforce development.[15] A growing number of cities have enacted this approach, including Chicago in 2016 under the leadership of Health Commissioner Julie Morita.

Actions needed to improve health equity, by contrast, should specifically address inequitable social conditions that sustain the inequities. Initiatives focused on the disadvantaged population (ironically, perhaps easiest to implement in the most geographically segregated cities) may also help to improve equity. Understanding that actions designed to improve overall outcomes differ from those designed to improve equity is important because efforts to simply improve health can sometimes exacerbate inequities.[16,17] Dr. David Williams and Dr. Lisa Cooper clarified this by noting that "reducing inequities in health requires dismantling the systems that initiate and sustain inequities in a broad range of social institutions" (p. 2).[18] Their review of effective initiatives for achieving equity included increasing investments in early childhood development, reducing child poverty, improving job opportunities for youth and adults, and enhancing environmental conditions in disadvantaged communities. Existing sources of health-related data at the neighborhood or census-tract level, such as USALEEP (and others reviewed in chapter 1), can help cities geographically target efforts to the areas needing the most support. Race equity tools can help cities evaluate policies for their impact on inequities (related to health or other outcomes).[19] Naming racism as a root cause of the inequities is an important step to acknowledge the historical roots of the problem and provide a foundation for subsequent actions toward equity. To this end, numerous government leaders or agencies have declared racism as a public health crisis, including those serving many of the largest cities studied here (e.g., Los Angeles, Denver, Boston, Columbus, Memphis, and Seattle).

Finally, several national organizations have been formed to provide support and guidance for those undertaking this important work. The National League of Cities, a 90-year-old organization that supports and advocates for US cities of all sizes, has a Race, Equity, and Leadership (REAL) initiative to provide training and resources to cities interested in working toward racial equity. Resources include valuable tools such as examples of policy and budgetary changes made at the local level to increase health equity. The group has also begun creating city profiles to explore the racial equity work being done around the country. The Boston profile, for instance, highlights that city's extensive efforts, including the Anti-racism Advisory Committee, mandatory racial justice training for all staff at the local health department, 5-year health equity goals, the Mayor's Office of Resilience and Racial Equity, a chief diversity officer, and the Office of Fair Housing and Equity.[20] Other resources, such as the Community-Driven Health Equity Action Plans from the National Academy of Medicine, have also helped cities to strategically address inequities like those documented here.[21]

Future Data and Research Needs

Race-specific data provided the impetus needed to take up the issue of inequities in Boston, as well as other states, cities, and counties. In addition to providing motivation and guidance for targeting efforts, data are needed at all geopolitical levels to help elected officials and agencies set and track goals. Public health officials at many levels set goals related to eliminating health inequities (including our national priorities as set forth in the Healthy People initiative). However, tracking equity goals is not always clear.

> *We often state that our national and local goals are improving overall health and reducing disparities. Unfortunately in measurement, policy, and research, we often emphasize the average or overall, such as setting future life expectancy targets, but without such attention and specificity to the disparity reduction component.*
> *David Kindig, 2015*[22]

Part of the problem observed by Kindig is that most sources of health data do not include explicit measures of inequities, such as the Black:white rate ratios or rate differences shown throughout this book. Adding specific equity-focused measures to public-facing websites such as County Health Rankings and City Health Dashboard would be valuable. Efforts to improve our ability to track inequities at the national level are already underway as part of the HP2030 initiative, which has an increased focus on health equity, through the "Closing the Gap" component of the framework.[23] At the very least, cities could follow the example of the Chicago Department of Public Health (CDPH), which makes public health data widely accessible through the Chicago Health Atlas website and includes data disaggregated by race/ethnicity. Notably, they display inequities not only by race/ethnicity but also by age, gender, and levels of economic hardship. More Chicago initiatives to address equity are discussed in the following section.

Although the importance of local data is increasingly recognized and is pushing researchers to examine ever-smaller geographic units (such as census tracts), we believe that city-level data like these are critical. As noted by Jacobson and Teutsch, "Geopolitical areas rather than simply geographic areas are recommended when measuring total population health since funding decisions and regulation are inherently political in nature."[24] However, we acknowledge that conducting this type of analysis is time-consuming and complex; many local departments of health do not have the resources to dedicate time to such an assessment of mortality in their jurisdictions.

City Spotlight: Chicago

Chicago's strengths and weaknesses related to mortality and equity have been highlighted throughout the book in the City Spotlight sections. Chicago struggled to attain even average levels of health and equity, as assessed by the various mortality outcomes and measures of racial inequities within (based on data from 2013 to 2017). The relatively bad news will not surprise those familiar with health in Chicago. In fact, statistics about the number of excess Black deaths (the result of a higher Black than white mortality rate) might seem familiar. Back in 2009, previous research from SUHI comparing Black and white mortality rates also resulted in widespread attention to the number of excess Black deaths in that city, which was actually slightly lower than our current estimate in chapter 3 (figure C.1).

In response to disheartening statistics such as 3,000-plus excess Black deaths a year, CDPH has been documenting and addressing health inequities at the city level for the past decade. This work has included collecting, analyzing, and disseminating data; enacting policies; promoting environmental changes; and fostering systems changes. Efforts are implemented in collaboration with other public health system partners and city departments to broaden the approach and strengthen the impact on populations most affected by inequities. Some examples of that work are summarized on the following page.

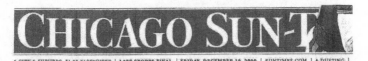

CHICAGO SUN-T

¢ CITY & SUBURBS $1.25 ELSEWHERE | LATE SPORTS FINAL | FRIDAY, DECEMBER 18, 2009 | SUNTIMES.COM | A DUSTING |

HEALTH CARE GAP KILLS

3,200

BLACK CHICAGOANS A YEAR — AND THE GAP IS GROWING

MONIFA THOMAS REPORTS ON PAGE 10

Figure C.1. Major Chicago Newspaper Headline Featuring the Number of Excess Black Deaths in 2009. *Source: Chicago Sun-Times*, December 18, 2009.

- Healthy Chicago 2.0, the City's 2016–2019 community health improvement plan, prioritized equity with the goal of allocating resources to areas with the greatest inequities.[25]
- Chicago's current community health improvement plan, Healthy Chicago 2025, moved further upstream with its vision of Chicago as "a city where all people and all communities have power, are free from oppression and strengthened by equitable access to resources, environments, and opportunities that promote optimal health and well-being." As part of this plan, strategies must adhere to 10 guiding principles, including a call to challenge and redress structural racism, promote equitable wealth and income building, and institutionalize community power.

- The city's online portal for health data, Chicago Health Atlas (www .chicagohealthatlas.org), provides easy access to citywide and community area data on 160 health, demographic, and social determinants of health indicators to assist coalitions, researchers, and community members in community planning and advocacy. It also tracks inequities, as data permit.

More broadly, the city of Chicago is also focused on racial equity and is implementing innovative approaches to strengthen communities. For example, in 2019 Mayor Lori Lightfoot instituted several administrative changes to forward equity goals, including appointment of Chicago's first chief equity officer and establishment of the Office for Equity and Social Justice. This office is responsible for understanding, tracking, and addressing inequity in all sectors and city departments, including employment, housing, economic development, and education.

As with each city included in this book, Chicago leaders, residents, and other stakeholders can use the data provided herein as a starting point for examining outcomes and equity in other health indicators, launching conversations with community groups, and targeting areas in most urgent need of attention. Importantly, these data can also serve as a baseline for assessing changes over time.

COVID-19: Adding a Major Driver of Inequality to an Already Unequal Landscape

In 2020, racial inequities in mortality leapt into the national spotlight as a result of the twin public health crises of the COVID-19 pandemic and police violence against Black people. Early data first revealed racial gaps in the number of COVID-19 cases and deaths among communities of color at the city level. In Chicago, the first wave of results revealed that 70% of COVID-19 deaths were among Black people (a disproportionate toll, as less than one-third of the city's population is Black). When discussing these results, Mayor Lightfoot was clear: "Those numbers take your breath away. . . . This is a call-to-action moment for all of us. . . . It is unacceptable, no one should think that this is OK."[26] In response, she quickly established a Racial Equity Rapid Response Team to coordinate efforts across the city, emphasizing community outreach, data sharing among researchers, and coordination among health systems. Similar inequities and responses were seen in cities across the United States.

Calls for more transparency on COVID-19 inequities at the national level quickly followed, and when the federal government refused to publish data revealing racial/ethnic inequities, journalists and researchers took the lead. Like our book, data revealed not only that COVID-19 mortality rates vary across racial/ethnic groups and localities but also that racial/ethnic inequities in the outcomes of this virus varied by geography as well.[27,28] The overall burden has been devastating to many communities. But it has not been uniform; again, local policies and actions matter.

Simultaneously, the murders of a growing number of Black individuals (including Breonna Taylor, George Floyd, Atatiana Jefferson, and others) at the hands of police sparked nationwide protests, increased awareness of these and other social injustices, and kindled support for movements such as Black Lives Matter. The urgency for individuals, organizations, and policies to become specifically anti-racist has never been clearer.[29] While the disproportionate risk of dying at the hands of police for people of color is particularly troubling (not to mention traumatic), having this same population be more likely to die of other causes of death compared to whites should also be an issue of grave concern for the US population.

The root cause of each of these inequities is racism, not race. Black individuals are more likely to contract COVID-19 because of the structural elements that increase their exposure to the virus, including working in essential occupations like food service, needing to take public transportation, and not having access to paid sick leave. Black individuals are also more likely to die from COVID-19 because similar structural elements have led them to have higher rates of chronic diseases that are linked to mortality, including heart disease and diabetes. The upstream determinants of this elevated risk among communities of color start with racism. This is why Link and Phelan call these structural factors "fundamental" causes of death.[30] That is, more proximal risk factors may change (or be eliminated), but the underlying patterns between racial groups and health outcomes remain. Unless we make substantial changes in our policies and practices to make them "anti-racist," all new health problems (like COVID-19) will continue to be marked by glaring racial inequities, mirroring the inequities in all-cause mortality, life expectancy, premature mortality, and mortality from other causes of death seen here. Thus, the historical context, the theoretical framework, the empirical patterns, and the examples for moving toward equity outlined in this book are not only relevant but also vitally important to understand as we work to address emerging public health crises.

Conclusion

Although the Black:white gap in life expectancy has been decreasing since 1990 across the United States,[31] inequities remain. When we examine health outcomes at the city level, previously hidden inequities emerge and the public health challenge becomes clearer: the country has a long way to go in reaching its goal of health equity.

However, if you take just one thing from this book, let it be that our data show that racial inequities in mortality *are not inevitable*. If health equity can be achieved in some cities, and across multiple causes of death, why not all cities and all causes of death? This is arguably the most important health equity issue of our time. We hope these city-level statistics and examples find their way to stakeholders in our largest urban areas to motivate and empower them to address the upstream factors that have led to the striking inequities seen here. Together, we can and must bring equity to all of our unequal cities.

References
 1. Benz JK, Espinosa O, Welsh V, Fontes A. Awareness of Racial and Ethnic Health Disparities Has Improved Only Modestly over a Decade. *Health Affairs.* 2011;30(10):1860–1867.
 2. Whitman S. Racial Disparities in Health: Taking It Personally. *Public Health Reports.* 2001;116(5):387–389.

3. Purtle J, Henson RM, Carroll-Scott A, Kolker J, Joshi R, Diez Roux AV. U.S. Mayors' and Health Commissioners' Opinions about Health Disparities in Their Cities. *American Journal of Public Health*. 2018;108(5):634–641.

4. Berkeley Media Studies Group and The Praxis Project. Meta Messaging: Framing What You Say to Make Your Case and Reinforce Your Allies. 2005. http://www.bmsg.org/resources/publications/meta-messaging-framing-your-case-and-reinforcing-your-allies/.

5. Gamble VN, Stone D. U.S. Policy on Health Inequities: The Interplay of Politics and Research. *Journal of Health Politics, Policy, and Law*. 2006;31(1):93–126.

6. LaVeist TA, Gaskin D, Richard P. Estimating the Economic Burden of Racial Health Inequalities in the United States. *International Journal of Health Services*. 2011;41(2):231–238.

7. Nanney MS, Myers SL, Xu M, Kent K, Durfee T, Allen ML. The Economic Benefits of Reducing Racial Disparities in Health: The Case of Minnesota. *International Journal of Environmental Research and Public Health*. 2019;16(5):742.

8. Grubbs SS, Polite BN, Carney J Jr, et al. Eliminating Racial Disparities in Colorectal Cancer in the Real World: It Took a Village. *Journal of Clinical Oncology*. 2013;31(16):1928–1930.

9. Rust G, Zhang S, Malhotra K, et al. Paths to Health Equity: Local Area Variation in Progress toward Eliminating Breast Cancer Mortality Disparities, 1990–2009. *Cancer*. 2015;121(16):2765–2774.

10. Rust G, Zhang S, Yu Z, et al. Counties Eliminating Racial Disparities in Colorectal Cancer Mortality. *Cancer*. 2016;122(11):1735–1748.

11. Centers for Disease Control and Prevention. Health Impact in 5 Years. 2019. https://www.cdc.gov/policy/hst/hi5/index.html.

12. Roy B, Stanojevich J, Stange P, Jiwani N, King R, Koo D. Development of the Community Health Improvement Navigator Database of Interventions. *MMWR Supplements*. 2016;65(2):1–9.

13. The BUILD HEALTH Challenge. *Community Approaches to Systems Change: A Compendium of Practices, Reflections, and Findings*. 2019.

14. Koo D, O'Carroll PW, Harris A, DeSalvo KB. An Environmental Scan of Recent Initiatives Incorporating Social Determinants in Public Health. *Preventing Chronic Disease*. 2016;13:E86.

15. Rudolph L, Caplan J, Ben-Moshe K, Dillon L. *Health in All Policies: A Guide for State and Local Governments*. Washington, DC: American Public Health Association; 2013. https://www.apha.org/-/media/files/pdf/factsheets/health_inall_policies_guide_169pages.ashx?la=en&hash=641B94AF624D7440F836238F0551A5FF0DE4872A.

16. Tabuchi T, Iso H, Brunner E. Tobacco Control Measures to Reduce Socioeconomic Inequality in Smoking: The Necessity, Time-Course Perspective, and Future Implications. *Journal of Epidemiology*. 2017:JE20160206.

17. Gebo KA, Fleishman JA, Conviser R, et al. Racial and Gender Disparities in Receipt of Highly Active Antiretroviral Therapy Persist in a Multistate Sample of HIV Patients in 2001. *JAIDS Journal of Acquired Immune Deficiency Syndromes.* 2005;38(1):96–103.

18. Williams DR, Cooper LA. Reducing Racial Inequities in Health: Using What We Already Know to Take Action. *International Journal of Environmental Research and Public Health.* 2019;16(4):606.

19. Racial Equity Tools. 2020. https://www.racialequitytools.org/home.

20. National League of Cities. *City Profile on Racial Equity: Boston, Massachusetts.* 2017. https://www.nlc.org/sites/default/files/2017-10/Boston%20 City%20Profile%20Racial%20Equity.pdf.

21. National Academy of Medicine. Community-Driven Health Equity Action Plan. Culture of Health website. https://nam.edu/programs/culture-of-health /community-driven-health-equity-action-plans/.

22. Kindig DA. What Are We Talking about When We Talk about Population Health? *Health Affairs* (blog), April 6, 2015.

23. National Academies of Sciences, Engineering, and Medicine. *Leading Health Indicators 2030: Advancing Health, Equity, and Well-Being.* Washington, DC: National Academies Press; 2020.

24. Jacobson DM, and Teutsch, S. An Environmental Scan of Integrated Approaches for Defining and Measuring Total Population Health. *National Quality Forum,* 2012. https://www.improvingpopulationhealth.org/PopHealthP haseIICommissionedPaper.pdf.

25. Dircksen J, Prachand, NG, Adams D, et al. *Healthy Chicago 2.0: Partnering to Improve Health Equity (2016–2020).* Chicago: Chicago Department of Public Health; March 2016.

26. Flynn M. "Those Numbers Take Your Breath Away": Covid-19 Is Hitting Chicago's Black Neighborhoods Much Harder Than Others, Officials Say. *Washington Post.* April 7, 2020.

27. APM Research Lab. The Color of Coronavirus: COVID-19 Deaths by Race and Ethnicity in the US. https://www.apmresearchlab.org/covid/deaths-by -race.

28. Millett GA, Jones AT, Benkeser D, et al. Assessing Differential Impacts of COVID-19 on Black Communities. *Annals of Epidemiology.* 2020;47:37–44.

29. Kendi IX. *How To Be an Anti-racist.* New York: One World; 2019.

30. Link BG, Phelan J. Social Conditions as Fundamental Causes of Disease. *Journal of Health and Social Behaviour.* 1995;Spec No:80–94.

31. Harper S, MacLehose RF, Kaufman JS. Trends in the Black-White Life Expectancy Gap among U.S. States, 1990–2009. *Health Affairs.* 2014;33(8): 1375–1382.

1. Methodology of Part II (Racial Inequities in US Cities: An Analysis of Mortality Data)
2. Methodology of Part III (Epidemiological Patterns and Sociological Explanations)
3. Methodological Limitations

1. Methodology of Part II (Racial Inequities in US Cities: An Analysis of Mortality Data)

Study Population

We identified the 30 most populous cities using 2013 US Census Bureau data (figure A.1). We used county data in places with consolidated city-county governments where some semi-independent areas remain (Louisville/Jefferson County, KY, Nashville/Davidson County, TN, and Indianapolis/Marion County, IN). Sociodemographic characteristics of the 30 cities are described in tables A.1 and A.2, drawing on the American Community Survey, City Health Dashboard, and Brown University's Diversity and Disparities Project website. Summary statistics of these variables and an analysis of their association with mortality data are provided in chapter 6.

Data Sources

MORTALITY DATA

All mortality data in the United States originate from death certificates. These documents are completed by the attending physician at the time of death and include information on the decedent (including name, sex, date of birth, race/ethnicity, marital status, place of residence, birthplace, occupation, and education level) and details about the death (immediate and underlying causes, date, and location), among other variables. In the United States, all deaths are legally required to be reported to health departments in the state where they occur. These data, which are compiled at the state and local levels, are then shared voluntarily with the National Center for Health Statistics

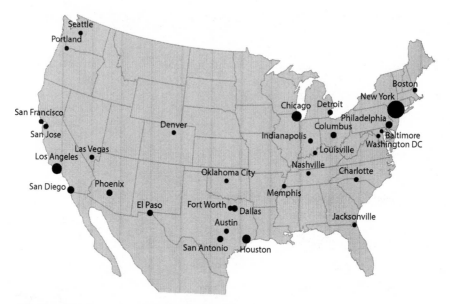

Figure A.1. The 30 Most Populous US Cities. *Note:* Area of circle represents population size. *Source:* Based on 2013 US Census Bureau data.

(NCHS).[1] The National Vital Statistics System (NVSS), part of the NCHS, works with these state offices and the National Association for Public Health Statistics and Information Systems to standardize and collect the data for national and state reporting. Although the system for collecting data on births has been fully electronic since 2013, the system for death data has evolved more slowly.[2] There is generally a 1-year lag from the end of the year until that year's mortality data are released.

We obtained these data from the Multiple Cause of Death data files from the NVSS for 2013–2017.[3] In part II, we examined how mortality rates and inequities differed within and across America's largest cities. In chapter 3, we assessed inequities in all-cause mortality, life expectancy, and years of life lost. In chapter 4, we provided race-specific mortality rates and related measures of inequities at the city level for the 10 leading causes of death. In chapter 5, we examined three other causes of death with notable inequity. We extracted race-specific deaths by place of residence, cause of death (for chapters 4 and 5), and age group. To calculate mortality rates and years of life lost, we used 10 age groups (0–4 years, 5–14 years, 15–24 years, 25–34 years, 35–44 years, 45–54 years, 55–64 years, 65–74 years, 75–84 years, and 85 years and over). To calculate life expectancy, we used 13 age groups (0–4 years, 5–9 years, 10–14 years, 15–19 years, 20–24 years, 25–29 years,

Table A.1. Selected City-Level Sociodemographic Characteristics for the United States and the 30 Largest US Cities

City, State	Population	Percent NH White	Percent NH Black	Percent Hispanic	Median Household Income	Percent Poverty	Percent HS Degree	Percent Unemployed	Percent Excessive Housing Cost
United States	311,536,594	63	12	17	$53,046	15	86	10	37
Austin, TX	836,800	49	8	35	$53,946	19	87	7	36
Baltimore, MD	621,445	28	63	4	$41,385	24	80	14	40
Boston, MA	629,182	47	23	18	$53,601	21	85	11	43
Charlotte, NC	757,278	44	35	13	$52,375	17	88	11	33
Chicago, IL	2,706,101	32	32	29	$47,270	23	81	14	41
Columbus, OH	800,594	59	27	6	$44,072	22	88	10	34
Dallas, TX	1,222,167	29	24	42	$42,846	24	74	9	37
Denver, CO	619,297	53	10	31	$50,313	19	85	9	35
Detroit, MI	706,663	8	81	7	$26,325	39	78	29	43
El Paso, TX	660,795	15	3	80	$41,406	22	76	9	32
Fort Worth, TX	761,092	41	19	34	$51,315	19	80	9	32
Houston, TX	2,134,707	26	23	44	$45,010	23	75	9	36
Indianapolis, IN	828,841	58	28	9	$41,962	21	84	12	34
Jacksonville, FL	829,721	49	8	8	$47,557	17	88	12	35
Las Vegas, NV	591,496	47	11	32	$51,143	17	83	14	37
Los Angeles, CA	3,827,261	29	9	49	$49,497	22	75	12	51
Louisville, KY	601,611	68	23	5	$44,159	18	87	11	29
Memphis, TN	650,932	27	63	6	$36,912	27	83	14	40
Nashville, TN	614,908	56	28	10	$46,686	19	86	9	34
New York, NY	8,268,999	33	23	29	$52,259	20	80	11	46
Oklahoma City, OK	590,995	56	14	18	$45,824	18	85	7	29
Philadelphia, PA	1,536,704	37	42	13	$37,192	27	81	15	39
Phoenix, AZ	1,473,639	47	6	40	$47,139	23	81	11	34
Portland, OR	594,687	72	6	9	$52,657	18	91	10	39
San Antonio, TX	1,359,033	27	6	63	$45,722	20	81	9	33
San Diego, CA	1,322,838	44	6	29	$64,058	16	87	10	43
San Francisco, CA	817,501	42	6	15	$75,604	14	86	8	36
San Jose, CA	968,903	28	3	33	$81,829	12	82	11	39
Seattle, WA	624,681	67	7	6	$65,277	14	93	7	35
Washington, DC	619,371	35	49	10	$65,830	19	88	11	37

Sources: American Community Survey, 2013, downloaded from American Fact Finder (second through ninth columns); City Health Dashboard, 2017 (tenth column).

Notes: NH = non-Hispanic; HS = high school.

Table A.2. Selected City-Level Segregation, Inequality, and Health Care Characteristics for the United States and the 30 Most Populous US Cities

City, State	Residential Segregation			Income and Racial Inequality				Health and Health Care			
	IOI White	IOI Black	Index of Dissimilarity	Gini Index	ICE Income	ICE Race	ICE Combined	Percent Disability Status	Percent Uninsured	FQHCs per 100,000	PCPs per 100,000
United States	74	46	58	0.48	—	—	—	12	15	—	11
Austin, TX	61	17	54	0.48	0.03	0.41	0.13	9	21	3	41
Baltimore, MD	58	83	69	0.53	-0.16	-0.35	-0.14	15	13	7	18
Boston, MA	65	51	69	0.53	-0.03	0.22	0.10	12	5	6	10
Charlotte, NC	62	52	53	0.51	-0.01	0.08	0.04	9	18	1	30
Chicago, IL	60	80	83	0.53	-0.09	0.03	-0.01	11	20	7	22
Columbus, OH	69	52	54	0.46	-0.14	0.29	-0.02	12	15	2	24
Dallas, TX	57	50	66	0.55	-0.11	0.05	0.00	10	31	1	17
Denver, CO	66	25	55	0.51	0.00	0.44	0.14	10	17	7	48
Detroit, MI	22	92	59	0.51	-0.42	-0.69	-0.37	20	19	4	4
El Paso, TX	23	7	31	0.47	-0.19	0.10	0.02	12	27	2	17
Fort Worth, TX	57	38	55	0.47	-0.06	0.22	0.04	10	24	0	22
Houston, TX	51	49	69	0.53	-0.09	0.03	0.02	10	29	3	25
Indianapolis, IN	71	51	56	0.50	-0.17	0.28	-0.03	13	17	8	32
Jacksonville, FL	64	53	48	0.47	-0.11	0.22	-0.01	12	17	1	31
Las Vegas, NV	57	18	32	0.54	-0.09	0.33	0.05	12	23	1	36
Los Angeles, CA	55	30	67	0.50	-0.05	0.20	0.08	10	26	4	8
Louisville, KY	78	53	55	0.52	-0.12	0.44	0.02	15	14	—	15
Memphis, TN	58	80	68	0.46	-0.25	-0.38	-0.19	14	19	2	—
Nashville, TN	67	50	49	0.55	-0.08	0.28	0.02	11	14	—	15
New York, NY	62	58	81	0.55	-0.04	0.10	0.06	10	14	1	—
Oklahoma City, OK	65	39	47	0.46	-0.08	0.40	0.05	13	21	1	3
Philadelphia, PA	66	73	73	0.52	-0.23	-0.06	-0.10	16	15	3	25
Phoenix, AZ	64	12	50	0.48	-0.09	0.37	0.08	9	22	4	15
Portland, OR	74	13	39	0.49	-0.02	0.65	0.14	12	16	3	19

San Antonio, TX	41	17	43	0.46	-0.13	0.19	0.04	14	21	1	34
San Diego, CA	61	14	55	0.48	0.09	0.37	0.15	9	17	4	34
San Francisco, CA	53	19	53	0.53	0.21	0.36	0.22	11	11	8	31
San Jose, CA	44	5	37	0.46	0.26	0.24	0.15	8	14	5	16
Seattle, WA	73	19	52	0.49	0.14	0.58	0.22	9	11	9	99
Washington, DC	63	77	72	0.53	0.10	-0.11	0.06	11	7	8	21

Sources: Brown University's Diversity and Disparities Project (Residential Segregation); 2013 American Community Survey 1-Year Estimates, downloaded from American Fact Finder (Gini index, Percent Disability Status, and Percent Uninsured); calculated using 2013–2017 American Community Survey data (ICE Income, ICE Race, and ICE Combined); Hunt BR, Silva A, Lock D, Hurlbert M, Predictors of Breast Cancer Mortality among White and Black Women in Large United States Cities: An Ecologic Study, *Cancer Causes Control* 2019;30(2):149–164 (FQHCs per 100,000 and PCPs per 100,000).

Note: Dash indicates that data were not available.

30–34 years, 35–44 years, 45–54 years, 55–64 years, 65–74 years, 75–84 years, and 85 years and over). As of this writing, 2017 was the most recent year of mortality data available.

POPULATION DATA

For each city, race- and age-specific population-based denominators were obtained using data from the US Census Bureau. Denominator data for the non-Hispanic white and total populations for 2013–2017 were obtained from the American Community Survey (ACS, 5-year estimates for 2015). For the ACS, approximately 250,000 households are interviewed monthly, and the survey responses are then released in annual, 3-year, and 5-year data cycles. The process for obtaining non-Hispanic Black denominator data was slightly different owing to the fact that the ACS only provides population estimates for the total Black population although *non-Hispanic* Black is reported in the 2010 Census. We therefore calculated the age-specific proportion of the Black population that was non-Hispanic in 2010 in each city and applied this proportion to the Black population data from the ACS (5-year estimates for 2015) to determine the non-Hispanic Black population for this period.[4,5] To calculate all-cause and cause-specific mortality rates and years of life lost, we used 10 age groups (0–4 years, 5–14 years, 15–24 years, 25–34 years, 35–44 years, 45–54 years, 55–64 years, 65–74 years, 75–84 years, and 85 years and over) from the ACS. To calculate life expectancy, we used all 13 age groups available in the ACS (0–4 years, 5–9 years, 10–14 years, 15–19 years, 20–24 years, 25–29 years, 30–34 years, 35–44 years, 45–54 years, 55–64 years, 65–74 years, 75–84 years, and 85 years and over). We applied a multiplier of five to the ACS population estimates in order to approximate the population over the 5 years of mortality data used. Note that the *total city* outcomes include *all* race/ethnic groups (not just Black and white).

The ACS population 5-year estimates for 2015 (i.e., 2013–2017) were used to calculate mortality rates, life expectancy, and years of life lost for the United States and its 30 largest cities.

Mortality Rates

Age-adjusted overall and race-specific mortality rates were calculated for all cities and the United States as a whole. Five-year age-adjusted rates per 100,000 population were calculated employing the year 2000 standard US population.[6] Data for Las Vegas were suppressed, as discussed in the limitations section.

For cause-specific mortality, cases were classified according to the *International Classification of Diseases* (ICD-10).[7] Specifically, we analyzed the following causes of death using code groups published by the US Centers for Disease Control and Prevention: heart disease, cancer, chronic lower respiratory diseases, accidents, stroke, Alzheimer's disease, diabetes, influenza and pneumonia, kidney disease, suicide, HIV, homicide, and opioid-related deaths.[8] All causes of death were based on the underlying cause except opioid-related deaths, which also included contributing causes of death. The use of contributing causes of death for opioid-related deaths means that some opioid-related deaths may also be included in another category (e.g., accidents or suicide), so these categories should not be considered mutually exclusive. Table A.3 lists the ICD-10 code groups for each cause of death included in the analysis. The NVSS uses a computerized system to select the underlying cause when multiple causes of death are listed on a death certificate, following the process outlined by the World Health Organization. If cities had fewer than 20 cause-specific deaths for any racial group, they were excluded, in accordance with research on the reliability of mortality rates.[9]

As recommended, we use multiple measures to assess levels of inequity in the summary mortality measures.[10,11] For example, the use of both an absolute and relative measure allows for a fuller understanding of the magnitude of the difference between groups. Other measures, such as excess deaths, quantify the additional (potentially preventable) deaths due to inequities.[12,13]

Table A.3. ICD-10 Codes for Specific Causes of Death

Cause of Death	ICD-10 Code Groups[a]
Heart disease	I00–I09, I11, I13, I20–I51
Cancer	C00–C97
Chronic lower respiratory diseases	J40–J47
Accidents	V01–X59, Y85–Y86
Stroke	I60–I69
Alzheimer's disease	G30
Diabetes	E10–E14
Influenza and pneumonia	J09–J18
Kidney disease	N00–N07, N17–N19, N25–N27
Suicide[b]	*U03, X60–X84, Y87.0
HIV	B20–B24
Homicide[b]	*U01–*U02, X85–Y09, Y87.1
Opioid-related deaths	X40–X44, X60–X64, X85, Y10–Y14 + Contributing Cause T40.0–T40.4, T40.6

[a] ICD-10 codes are published by the World Health Organization, and the code groups used here were published by the CDC in "ICD-10 Cause-of-Death Lists for Tabulating Mortality Statistics."
[b] *U codes, representing terrorism-related deaths, were created by the US government and therefore do not have a comparable World Health Organization code.

All measures of inequities were calculated using the age-adjusted, 5-year average (2013–2017) mortality rates as described above.

Relative inequities were assessed by calculating Black:white rate ratios (RR). These provide the proportional disparity in Black and white deaths. *Absolute inequities* were calculated using the risk difference (RD) in rates. Specifically, we subtract the white rate from the Black rate. This measure provides insight into potential excess risks of mortality among the Black population. Finally, the number of *excess deaths* due to differences in mortality rates was calculated. Excess Black deaths are deaths that occur because of the racial disparity in mortality. Excess deaths were calculated by multiplying the age-specific white mortality rates by the corresponding Black populations in each age category. The sum of these products is the number of Black deaths that would be expected if white death rates were applied to this population. We then subtracted the number of expected deaths from the number of observed deaths to obtain the excess number of deaths annually for the United States and each city. For all of these, we use whites as the reference group both because they are the largest racial group in our country and because they generally have more favorable health outcomes.[10]

Life Expectancy

Life expectancy measures the average number of years from birth a person can expect to live, according to the current mortality experience (age-specific death rates) of the population. This measure takes into account the number of deaths in a given time period and the average number of people at risk of dying during that period, allowing us to compare data across cities with different population sizes. We used the mortality and the 5-year ACS population estimates to calculate the total and race-specific life expectancy at birth for the United States and its largest cities.

We calculated life expectancy at birth using a modified version of the life expectancy calculation developed by Chiang.[14] To calculate life expectancy using the ACS population estimates, we were required to modify the standard method of calculating life expectancy to fit the 13 age groups available in ACS (0–4 years, 5–9 years, . . . , 30–34 years, 35–44 years, . . . , 75–84 years, 85+ years), compared to the 19 age groups used in Chiang's original formula.[14] We compared results of both the original formula and our modified formula using US 2010 Census data, which could be separated into 13 or 19 age groups, and found minimal differences in the life expectancies calculated by the two methods (less than 0.1 years in most cases). We therefore concluded that the reduction in the number of age groups was a reasonable modification to Chiang's method and opted to use the ACS data in order to be consistent with the population denominators used for other outcomes in this book.

To assess inequities in life expectancy, we calculated an absolute difference in life expectancy between Black and white populations by subtracting the Black life expectancy from the white life expectancy.

Years of Life Lost

To calculate the age-adjusted years of life lost (YLL) rate, we divided the total number of years of life lost in a population before the age of 75 by the total population under age 75 as follows:

$$\text{YLL rate} = \left[\sum_{i=1}^{8} (75 \text{ years} - \text{midpoint}_i) \times \text{death rate}_i \times \text{weight}_i \right] \times 100{,}000,$$

where i represents the age group (eight groups included, from 0–4 through 65–74), midpoint$_i$ is the middle of each age group, death rate$_i$ is calculated as the number of deaths divided by the population of each age group, and weight$_i$ is the population weight for the age group derived from the US 2000 standard population under age 75. We used the mortality data and 5-year ACS population estimates to calculate the YLL rate.

For each age group, we estimated that the average decedent lived until the midpoint of the age group (e.g., until age 12.5 for the 10–14 age group and until age 49.5 for the 45–54 age group). For each age group, we calculated the age-specific YLL as 75 years minus the average age at death, multiplied by the number of deaths and divided by the total population. Similar to the mortality rates, we used the ACS population estimates. We multiplied this number by 100,000 to get the age-specific YLL rate per 100,000 population. We used the US 2000 standard population under the age of 75 to create weights for age standardization, which were applied to each age-specific YLL rate before calculating the sum to find the age-standardized YLL rate.

To assess inequities in YLL, we calculated the YLL rate difference between Black and white populations (by subtracting the white YLL from the Black YLL) for the United States and for each of the largest cities.

Assessing Statistical Significance

For all of the measures described above, we calculated 95% confidence intervals, which define the range of values that we are reasonably certain include the correct value of the measure. To define statistical significance, we looked for two measures whose confidence intervals did not overlap.

For life expectancy, confidence intervals (CI) were calculated using the life tables formulated by Chiang.[14] Confidence intervals for the RRs and RDs for age-adjusted mortality rates and YLL rates were calculated using a Taylor series expansion technique[15] as follows:

$$95\% \text{ CI for RR}: \left(\left[RR_{B:W} * e^{-z^* \sqrt{\frac{var_B}{(r_B)^2} + \frac{var_W}{(r_W)^2}}} \right], \left[RR_{B:W} * e^{z^* \sqrt{\frac{var_B}{(r_B)^2} + \frac{var_W}{(r_W)^2}}} \right] \right),$$

$$95\% \text{ CI for RD}: \left(\left[RD_{B-W} - z^* \sqrt{var_B + var_W} \right], \left[RD_{B-W} + z^* \sqrt{var_B + var_W} \right] \right),$$

where B and W refer to metrics for the non-Hispanic Black and non-Hispanic white populations, respectively, z is set to 1.96, RR refers to the rate ratio, RD refers to the risk difference, r refers to the age-adjusted mortality rate, and var refers to the variance of the age-adjusted mortality rate or YLL rate, as appropriate. Note: rate ratios were only calculated for age-adjusted mortality rates, while risk differences were calculated for both age-adjusted mortality rates and YLL rates.

2. Methodology of Part III (Epidemiological Patterns and Sociological Explanations)

We examined the ecological association between city-level characteristics and mortality outcomes. The cornerstone variables (poverty, median household income, and educational attainment) are described in chapter 6. Racial composition (percent non-Hispanic Black, percent non-Hispanic white) and the index of isolation are also described in chapter 6. Here we provide additional details on two of the more nuanced measures, the index of concentration at the extremes (ICE, which we used to quantify racial segregation) and income inequality, as well as the combined effect of both. City-level values for all variables are first presented in tables A.1 and A.2.

ICE was computed using data from the 2013–2017 ACS 5-year estimates. ACS tables were downloaded by the geographic type "place within state" to obtain city-specific data. Consistent with previous research, ICE was calculated as follows:

$$ICE_i = \frac{(A_i - P_i)}{T_i}.$$

Here A_i is the number of privileged people in city i, P_i represents the number of deprived people in the city i, and T_i represents the population of city i.[16,17] For ICE(race), the advantaged group was non-Hispanic white and the disadvantaged group was non-Hispanic Black, derived from table B03002 (Hispanic or Latino Origin by Race) from the American FactFinder web portal. B19001 (household income) from the American FactFinder web portal was used to calculate ICE(income). Affluence represented household incomes greater than or equal to $125,000 USD. Conversely, deprivation was considered as household incomes less than $25,000 USD. For the combined measure, ICE(combined), ACS tables for household income by race/ethnicities were used, specifically B19001H for household income of white alone, not Hispanic or Latino, and B19001B for Black or African American alone. The extremes for the combined measure were non-Hispanic white and household income ≥$125,000 USD (privilege) and Black or African American and household income < $25,000 USD (deprivation).

A second measure that we utilized in chapter 6 that warrants additional detail is the Gini coefficient. It is a commonly used measure of income inequality. The Gini coefficient is derived from a "Lorenz curve," illustrated in figure A.2. The Lorenz curve shows the percentage of total income earned by cumulative percentage of the population.[18] In a perfectly equal society, the poorest 25% of the population would earn 25% of the total income, the poorest 50% of the population would earn 50% of the total income, and

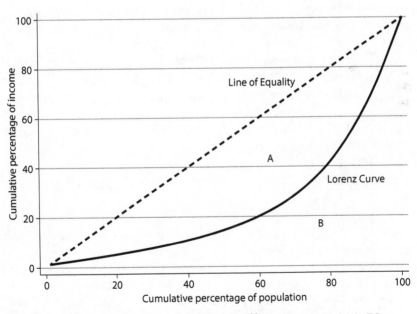

Figure A.2. The Lorenz Curve and the Gini Coefficient. *Source:* De Maio FG. Income Inequality Measures. *Journal of Epidemiology and Community Health.* 2007;61(10):849–852. Used with permission.

the Lorenz curve would follow the path of the 45° line of equality. However, as inequality increases, the Lorenz curve deviates from the line of equality: the poorest 25% of the population may earn 10% of the total income, the poorest 50% of the population may earn 20% of the total income, and so on. This framework can be used to generate a single summary statistic of the income distribution, the Gini coefficient.

The Gini coefficient is equivalent to the size of the area between the Lorenz curve and the 45° line of equality divided by the total area under the 45° line of equality. In figure A.2, it is depicted as area A divided by area A+B. The Gini coefficient can be presented as a value between 0 and 1 or as a percentage. A coefficient of 0 reflects a perfectly equal society in which all income is equally shared; in this case, the Lorenz curve would follow the line of equality. The further that the Lorenz curve deviates from the line of equality, the higher the Gini coefficient. A coefficient of 1 (or 100%) represents a perfectly unequal society wherein all income is earned by one individual.[19-22] Gini values were obtained from 2013 ACS 1-year estimates. City-specific values are presented in table A.2.

3. Methodological Limitations

As noted previously, this book focuses on mortality differences between Blacks and whites. Although we recognize that disparities likely exist among several other racial and ethnic groups for some outcomes, we did not expand our analyses for several reasons. For one, in the United States, mortality inequities primarily affect the Black population, while Hispanic and Asian populations tend to have better mortality outcomes than both Blacks and whites.[23] In addition, the historical and sociopolitical context of the racial inequities differs for each group. Moreover, the smaller number of deaths within these subpopulations, particularly for the less common causes of death, would greatly limit the number of cities we could assess. However, these are important analyses that should be pursued in cities with sufficiently large populations.

Our analyses also have several methodological limitations to acknowledge. To begin, reporting errors on the death certificate are common[24] and may lead to inaccurate estimates of certain causes of death, such as heart disease.[25] In addition, communications with Las Vegas health department leaders and its local researchers, combined with careful comparisons with county and zip code data, identified a likely error in the mortality estimates for Las Vegas. Although the extent of this bias cannot be directly calculated, it appears that an unknown number of deaths of residents of unincorporated areas were misclassified as having occurred to residents of Las

Vegas. Thus, we excluded data for this city from our results. No concerns regarding other cities were raised by our data checking processes or outside experts following earlier publications.[26] Furthermore, using the ACS to estimate the population size for each racial group in each city is a limitation, as the ACS is itself subject to sampling error. However, during years in which the Census is not conducted, the ACS is the only publicly available data source with population estimates at the city level. Finally, as noted in chapters 4 and 5, there were insufficient deaths within certain causes to provide race-specific rates and/or to analyze inequities for all cities. For each outcome, the maximum number of cities was included in the analyses.

References

1. Ventura S. The U.S. National Vital Statistics System: Transitioning into the 21st Century, 1990–2017. *Vital and Health Statistics. Series 1*. 2018;(62):1–84.

2. National Center for Health Statistics. *National Vital Statistics System Improvements*. Hyattsville, MD: NCHS Fact Sheet; 2020.

3. National Center for Health Statistics. *All County (Micro-Data2), 2007–2017, as Compiled from Data Provided by the 57 Vital Statistics Jurisdictions through the Vital Statistics Cooperative Program*. Hyattsville, MD: National Center for Health Statistics. 2020.

4. US Census Bureau. *American Community Survey, 2015 5-Year Estimates. Tables B01001, B01001h, B01001b*. http://data.census.gov/cedsci/.

5. US Census Bureau. *2010 Census. Tables Pct12b, Pct12j*. http://data.census .gov/cedsci/.

6. Klein RJ, Schoenborn CA. Age Adjustment Using the 2000 Projected U.S. Population. *Healthy People 2010 Statistical Notes*. 2001;20:1–10.

7. World Health Organization. *International Statistical Classification of Diseases and Related Health Problems, Tenth Revision (ICD-10)*. 5th ed. Geneva: World Health Organization; 2016.

8. Centers for Disease Control and Prevention. *ICD-10 Cause-of-Death Lists for Tabulating Mortality Statistics*. Hyattsville, MD: National Center for Health Statistics; 2018.

9. Hoyert DL, Heron MP, Murphy SL, Kung HC. Deaths: Final Data for 2003. *National Vital Statistics Report*. 2006;54:1–120.

10. Keppel K, Pamuk E, Lynch J, et al. Methodological Issues in Measuring Health Disparities. *Vital and Health Statistics. Series 2*. 2005;(141):1–16.

11. Harper S, Lynch J, Burris S, Davey Smith G. Trends in the Black-White Life Expectancy Gap in the United States, 1983–2003. *Journal of the American Medical Association*. 2007;297(11):1224–1232.

12. McCord C, Freeman HP. Excess Mortality in Harlem. *New England Journal of Medicine*. 1990;322(3):173–177.

13. Geronimus A, Bound J, Waidmann TA, Hillemeier MM, Burns PB. Excess Mortality among Blacks and Whites in the United States. *New England Journal of Medicine.* 1996;335:1552–1558.

14. Chiang CL. The Life Table and Its Construction. In: *Introduction to Stochastic Processes in Biostatistics.* New York: John Wiley & Sons; 1968:189–214.

15. Kleinbaum D, Kupper L, Morgenstern H. *Epidemiologic Research Principles and Quantitative Methods.* Belmont: California Lifetime Learning Publications; 1982.

16. Krieger N, Waterman PD, Spasojevic J, Li W, Maduro G, Van Wye G. Public Health Monitoring of Privilege and Deprivation with the Index of Concentration at the Extremes. *American Journal of Public Health.* 2016;106(2): 256–263.

17. Lange-Maia BS, De Maio F, Avery EF, et al. Association of Community-Level Inequities and Premature Mortality: Chicago, 2011–2015. *Journal of Epidemiology and Community Health.* 2018;72(12):1099–1103.

18. De Maio FG. Income Inequality Measures. *Journal of Epidemiology and Community Health.* 2007;61(10):849–852.

19. Gillis M, Perkins DH, Roemer M, Snodgrass DR. *Economics of Development.* New York: W. W. Norton; 1996.

20. Atkinson AB. *The Economics of Inequality.* Oxford: Claredon; 1975.

21. Champernowne DG, Cowell FA. *Economic Inequality and Income Distribution.* Cambridge: Cambridge University Press; 1998.

22. Campano F, Salvatore D. *Income Distribution.* Oxford: Oxford University Press; 2006.

23. Xu J, Murphy SL, Kochanek KD, Bastian B, Arias E. Deaths: Final Data for 2016. *National Vital Statistics Reports.* 2018;67(5):1–76.

24. McGivern L, Shulman L, Carney JK, Shapiro S, Bundock E. Death Certification Errors and the Effect on Mortality Statistics. *Public Health Reports.* 2017;132(6):669–675.

25. Sington JD, Cottrell BJ. Analysis of the Sensitivity of Death Certificates in 440 Hospital Deaths: A Comparison with Necropsy Findings. *Journal of Clinical Pathology.* 2002;55(7):499–502.

26. Benjamins MR, Silva A, Saiyed NS, De Maio FG. Comparison of All-Cause Mortality Rates and Inequities between Black and White Populations across the 30 Most Populous US Cities. JAMA Network Open. 2021;4(1):e2032086.

Editors

Maureen R. Benjamins, PhD, is a Senior Research Fellow at the Sinai Urban Health Institute (SUHI) in Chicago, Illinois. Her research interests pertain to health inequities and the influence of social factors on these inequities. She has led several initiatives to study health equity nationally and in Chicago, including the Sinai Community Health Survey 2.0, of which she was the co-Principal Investigator. She coedited *Urban Health: Combating Disparities with Local Data* (Oxford University Press, 2011), a book that describes a broad Chicago initiative to translate public health data into community-based interventions and policy changes. Dr. Benjamins is an adjunct faculty member at the Parkinson School of Health Sciences and Public Health at Loyola University Chicago and at Rosalind Franklin University of Medicine and Science. She also directs the SUHI Research Fellows program.

Fernando De Maio, PhD, is a Professor in the Department of Sociology at DePaul University and Director of Health Equity Research and Data Use at the Center for Health Equity, American Medical Association. His research and teaching interests lie primarily within medical sociology and social epidemiology. Much of his work has focused on the income inequality hypothesis and the concept of structural violence. He is the author of *Health and Social Theory* (Palgrave Macmillan, 2010) and *Global Health Inequities* (Palgrave Macmillan, 2014), and coeditor of *Latin American Perspectives on the Sociology of Health and Illness* (Routledge, 2018) and, most recently, *Community Health Equity: A Chicago Reader* (University of Chicago Press, 2019). Dr. De Maio is a founding codirector of the Center for Community Health Equity. In 2019, he was a Research Fellow at the Sinai Urban Health Institute.

Contributors

David Ansell, MD, MPH, is Senior Vice President for Community Health Equity at Rush University Medical Center and Associate Provost for

Community Health Equity at Rush University. Dr. Ansell leads Rush University's strategy to be a catalyst for community health and economic vitality on Chicago's West Side. He helped found West Side United (WSU) and also serves as an Executive Committee Member of the WSU Leadership Council. Dr. Ansell is known for his establishment of the not-for-profit Metropolitan Chicago Breast Cancer Taskforce and his role in the creation of the Center for Community Health Equity, a Chicago-based educational and research center jointly run by Rush and DePaul Universities. Dr. Ansell is the author of *County: Life, Death and Politics at Chicago's Public Hospital* and *The Death Gap: How Inequality Kills*, as well as numerous papers and book chapters on health inequities.

Darlene Oliver Hightower, JD, is Vice President of Community Health Equity at Rush University Medical Center, where she is responsible for a team of 40 staff who oversee the implementation and evaluation of community programs. She is a member of the senior leadership team for West Side United and has served as a Chicago Community Trust Leadership Fellow, a University of Chicago Civic Leadership Academy Fellow, and an Administrative Law Judge for the Chicago Department of Human Relations. She was recently named a Culture of Health Leader Fellow with the Robert Wood Johnson Foundation.

Jana Hirschtick, PhD, MPH, is a social epidemiologist at the Center for Social Epidemiology and Population Health, University of Michigan School of Public Health. Formerly, she was the director of the Health Equity and Assessment Research strategy at the Sinai Urban Health Institute and a Principal Investigator of the Sinai Community Health Survey, one of the largest community-driven health surveys ever conducted in Chicago.

Sharon Homan, PhD, was the President of the Sinai Urban Health Institute. She is a biostatistician and maternal child mental health epidemiologist. Her prior experience includes public health leadership and faculty positions with the University of North Texas School of Public Health (Professor and Chair of the Department of Biostatistics and Epidemiology and Associate Dean for Research), the Kansas Health Institute (Vice President for Public Health), and Saint Louis University (Professor of Biostatistics). Her research on health disparities, maternal and child health, violence prevention, and community health improvement initiatives has been funded by NIH, HRSA, CDC, DOJ, state contracts, and foundations.

Ayesha Jaco, MAM, is the Executive Director of West Side United and a faculty member at Northeastern University's Jacob Carruthers Center for Inner-City Studies. In 2008, she founded the youth dance company Move Me Soul, which has provided over 1,000 Chicago teens and young adults with training and life skill development. She has partnered with Chicago organizations to provide social services, substance abuse prevention, food equity, study abroad, and artistic programming for over 18,500 inner-city youth and their families. She was awarded the Power 25 Chicago Award by Walker's Legacy for her commitment to excellent leadership, community, and philanthropic contributions.

Emily LaFlamme, MPH, is a senior epidemiologist at the Chicago Department of Public Health, focused on the intersection of community development and health equity. Using tools such as health impact assessment, community health assessment, and qualitative analysis, she leverages data to advocate for and evaluate the impact of environments that promote community well-being.

Brittney S. Lange-Maia, PhD, MPH, is an Assistant Professor in Preventive Medicine at Rush University Medical Center. She is an epidemiologist with specialized training in aging research and health disparities. Her work specifically focuses on physical activity and physical function, and she has a strong interest in promoting health throughout the life span. Brittney is also a co-Chair of the West Side United Metrics Working Group.

Kristin Monnard, MPH, leads community engagement efforts at the Sinai Urban Heath Institute. Her professional interests include social determinants of health, participatory action research, translational communication, and qualitative research.

Nikhil G. Prachand, MPH, is the Director of Epidemiology at the Chicago Department of Public Health. He has more than 25 years of experience analyzing and interpreting health-related data in Chicago beginning as a graduate student in epidemiology investigating the 1995 Chicago heat wave. He served as the Director of HIV/STI Surveillance before taking on his current role. He is actively involved in overseeing the Healthy Chicago Survey and the Chicago Health Atlas (chicagohealthatlas.org) and working with stakeholders on the development of Healthy Chicago 2025, the city's health improvement plan.

Pamela T. Roesch, MPH, is a senior epidemiologist at the Sinai Urban Health Institute (SUHI) and serves as co-Chair of the West Side United Metrics Working Group. She directs the Health Equity and Assessment Research (HEAR) strategy for SUHI. Pam is currently leading the dissemination of Sinai Community Health Survey 2.0 data as well as various community-driven assessment projects across Chicago's West and Southwest Sides. She serves in a leadership role on numerous Chicago collaboratives, including the East Garfield Park Best Babies Zone.

Michael Rozier, SJ, PhD, is an Assistant Professor in the Department of Health Management and Policy, Saint Louis University, with a secondary appointment to the Gnaegi Center for Health Care Ethics. He earned his doctorate from University of Michigan and completed graduate studies at University of Toronto (philosophy), Johns Hopkins University (international health), and Boston College (moral theology). Michael's research interests include the ethics of population health, moral rhetoric in policy discourse, and hospital-community partnerships.

Nazia Saiyed, MPH, is an epidemiologist at the Sinai Urban Health Institute (SUHI). She leads the research and evaluation of numerous projects designed to address diabetes, asthma, and lead poisoning in underserved communities. Prior to joining SUHI, Nazia worked with the New York State Department of Health contributing to research on the impact of environmental conditions on population health. Her research interests include health disparities, chronic disease epidemiology, environmental epidemiology, and children's health.

Eve Shapiro, MPH, is the Director of Data and Evaluation at West Side United. She is a health researcher and evaluator focused on programs that reduce health disparities. She is passionate about health equity and access to quality health care, education, and livelihoods for Chicagoans. Prior to her work at West Side United, she was an analyst with NORC at the University of Chicago and a community and labor organizer. Eve holds a Master of Public Health from Emory University and a Bachelor of Arts in Psychology from the University of Minnesota.

Abigail Silva, PhD, is an Assistant Professor in the Department of Public Health Sciences at Loyola University Chicago and a Research Health Scientist at the Hines VA Hospital. As a former epidemiologist at the

Chicago Department of Public Health and one of the founding members of the Sinai Urban Health Institute (SUHI), she has a long history of using public health surveillance data and local data to bring attention to racial health disparities to help effect change. The broad focus of her research is in identifying and explaining inequities in health care and outcomes, particularly related to cancer, with the goal of informing policy and interventions. In 2019, Dr. Silva served as a SUHI Research Fellow.

Veenu Verma, MS, MPP, is Principal at the Civic Consulting Alliance, working in the Education and Community and Neighborhood Change program areas. Prior to joining Civic Consulting, Veenu spent 11 years at Chicago Public Schools, where she served as the Executive Director of Early College and Career Education and led the district's portfolio of career-related high school programming for 18,000 students. Veenu holds a master's degree in economics from the University of Illinois Urbana-Champaign and a master's degree in public policy from the University of Chicago.

West Side United Metrics Working Group members who contributed substantially to the development of the West Side United Assessment Framework and provided a review of chapter 9 include Marie Heffernan, PhD, Associate Director, Surveys of Child Health in Chicago at the Mary Ann and J. Milburn Smith Child Health Research, Outreach, and Advocacy Center, Ann & Robert H. Lurie Children's Hospital of Chicago; Jacquelyn Jacobs, MPH, Director of Evaluation Technical Assistance at the Sinai Urban Health Institute; Charlotte Picard, MS, Epidemiologist at the Sinai Urban Health Institute; Elizabeth Lynch, PhD, Associate Professor in the Department of Preventive Medicine and Center for Community Health Equity at Rush University Medical Center; Elena Jimenez, Former Program Manager at West Side United; and coauthors Pamela Roesch, Dr. Brittney Lange-Maia, Eve Shapiro, Veenu Verma, Nikhil Prachand, and Dr. Sharon Homan.

Ruqaiijah Yearby, JD, MPH, is a Professor of Law and Executive Director of the Institute for Healing Justice and Equity at Saint Louis University. She evaluates the effectiveness of processes implemented by local governments across the country to achieve racial equity as co-Principal Investigator of the Robert Wood Johnson Foundation grant, "Are Cities and Counties Ready to Use Racial Equity Tools to Influence Policy?" Her work has been cited in *The Oxford Handbook of Public Health* (2019) and Mark Hall et al., *Health Care Law and Ethics* (2018). She earned her BS in Honors Biology from the University of Michigan, MPH from Johns Hopkins School of Public Health, and JD from Georgetown University Law Center.

Boxes, figures, and tables are indicated by b, f, and t following page numbers respectively.

National Center for Health Statistics (NCHS) mortality data, 22*f*, 34*t*, 285–86

National Center of Minority Health and Health Disparities, 24*t*, 25

national data, 21, 30–35, 31–34*t*, 40–41

National Healthcare Quality and Disparities report, 24*t*, 36

National Immunization Survey, xi

National Institute on Minority Health and Health Disparities (NIMHD), 25*t*, 27, 31*t*

National Institutes of Health (NIH), 23–25, 24–25*t*

National Leadership Summit on Eliminating Racial and Ethnic Disparities, 24*t*, 26

National Negro Health Week, 14–15

National Partnership for Action to End Health Disparities, 24*t*, 26

National Stakeholder Strategy for Achieving Health Equity, 25*t*, 26

National Standards for Culturally and Linguistically Appropriate Services in Health and Health Care (CLAS), 24*t*, 25

National Vital Statistics System (NVSS), 29–30, 31*t*, 35, 36, 41, 82, 286

neighborhood- and community-level data: CDPH and, xi; Chicago as focus, 169–72, 170–71*f*, 237; on mortality, 31–34*t*, 38–41, 39*f*, 80, 159; West Side United and, 247–53, 250*t*, 259–60

neoliberalism, 57*f*, 59

obesity, 55, 255*t*, 256

Office of Minority Health (OMH), 23–27, 24–25*t*, 28

opioid-related mortality, 124, 128*f*, 129–34, 129*f*, 166–68, 167*t*, 194, 250–51, 254*f*, 264–65, 270*b*

Patient Protection and Affordable Care Act (ACA) of 2010, 17–18, 25*t*

personal responsibility narratives, 8, 54–56, 60, 273

place: ecological analysis and, 148; mortality inequities and, 20–22, 80–81, 269; personal responsibility

narratives vs., 55–56; in psychosocial tradition, 62–65, 145; social justice framework through, 185, 198–99, 260–61; in sociopolitical tradition, 65–68; in West Side United's approach, 229, 234–35, 264–65

pneumonia. *See* influenza and pneumonia

policing and police brutality, 1, 2, 228, 281

population size, 147, 149, 152, 163, 165, 166, 168, 286*f*

poverty: all-cause mortality and, 152, 153*t*, 154, 271; Black:white mortality rates and, 153*t*, 154, 160–62*t*, 163; cause-specific mortality and, 160–62*t*, 163, 165; Chicago's Black population and, 43; differences across cities in, 149; health inequity from, 12–13, 54, 60, 139, 168, 176; HIV, homicide, and opioids, 166–68, 167*t*; life expectancy and, 152, 153*t*, 154; as variable characterizing cities, 143–44, 150*t*

Practitioner's Guide for Advancing Health Equity (CDC), 197

praxis approach: action in, 195–96; "Circle of Praxis" and, 188, 189*f*, 191; defined, 183–84; evaluation in, 196–98, 197*b*; experience in, 184, 189–91; hope in, 186–88, 198–99; reflection in, 194–95, 197*b*; social analysis in, 191, 193; social justice orientation of, 188–89; stance of commitment in, 186, 191; structural change through, 184–86, 198–99. *See also* community engagement; social justice

premature death, 80, 133, 169–72, 170–71*f*. *See also* years of life lost

Principles of Community Engagement, 184–85, 191, 192*b*, 199

proximal vs. distal causes of disease, 54–56, 57*f*, 60

psychosocial theoretical tradition, 60–65, 68–69, 145, 158–59

Public Health Service Act (1944), 23

public policy: best- and worst-performing cities in, 172–75, 173*t*, 174–75*f*; cause-specific mortality and,

101; city-level data spurring, 41–44, 82, 96–97, 108, 117–18, 133–34, 272–73; "Health in All Policies" approach to, 66–67, 275; in social epidemiological models of health, 56–59, 57*f*

racism. *See* structural racism
redlining, 14–16, 67, 190, 225
Robert Wood Johnson Foundation (RWJF), 28, 33*t*, 34*t*, 37–39, 146, 214*b*
Roesch, Pamela, 246
Rush University Medical Center, 224, 227*f*, 235–37, 261, 263

segregation: all-cause mortality and, 153*t*, 155, 159, 271; Black:white mortality rate ratios and, 153*t*; cause-specific mortality and, 160–62*t*, 163, 165; differences across cities in, 151, 288–89*t*; health inequity and, 12, 27, 185; HIV, homicide, and opioids, 167*t*, 168; of hospitals and care facilities, 14, 17; housing policy and, 16, 225–26; life expectancy and, 153*t*, 155; in social epidemiological models of health, 60, 145, 168; as variable characterizing cities, 63, 143–47, 150*t*, 171–72
Shapiro, Eve, 246
shared values, 183, 188, 192*b*, 193, 199, 273
Sinai Community Health Survey, 195–96, 210–20, 211*b*, 213*t*
Sinai Urban Health Institute (SUHI), 146, 147, 170
small area estimation methodology, 22, 37
Small Business Grant (SBG) program, 242–44, 256, 257*t*
social and structural determinants: cause-specific mortality and, 101; health data and, xii, 10, 185, 205–7; health inequities from, 8, 11–17, 185; income inequality as, 60, 62–63, 65, 66, 139, 142, 158–59, 168–69, 176, 203, 271; modifiability of, xi, 2; psychosocial tradition on, 60–65, 68–69; racism

as, 56–61, 145–46, 185, 194, 205, 219, 269, 276; social epidemiological framework for, 54, 56–61, 57*t*; sociopolitical tradition on, 60–61, 65–69. *See also* structural change
social epidemiologic theory, 54, 56–61, 57*f*, 139–40, 142
social justice: as framework for health equity, 5, 183–84, 188–89, 198–99, 273; hope and, 186–87, 198; principles of, 185; reflection and, 194; social analysis driving, 184–86; West Side United and, 234–35, 260–61. *See also* praxis approach
sociodemographic characteristics of US and 30 largest cities, 287*t*
sociopolitical tradition, 60–61, 65–69, 158–59
solutions-focused communication: community engagement through, 203–4, 206–9, 208*f*; data requiring, 205; knowledge cocreation and, 207–9; resources for, 214*b*; Sinai Community Health Survey 2.0 and, 212, 213*t*; traditional communication vs., 205–6; West Side United and, 228–29
Spearman's rank-order coefficient, 148
State and Territorial Efforts to Reduce Health Disparities (2018), 28, 35
state-level data, 21, 28–29, 30, 35–36, 40–41, 81
stress responses, 61–62, 64, 65, 67, 69, 155
stroke, 20, 76, 100, 103*f*, 104*t*, 105, 106*t*, 107*t*, 108, 113*f*, 114–17, 115*f*, 160*t*, 163
structural change, x–xi, 183, 184–86, 188, 190, 193, 203–5, 272
structural racism: ACA and, 18; biological vs. social framework for, 13, 53–54, 69, 96; community engagement against, 207–9, 215, 238; data gaps in quantifying, 80–82, 92, 124; defined, 66, 67, 185; differences across cities in, 149, 151; health inequity and, 12; hospitals and, 15–17; life expectancy and, 89, 90*t*, 93*f*; mortality rates and, 83–87, 84*t*,

MORE BOOKS *in* PUBLIC HEALTH *from* HOPKINS PRESS

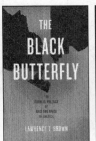
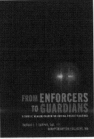
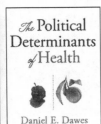
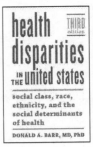
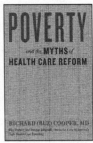

The Black Butterfly
The Harmful Politics of Race and Space in America

Lawrence T. Brown

"*The Black Butterfly* dissects American apartheid with unflinching precision and poignancy, weaving together fresh historical accounts with undiluted analysis of our present moment."—Ruha Benjamin, author of *Race After Technology: Abolitionist Tools for the New Jim Code*   **$29.95 hardcover/ebook**

From Enforcers to Guardians
A Public Health Primer on Ending Police Violence

Hannah L. F. Cooper, ScD, and Mindy Thompson Fullilove, MD

A public health approach to understanding and eliminating excessive police violence.

$34.95 hardcover/ebook

The Political Determinants of Health

Daniel E. Dawes
foreword by David R. Williams

"Arguably the most important book written on the driving force that has prevented us from realizing health equity in America and around the world."—Patrick J. Kennedy, author of *A Common Struggle: A Personal Journey through the Past and Future of Mental Illness and Addiction*   **$29.95 paperback/ebook**

Health Disparities in the United States
Social Class, Race, Ethnicity, and the Social Determinants of Health
third edition

Donald A. Barr, MD, PhD

"Will serve well as a foundational text for courses on the subject and for individuals looking for a well-organized, highly researched text."—*JAMA*   **$57.95 paperback/ebook**

Poverty and the Myths of Health Care Reform

Richard (Buz) Cooper, MD

"Offers helpful information for every American interested in improving the country's health care system. Recommended."—*Choice*

$28.95 paperback/ebook

JOHNS HOPKINS UNIVERSITY PRESS

@JHUPress

@JohnsHopkins UniversityPress

@JHUPress

For more Public Health books, visit **press.jhu.edu**